Molecular Mechanisms of Dementia

Contemporary Neuroscience

Molecular Mechanisms of Dementia

Edited by

Wilma Wasco
Rudolph E. Tanzi

Massachusetts General Hospital, Charlestown, MA

Humana Press ✳ Totowa, New Jersey

This publication is printed on acid-free paper. ∞
ANSI Z39.48-1984 (American Standards Institute) Permanence of Paper for Printed Library Materials.

Cover illustration: Modified from Fig. 2A, Chapter 12, "τ Protein and the Neurofibrillary Pathology of Alzheimer's Disease," by Michel Goedert, John Q. Trojanowski, and Virginia M.-Y. Lee.

Cover design by Patricia F. Cleary.

For additional copies, pricing for bulk purchases, and/or information about other Humana titles, contact Humana at the above address or at any of the following numbers: Tel: 201-256-1699; Fax: 201-256-8341; E-mail: humana@interramp.com

Printed in the United States of America. 10 9 8 7 6 5 4 3 2 1

Library of Congress Cataloging in Publication Data

Molecular mechanisms of dementia/edited by Wilma Wasco and Rudolph E. Tanzi.
      p. cm.—(Contemporary neuroscience)
   Includes index.
   ISBN 0-89603-371-6 (alk. paper)
   1. Dementia—Molecular aspects.   I. Wasco, Wilma.   II. Tanzi, Rudolph E.
   [DNLM: 1. Alzheimer's Disease—etiology. WT 155 M718 1997]
RC521.M65 1997
616.8'3—dc20
DNLM/DLC
for Library of Congress
96-38858
CIP

Preface

The past decade has witnessed a revolution in the attempts of scientists to understand the molecular basis of dementia. Although dementia, as defined by global cognitive decline involving gradual loss of memory, reasoning, judgment, and orientation, presents most commonly in the form of Alzheimer's disease (AD), an assortment of other less common disorders, such as prion and Pick's disease, can also lead to symptoms that are similar to those observed in patients with AD. The primary goal of *Molecular Mechanisms of Dementia* is to address the various mechanisms and multifaceted approaches currently being employed to more clearly delineate the etiological and pathogenic events responsible for the onset of dementia.

Perhaps the greatest boon to obtaining a clearer understanding of the causes of AD has come from genetic and molecular biological studies carried out over the past decade. At the genetic level, it has become increasingly clear that AD is a heterogeneous disorder that can be broadly classified into two categories. "Late onset" (>60 yr) cases, which account for the vast majority of AD, genetically involve "susceptibility" genes representing risk factors for the disease (e.g., inheritance of the ε4 allele of the Apolipoprotein E gene). In many cases, the susceptibility gene can act as a "modifier" that modulates the pathogenic cascade occurring subsequent to a separate etiological event "initiating" or "causing" the disorder. "Early-onset" (<60 yr) cases account for 15–20% of AD and appear to involve "causative" or "deterministic" gene defects sufficient to cause the disorder (e.g., mutations in the amyloid β protein precursor gene and the presenilin genes). Following the identification of gene defects associated with dementia, a logical next step involves attempts to establish cell culture-based models and transgenic animals as experimental models for dementia. This strategy has already proven successful for prion disease, and a great deal of progress has recently been made in developing a viable animal model for AD.

Though genetic studies aimed at identifying gene defects leading to dementia do not require a biological hypothesis to arrive at the end result, a large volume of literature exists in which molecular biological strategies have been implemented to test a wide variety of models for the etiological and pathogenic mechanisms of dementia. Topics addressed in *Molecular Mechanisms of Dementia* include apoptosis, energy metabolism, excitotoxicity and calcium-mediated cell death, free radicals, electrophysiological abnormalities, inflammatory and complement activation pathways, environmental toxins, degeneration of neural networks, and modifications of the cytoskeleton. Additionally, a common phenocopy for AD and related disorders is onset of dementia owing to the occurrence of multiple infarctions; thus, mechanisms by which ischemia and hypoxia result in dementia are also covered here.

The powerful combination of genetic studies leading to the identification of gene defects associated with dementia and molecular biological, biochemical, and immuno-histochemical strategies for testing possible mechanisms underlying neuronal cell death has already provided a much more lucid understanding of the molecular basis of dementia. The goal of *Molecular Mechanisms of Dementia* is to review the tremendous progress that has been made in developing testable models of the molecular mechanisms of dementia, as well as to provide direction for future investigations of dementia.

Wilma Wasco
Rudolph E. Tanzi

Contents

Contributors

MICHAEL AKSENOV • *Department of Pharmacology, University of Kentucky, Lexington, KY*

MARINA AKSENOVA • *Department of Pharmacology, University of Kentucky, Lexington, KY*

DANIEL L. ALKON • *Laboratory of Adaptive Systems-NINDS, National Institutes of Health, Bethesda, MD*

AILEEN J. ANDERSON • *Institute of Brain Aging and Dementia, University of California, Irvine, CA*

CRAIG S. ATWOOD • *Genetics and Aging Unit, Massachusetts General Hospital, Charlestown, MA*

GIULIANO BINETTI • *Massachusetts Alzheimer Disease Research Center, Massachusetts General Hospital, Boston, MA; and Departments of Neurology and Alzheimer's Disease Unit, S. Cuore Fatebenefratelli, Brescia, Italy*

EMMANUELLE BLANC • *Sanders-Brown Research Center on Aging and Department of Anatomy and Neurobiology, University of Kentucky, Lexington, KY*

JOHN P. BLASS • *Altschul Laboratory for Dementia Research, Burke Medical Research Institute, Cornell University Medical College, White Plains, NY*

ANNADORA J. BRUCE • *Sanders-Brown Research Center on Aging and Department of Anatomy and Neurobiology, University of Kentucky, Lexington, KY*

ASHLEY I. BUSH • *Genetics and Aging Unit, Massachusetts General Hospital, Charlestown, MA*

D. ALLAN BUTTERFIELD • *Department of Chemistry and Center of Membrane Sciences, University of Kentucky, Lexington, KY*

JOHN M. CARNEY • *Department of Pharmacology, University of Kentucky, Lexington, KY*

RAYMOND T. F. CHEUNG • *Department of Clinical Neurological Sciences, University of Western Ontario, London, Ontario, Canada*

PAMELA COLE • *Department of Chemistry and Center of Membrane Sciences, University of Kentucky, Lexington, KY*

CARL W. COTMAN • *Institute of Brain Aging and Dementia, University of California, Irvine, CA*

DAVID H. CRIBBS • *Institute of Brain Aging and Dementia, University of California, Irvine, CA*

RENÉ ETCHEBERRIGARAY • *Laboratory of Applied Neuroscience, Institute of Cognitive and Computational Sciences, Georgetown University Medical Center, Washington DC*

KATSUTOSHI FURUKAWA • *Sanders-Brown Research Center on Aging and Department of Anatomy and Neurobiology, University of Kentucky, Lexington, KY*

PIERLUIGI GAMBETTI • *Division of Neuropathology, Institute of Pathology, Case Western Reserve University, Cleveland, OH*

MICHEL GOEDERT • *Medical Research Council Laboratory of Molecular Biology, Cambridge, UK*

W. SUE T. GRIFFIN • *Departments of Pediatrics, Pathology, Anatomy, and Physiology, University of Arkansas for Medical Sciences, Department of Veterans' Affairs Medical Center, Arkansas Children's Hospital Research Institute, Little Rock, AR*

VLADIMIR HACHINSKI • *Department of Clinical Neurological Sciences, University of Western Ontario, London, Ontario, Canada*

NATHAN HALL • *Department of Chemistry and Center of Membrane Sciences, University of Kentucky, Lexington, KY*

MARNI E. HARRIS • *Department of Pharmacology, University of Kentucky, Lexington, KY*

KENNETH HENSLEY • *Department of Chemistry and Center of Membrane Sciences, University of Kentucky, Lexington, KY*

BEVERLY J. HOWARD • *Department of Chemistry and Center of Membrane Sciences, University of Kentucky, Lexington, KY*

KAREN K. HSIAO • *Department of Neurology, University of Minnesota, Minneapolis, MN*

XUDONG HUANG • *Genetics and Aging Unit, Massachusetts General Hospital, Charlestown, MA*

BRADLEY T. HYMAN • *Neurology Service, Massachusetts General Hospital, Boston, MA*

LYNNE M. KELLEY • *Laboratory for Molecular Neuropathology, Massachusetts General Hospital, Charlestown, MA; and Massachusetts Alzheimer Disease Research Center, Massachusetts General Hospital, Boston, MA*

MICHAEL LAFONTAINE • *Department of Chemistry and Center of Membrane Sciences, University of Kentucky, Lexington, KY*

ANDRÉA LEBLANC • *Department of Neurology and Neurosurgery, McGill University; The Bloomfield Center for Research in Aging, Lady Davis Institute for Medical Research, The Mortimer B. Davis Jewish General Hospital, Montréal, Québec, Canada*

VIRGINIA M.-Y. LEE • *Department of Pathology and Laboratory Medicine, University of Pennsylvania School of Medicine, Philadelphia, PA*

ROBERT J. MARK • *Sanders-Brown Research Center on Aging and Department of Anatomy and Neurobiology, University of Kentucky, Lexington, KY*

MARK P. MATTSON • *Sanders-Brown Research Center on Aging and Department of Anatomy and Neurobiology, University of Kentucky, Lexington, KY*

ROBERT D. MOIR • *Genetics and Aging Unit, Massachusetts General Hospital, Charlestown, MA*

ROBERT E. MRAK • *Departments of Pediatrics, Pathology, Anatomy, and Physiology, University of Arkansas for Medical Sciences, Department of Veterans' Affairs Medical Center, Arkansas Children's Hospital Research Institute, Little Rock, AR*

STEPHEN O'BARR • *L. J. Roberts Center, Sun Health Research Institute, Sun City, AZ*

PIERO PARCHI • *Division of Neuropathology, Institute of Pathology, Case Western Reserve University, Cleveland, OH*

G. WILLIAM REBECK • *Alzheimer's Research Center, Massachusetts General Hospital (East), Boston, MA*

JOSEPH ROGERS • *L. J. Roberts Center, Sun Health Research Institute, Sun City, AZ*

JIN G. SHENG • *Departments of Pediatrics, Pathology, Anatomy, and Physiology, University of Arkansas for Medical Sciences, Department of Veterans' Affairs Medical Center, Arkansas Children's Hospital Research Institute, Little Rock, AR*

RAMACHANDRAN SUBRAMANIAM • *Department of Chemistry and Center of Membrane Sciences, University of Kentucky, Lexington, KY*

RUDOLPH E. TANZI • *Genetics and Aging Unit, Department of Neurology, Massachusetts General Hospital, Harvard Medical School, Charlestown, MA*

JOHN Q. TROJANOWSKI • *Department of Pathology and Laboratory Medicine, University of Pennsylvania School of Medicine, Philadelphia, PA*

VLADIMIR VOLLOCH • *Boston Biomedical Research Institute, Boston, MA*

JEAN PAUL G. VONSATTEL • *Laboratory for Molecuar Neuropathology, Massachusetts General Hospital, Charlestown, MA; Brain Tissue Resource Center, McLean Hospital, Belmont, MA; C. S. Kubik Laboratory for Neuropathology, James Homer Wright Pathology Laboratories; Massachusetts Alzheimer Disease Research Center, Massachusetts General Hospital, Boston, MA; and Departments of Pathology and Neurology, S. Cuore Fatebenefratelli Institute, Brescia, Italy*

WILMA WASCO • *Genetics and Aging Unit, Department of Neurology, Massachusetts General Hospital, Harvard Medical School, Charlestown, MA*

SERVET YATIN • *Department of Chemistry and Center of Membrane Sciences, University of Kentucky, Lexington, KY*

Etiological Clues from Gene Defects Causing Early Onset Familial Alzheimer's Disease

Wilma Wasco and Rudolph E. Tanzi

1. INTRODUCTION

Alzheimer's disease (AD) is a progressive neurodegenerative disorder of the central nervous system that is invariably associated with and defined by the presence of intracellular neurofibrillary tangles (NFT), and extracellular deposits of β-amyloid in senile plaques and cerebral blood vessels in the brain. The etiologic events that lead to the generation of these pathological hallmarks and ultimately to synaptic loss, neurodegeneration, and cognitive decline are not well understood. However, it is clear that a significant portion of AD has a genetic basis (for review, *see* ref. *1*). These familial forms of Alzheimer's disease (FAD) have been classified based on both the age of onset and the type of gene defect inherited. Within recent years, molecular genetic analyses have successfully led to the identification of three "causative" early onset (<60 yr) FAD genes located on chromosomes 1, 14, and 21, and, additionally, to the identification of an inherited "risk factor" for late-onset FAD (>60 yr old) on chromosome 19. In this chapter, we will concentrate on the causative defects in the three early onset FAD genes with an emphasis on the clues gained regarding the etiology and neuropathogenesis of the disease. The putative role of the fourth FAD gene, Apolipoprotein E (ApoE), and how it contributes to the disease process as a genetic risk factor will be covered in Chapter 2.

In considering a potential common mechanism by which early onset FAD gene defects lead to AD, a growing collection of data support a central role for the generation of β-amyloid, and its chief component, the Aβ peptide in all cases of the disease *(2)*. In addition, the accelerated production of β-amyloid also occurs in middle-aged patients with Down's syndrome (DS; trisomy 21) who inevitably develop AD-related neuropathology. In the DS cases, the heightened production β-amyloid is most likely owing to the presence of three copies of the gene encoding the amyloid β-protein precursor (APP), which resides on chromosome 21. DS patients go on also to develop other Alzheimer-type lesions, such as NFT and neuropil threads. Perhaps the greatest support for the central role of β-amyloid in AD neuropathogenesis derives from the discovery of a series of mutations in the APP gene *(3–9)*; these were the first FAD gene defects to be described. The mutations in the APP gene appear to be 100% penetrant:

From: Molecular Mechanisms of Dementia Edited by: W. Wasco and R. E. Tanzi Humana Press Inc., Totowa, NJ and are thus considered to be "deterministic" for early onset FAD. However, since their discovery in 1991, APP mutations have been shown to be responsible for only a small proportion (2–3%) of reported cases of early onset FAD *(10)*. Meanwhile, the vast majority of early onset FAD appears to be caused by mutations in two recently identified genes, which have been termed presenilin 1 (PS1) and presenilin 2 (PS2), localized to chromosomes 14 and 1, respectively *(11–13)*. Plasma and fibroblasts obtained from carriers of these mutations have been reported to contain increased amounts of specific, more amyloidogenic forms of the Aβ peptide (Aβx-42; *14*). Finally, the inheritance of a specific allele (ε4) of a fourth gene, ApoE, which is located on chromosome 19, confers increased "risk" for late-onset FAD (for review, *see* ref. *15*), and is associated with increased amyloid burden in AD and DS patients who carry this allele. Thus, the most likely common event tying together AD-associated variants of these four genes is the increased generation of the Aβ peptide and the accumulation of β-amyloid in the brain. Although great strides have already been made in attempts to determine how alterations in the FAD genes lead to the increased presence of β-amyloid, the precise mechanisms underlying this process remain to be elucidated.

2. THE BIOLOGICAL ROLE OF THE APP GENE

APP is a type I integral membrane protein that exists as either a transmembrane or secreted protein with a variety of posttranslational modifications *(16–23)*. The main component of the AD-associated senile plaques, the 39–43 amino acid amyloidogenic peptide termed Aβ, is derived by the proteolytic processing of APP *(2)*. The APP gene is comprised of 18 exons, 3 of which can be alternatively transcribed to produce a variety of mRNA species that have been named according to the number of amino acids that they encode *(24–27)*. The three alternatively transcribed exons encode:

1. A 19 amino acid domain of unknown function that has homology to the MRC OX-2 antigen;
2. A 56 amino acid Kunitz protease inhibitor (KPI) domain; and
3. A 15 amino acid domain.

APP mRNA transcripts appear to be widely, if not ubiquitously, expressed. However, Northern blot analysis provides evidence for tissue-specific and developmental regulation of APP transcription. The expression of APP mRNA is relatively high in heart, brain, and kidney, and low in lung and liver *(19,26)*. All of the major APP transcripts have been shown to be expressed in brain. However, individual alternatively spliced transcripts appear to be expressed with some degree of cellular specificity. The predominant form of APP mRNA in neurons does not contain the KPI domain, whereas the majority of APP transcripts produced in astrocytes and microglia do; in peripheral tissues, KPI-containing APP transcripts are more abundant. Interestingly, in normal aging, a relative decrease in the production of APP695 transcripts relative to KPI-containing transcripts of APP has been reported *(28,29)*. This could be the result of increased production of APP-KPI forms by reactive astrocytes that appear with increasing frequency with age. The APP promoter lacks typical TATA and CAAT boxes, and has multiple transcriptional start sites, making it typical of a housekeeping gene promoter. Other elements localized to the promoter region of APP have been shown to be critical to the regulation of APP transcription. For example, the deletion of a combined AP1/AP4 site that is conserved in human, rat, and mouse APP promoters results in a 30% decrease in the transcription of APP in PC-12 cells, and recent evidence indicates that the factor that binds to the AP1/AP4 site in the human APP promoter is the basic helix-loop-helix protein known as the upstream stimulatory factor (USF; *30*). The factors regulating alternative transcription of APP have yet to be identified.

The APP gene has been shown to be a member of an evolutionarily conserved gene family, which includes two mammalian amyloid precursor-like proteins, APLP1 and APLP2 as well as APP-like proteins in *Drosophila* and *Caenorhabditis elegans (31– 36)*. The overall structure and the majority of APP's specific structural/functional domains are extremely well conserved in all five of these proteins. In fact, the only region of APP that is not well conserved in either of the mammalian APLPs or in the *Drosophila* or *C. elegans* homologues is the Aβ domain. The conspicuous absence of Aβ in the APLPs indicates that, although it is likely that APP and the APLPs possess similar physiological roles, only APP can directly give rise to Aβ, the main component of β-amyloid associated with AD.

The normal biological roles of APP and the APLPs remain unclear. The existence of secreted forms of APP in plasma and cerebral spinal fluid (CSF) as well as in growth conditioned media of cultured cells suggests a role for these molecules in vivo. APP has been demonstrated to have growth-promoting effects on fibroblasts, PC12 cells, and cortical and neuronal cells. Furthermore, a specific amino acid sequence (RERMS) within the N-terminal domain of APP has been shown to be responsible for some of these trophic effects *(37)*. Studies on hippocampal neurons suggest that secreted APP can protect cells from excitotoxic effects of glutamate by regulating intracellular levels of calcium *(38)*. To date, the most clearly defined role for APP is that of a secreted protease inhibitor. KPI-containing forms of APP have the ability to inhibit a number of serine proteases in vitro, and these forms of the molecule have been shown to be identical to protease nexin II, a molecule that was previously identified based on its tight association with proteases. Additionally, KPI-containing forms of APP have also been shown to be identical to factor XIa inhibitor, which is released from the α-granules of platelets and inhibits activated factor XIa at the late stages of the cascade *(39)*.

Another proposed role for APP involves its potential interaction with the extracellular matrix, where it is believed to be influential in the guidance of neurites in the developing nervous system and during regeneration of neurites following injury. APP preadsorbed to the culture dish promotes cell adhesion to the substratum, and has been shown to interact with heparan sulfate proteoglycan *(40,41)*, collagen *(42)*, and laminin *(43,44)*, all of which are major protein components of the extracellular matrix that have been localized in amyloid plaques. In addition, APP, APLP1, and APLP2 all bind heparin, a heparan analog, and this binding is promoted by the presence of zinc *(45)*. In B103 cells, a clonal CNS neuronal cell line that makes little or no endogenous APP, the ability of an APP695 transgene to promote neurite outgrowth as has been determined to lie within the 17 amino acids contained between amino acids 319 and 335 *(46)*. In this system, the effects of APP do not appear to be mediated by stimulation of cell adhesion. However, the addition of the 17 mer did increase the turnover of inositol polyphosphates, suggesting that, in these cells, APP may promote neurite extension through cell-surface interaction and subsequent activation of inositol phosphate signal transduction systems.

3. APP AND THE PRODUCTION OF β-AMYLOID IN AD

Attempts to delineate the events leading to the production of β-amyloid have led to the intensive investigation of the factors regulating the intracellular trafficking and processing of APP (for review, *see* refs. *47–49*). Particular emphasis has been placed on determining the exact pathways through which Aβ is liberated from APP. APP contains an N-terminal signal sequence that allows it to be inserted into the plasma membrane via constitutive secretory pathways subsequent to maturation in the endoplasmic reticulum and Golgi *(22)*. The molecule can then be metabolized via one of at least three pathways producing C-terminal fragments of APP that may or may not contain the "intact" Aβ domain, thereby permitting or precluding β-amyloid production, respectively. The majority of APP appears to be processed through the so-called α-secretase pathway, whereby full-length, mature APP is transported to the cell surface and is cleaved close to the plasma membrane, within the Aβ domain. Because α-secretase cleavage takes place within the Aβ domain, utilization of this pathway precludes the formation of β-amyloid. This cleavage also results in the secretion of the ectodomain of APP *(22,50,51)*, whereas the C-terminal membrane-bound fragment of APP is internalized via clathrin-coated pits or by other mechanisms, and subsequently enters the endosomal–lysosomal pathway *(51–55)*.

The ability to detect soluble Aβ in the CSF of individuals unaffected by AD as well as in a variety of APP-transfected cultured cell systems first indicated that alternative APP processing pathway(s) must exist. Indeed, in what has been termed the "β-secretase" pathway, cleavage of APP at the N-terminal amino acid of Aβ produces a C-terminal fragment that contains an intact Aβ domain. This fragment may then be further cleaved by γ-secretase to produce Aβ *(52,53,56–62)*. Clearly, a delicate balance between these processing pathways must be maintained in order to keep the amounts of secreted Aβ below concentrations that would foster the pathological development of β-amyloid.

Following the observations that APP can give rise to either a secreted ectodomain (APPs) or the Aβ peptide, the apparent interdependence of these processing pathways was illustrated by the observed decrease in the levels of Aβ generated in experimental systems that increase levels of APPs *(63)*. Internalization of APP has recently been implicated in the generation of Aβ based on the finding that attenuation of Aβ release is accompanied by a reduction in the amounts APP that are internalized *(64)*. Internalization of APP via clathrin-coated vesicles has been proposed as the pathway by which cell-surface APP gains entry into the endosomal/lysosomal pathway. Clathrin-coated pit-mediated internalization of APP occurs via the NPXY motif in the cytoplasmic domain of APP *(52,65)*. Deletion of this motif has been shown to not only impair endocytosis of cell-surface APP, but also to alter its intracellular trafficking, targeting APP into the endocytic pathway prior to reaching the cell surface *(66)*.

In a search for the cellular factors and mechanisms responsible for mediating the intracellular trafficking and the normal function of cell-surface APP, we have recently employed a two-hybrid system known as the "interaction trap" to isolate a gene encoding a protein that specifically binds to the cytoplasmic domain of APP (Guenette et al., submitted). The gene, hFE65L, encodes a homolog of the rat FE65 gene. We also identified two other human sequences that appear to represent additional human homologs of the rat FE65 gene. All three members of this human FE65/FE65L multigene family contain two motifs previously found in signal transduction proteins, a WW domain and phosphotyrosine-binding domains. These latter domains are known to bind to the consensus sequence NPXY in which the tyrosine is phosphorylated. This implies that hFE65L most likely binds to the clathrin-coated pit motif in the cytoplasmic domain of APP. We also confirmed the in vivo interaction of hFE65L with APP and its homolog APLP2 in mammalian cells. These studies raise the intriguing possibility that interaction of the C-termini of APP and APLP2 with hFE65L may serve to modulate the trafficking or even the function of these molecules.

Recent data indicating that the LDL receptor-related protein (LRP) binds secreted APP and mediates its internalization and degradation provides a biochemical link for APP and ApoE in a single metabolic pathway. LRP is a multifunctional, multiligand receptor that is a member of the LDL receptor family. Other members of this family include the VLDL receptor, glycoprotein 330, and the LDL receptor. One known function of LRP is to bind and mediate the uptake and degradation of proteinases (including tissue factor pathway inhibitor and urokinase-type plasminogen activator), proteinase–inhibitor complexes, and matrix proteins, such as ApoE-enriched lipoproteins. In the CNS, LRP is believed to be a major ApoE receptor and is thus used to deliver lipid to neurons especially during compensatory synaptogenesis following neuronal cell injury *(67)*. LRP also serves to clear proteases and protease–protease inhibitor complexes in the brain during neurite regeneration occurring subsequent to neuronal degeneration.

We have recently shown LRP to be localized to pre- and postsynaptic plasma membranes, where it may help to protect against synaptic degradation following neuronal cell injury by aiding in the clearance of glial and neuronal-derived proteases and their complexes *(68)*. The ligand-binding ability of LRP and other members of the family is blocked by the binding of a 39-kDa protein receptor-associated protein (RAP). Kounnas et al. *(69)* have demonstrated that LRP is responsible for the endocytosis of forms of secreted APP that contain the KPI domain. The degradation of internalized APP is inhibited by RAP and by LRP antibodies, and is significantly diminished in cell lines that are genetically deficient in LRP. Meanwhile, forms of APP lacking the KPI domain are poor LRP ligands. These data suggest that LRP serves as a receptor for APP and for ApoE, two of the four molecules that have been genetically linked to AD. These data also raise the possibility that LRP may play a role in internalizing full-length APP containing an intact Aβ domain. In view of the recent finding that internalization of APP precedes the secretion of Aβ, it will be important in future studies to determine whether LRP plays a role in the process and, more critically, whether specific variants of ApoE can differentially interfere with the internalization of APP.

All of the AD-associated APP mutations result in amino acid substitutions within or adjacent to the Aβ domain *(3–9)*, and certain of these mutations have been directly demonstrated to cause either quantitative or qualitative changes in the secretion of Aβ *(70–72)*. These mutations appear to affect the generation of Aβ by leading to overproduction of the peptide or by producing a longer version of Aβ, which contains two extra amino acids on the C-terminal end (Aβ1–42). The precise mechanism by which these mutation exert their effect remains unclear. However, a variety of data indicate that aggregated Aβ may be neurotoxic *(73–75)*. The exact mechanism by which Aβ exerts its apparently toxic effects is still unclear, although evidence for apoptosis has been reported (see *76,77*, and Chapter 2, this vol.). Studies of APP trafficking in polarized cells have revealed that 80–90% of α-secretase-cleaved APP is released from the basolateral surface of Madin-Darby canine kidney cells *(78)*. Expression of the "Swed-ish" mutant of APP leads to increased secretion of Aβ at the apical surface *(79,80)*. To date, these mutations and their location provide the strongest evidence for the genera-tion of Aβ and, in particular, specific forms of this peptide, as a central etiologic event in AD. It will be extremely important in future studies to isolate and identify the "secretase" enzymes involved in the generation of Aβ. The identification of these enzymes and factors involved in the trafficking, internalization, and degradation of APP should ultimately represent important new targets for drug discovery. The recent report of a transgenic mouse expressing an FAD variant of APP (APP V717F; *81*) carries the promise of becoming a valuable animal model for AD for testing new compounds aimed at attenuating β-amyloid production and its neuropathological consequences.

4. THE IDENTIFICATION AND CHARACTERIZATION OF THE PRESENILIN GENES

Both PS1 and PS2 were isolated in the latter half of 1995 *(11–13)*. PS1, which is located on chromosome 14 and is the major early onset FAD gene, was identified by classical "positional cloning" techniques *(11,83)*. PS2, which is located on chromo-some 1 *(12)*, was isolated based on its homology to PS1 and was then tested as a candi-date gene for the nonchromosome 14-linked form of FAD present in pedigrees of Volga German descent *(82)*. The identity of PS2 as a third early onset FAD gene was later confirmed by Rogaev et al. *(13)*. A multitude of apparently pathogenic mutations in both of these genes have now been identified, and it appears that mutations in these two genes, together with those in APP, account for the vast majority of early onset FAD. The existence of a number of early onset FAD kindreds that do not appear to harbor mutations in the coding regions of APP, PS1, or PS2 (St. George-Hyslop, P., American Academy of Neurology, 1996), indicates the probable existence of at least one more onset FAD gene.

Relatively little is known about the function of the presenilin proteins. The presence of six to nine hydrophobic domains indicates that both proteins share a "serpentine" membrane-spanning topology *(11–13)*. Although the actual number of membrane-span-ning domains remains unclear, we have recently chosen to use a seven-transmembrane domain model that dictates that both proteins have one large and five small hydrophilic loops. This model also predicts that, for both proteins, the N-terminus and the large hydrophilic loop between predicted transmembrane domains six and seven are located on the same side of the membrane, whereas the C-terminus is located on the other (*see* Fig. 1). Future studies utilizing PS1 and PS2 antibodies raised against specific domains should help to elucidate exactly how the presenilins are arranged within the membrane. Both PS1 and PS2 lack a traditional N-terminal signal sequence suggesting that they may be cotranslationally inserted into the endoplasmic reticulum by means of an as yet unidentified internal signal sequence. Such a process would result in the retention of the N-terminal amino acids. Interestingly, two specific regions of PS1 and PS2 — the first 80 amino acids and the single large hydrophilic loop — stand out because they are not particularly well conserved in the two mammalian presenilins. This lack of homol-ogy suggests that although the overall amino acid similarity and structure exhibited by PS1 and PS2 predict similar functions for these proteins, these nonhomologous regions most likely impart specificity of function or subcellular localization to PS1 and PS2.

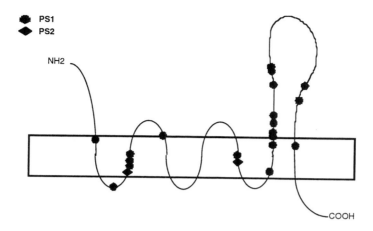

Fig. 1. Location of presenilin mutations. The positions of the presenilin 1 (PS1) and presenilin 2 (PS2) mutations (listed in Table 1) are shown.

Northern blot analysis indicates that both of the PS1 and PS2 genes produce two major transcripts. The PS1 messages migrate at approx 2.7 and 7.5 kb *(11)* and the PS2 transcripts at 2.3 and 2.6 kb *(12)*. To date, only the cDNA sequences for the smaller of the two messages from each gene have been reported. Whether the differences in size of the two major transcripts for each gene are the result of alternative splicing or of alternative polyadenylation remains to be determined. A number of minor alternative PS1 transcripts have been reported, including a form that lacks only four amino acids (VRSQ) encoded at the 3'-end of exon 3. Three of these four amino acids are conserved in PS2, where the analogous motif is WRSQ. However, PS2 transcripts lacking these four amino acids have not been identified. Interestingly, it has been reported that the human tyrosine hydroxylase gene and the chicken GABA receptor β4 subunit gene also contain alternatively transcribed VRSQ motifs *(84)*. Although it is not yet clear whether the alternative splicing of this motif has a physiological function in any or all of these genes, it has been noted by Clark et al. *(84)* that, in PS1, these four amino acids form part of a putative recognition site for casein kinase II and for protein kinase C.

Although PS1 and PS2 both appear to be ubiquitously expressed, there are some striking differences in their expression patterns. Most notably, PS2 transcripts appear to be far less abundant than PS1 transcripts in brain (Wasco and Tanzi, unpublished findings). In addition, although both of the PS1 transcripts are expressed in all tissues examined, it appears that there is clear tissue-specific regulation of the production of the two different PS2 transcripts; only the smaller of the two transcripts is detected in brain, placenta, lung, and liver, whereas both transcripts are detected in heart, skeletal muscle, and pancreas *(12,13)*. *In situ* hybridization analysis of rat brain sections with antisense oligonucleotides to the PS1 gene have shown that PS1 mRNA is predominantly in neurons *(85)*. The hippocampal formation and cerebellar granule cell layers contain more PS1 message than adjacent areas of cortex, striatum, or midbrain. White matter, including populations of fibrous astrocytes and oligodendrocytes, do not express detectable levels of PS1 mRNA. However, the choroid plexus contains relatively high levels of PS1 message. *In situ* hybridizations to sections of human temporal lobe have revealed similar patterns of hybridization for both PS1 and PS2 *(85)*, with both being expressed maximally in neuronal laminae of the parahippocampal gyrus and within the CA fields of the hippocampal formation. Choroid plexus adjacent to the hippocampal formation has also been shown to contain relatively higher levels of PS1 and PS2 mRNA *(85)*. These observations are consistent with the pattern of PS1 expression observed in rat brain *(85)* and indicate that the presenilins are largely, if not exclusively, of neuronal origin in the CNS.

The PS1 gene has been localized to a 75-kb region of chromosome 14, and the open reading frame has been found to be encoded by 10 exons *(84)*. Although it has been suggested that the homology between PS1 and PS2 can be extended to intron/exon boundaries *(84)*, no data about the genomic structure of PS2 or about the promoter sequences of either gene are currently available. The sequence of the mouse PS1 gene has been reported *(11)*, and it encodes a protein that is 92% identical to the human gene at the amino acid level. Although the full-length PS2 sequence is only available for the human gene, the isolation of the C-terminal portion of the mouse PS2 cDNA, which has recently been reported *(86)*, indicates that within these 103 amino acids, the mouse and human PS2 proteins are 98% identical.

5. THE BIOLOGICAL ROLE OF THE PRESENILINS

The normal biological role(s) of the presenilins and the mechanism(s) by which the FAD-associated mutations exert their effect remain unknown. To date, 24 apparently pathogenic mutations in 52 individual chromosome 14-linked pedigrees have been identified in PS1 and two such mutations have been detected in eight PS2 pedigrees *(11–13,87–92)*. All of these alterations are missense mutations, which result in single amino acid changes (*see* Table 1). Since the identified PS1 mutations are scattered throughout the protein, their positions provide no immediate mechanistic clues about their pathogenic nature. A number of PS1 mutations, however, do appear to cluster in exons 5 and 8, suggesting that the predicted transmembrane domain II and the large hydrophilic loop may be critical to proper functioning of the molecule (*see* Fig. 1). The two known PS2 mutations are an N to I substitution at amino acid 141 (in seven Volga-German pedigrees) and an M to V substitution at amino acid 239 (in an Italian pedigree). These mutations result in changes in positions within transmembrane domains 2 and 5 of PS2, presuming a seven-transmembrane domain structure (*see* Fig. 1).

Despite the fact that the average age of onset in specific chromosome 14 FAD pedigrees varies from 25 to 63 yr, to date, there have been no correlations between the location of mutations and specific AD phenotypic features. On the other hand, the average age of onset in the families with mutations in PS2 is slightly later than that of the PS1-linked families (44–84 yr; *12*; a member of an Italian pedigree with the M239V mutation in PS2 did not manifest symptoms of AD until the age of 84 yr [St. George-Hyslop, American Academy of Neurology, 1996]), supporting the notion that mutations in the PS2 gene may not be quite as severe as those in the PS1 gene, at least in terms of age of onset. It is unclear whether this difference is because mutations in PS1 have more profound consequences than mutations in PS2, or is owing to the specific type or location of the mutations identified in these genes thus far. Whether the degree of "amyloid burden" is correlated with specific mutations or with mutation location has also not yet been assessed.

Table 1
Presenilin Mutations

Mutation	Number of families	Ethnic origin	Mutation location
PS1			
V82L	1	Caucasian	TM-1/4
Y115H	1	Caucasian	HL-1/5
M139V	2	United Kingdom	TM-2/5
M139T	1	Caucasian	TM-2/5
I143T	2	Caucasian/Belgian	TM-2/5
M146L	10	Italian	TM-2/5
M146V	3	Italian/UK/Finnish	TM-2/5
H163Y	1	Swedish	HL-2/6
H163R	3	American/Canadian/Japanese	HL-2/6
G209V	1	Caucasian	TM-4/7
A23 IT	1	Caucasian	TM-5/7
A246E	1	Nova Scotian	TM-6/7
A260V	1	Japanese	TM-6/8
C263R	1	Caucasian	HL-6/8
P264L	1	Caucasian	HL-6/8
P267S	1	United Kingdom	HL-6/8
R269H	1	Caucasian	HL-6/8
E280G	2	United Kingdom	HL-6/8
E280A	4	Columbian	HL-6/8
A285V	1	Japanese	HL-6/8
L286V	1	German	HL-6/8
G384A	2	Caucasian/Belgian	HL-6/11
L392V	1	Italian	HL-6/11
C410Y	2	Ashkenazi Jewish	TM-7/11
PS2			
N141I	7	Volga German	TM-2
M239V	1	Italian	TM-5

TM, transmembrane domain; HL, hydrophilic loop.

Although none of the known mutations in the presenilins have been found in kindreds with late-onset FAD or cases of sporadic, late-onset AD, a polymorphism within the intron 3' of exon 8 of PS1 *(87)* has recently been shown to be associated with late-onset AD when homozygous for the 1 allele *(93)*. In the Caucasian population tested, homozygosity at this polymorphism was found to be associated with 22% of AD as compared to 35% for a single copy of ApoE 4, and 15% for a double dose of ApoE 4 *(93)*. Given the location of the intronic polymorphism, potential effects on the alternative splicing of PS1 associated with the appearance of the 1 allele would be worth investigating with regard to addressing a potential mechanism for this observation. Along these lines, Anwar et al. *(94)* have recently identified abnormal splice variants of PS1 (involving deletions and truncations throughout the gene) in sporadic cases of AD and in normal controls. It will be interesting to determine whether the 1 allele of the AD-associated, intronic polymorphism in PS1 correlates with the presence of any of the unusual splice variants observed in this study. Interestingly, the intronic polymorphism occurs in the intron next to the exon encoding the N-terminal portion of the large hydrophilic loop between predicted transmembrane domains 6 and 7, a region of PS1 in which the largest number of FAD-associated missense mutations appear to be clustered.

The full-length PS1 and PS2 genes encode predicted proteins of 463 and 448 amino acids, respectively. We have demonstrated that by Western blot analysis of presenilin protein extracts derived from COS cells transiently transfected with the PS1 and PS2 FLAG-tagged that PS2 exists as either a 50–55 kDa full-length form or as a high-mol-wt species *(85)*. We have also found that PS2 is proteolytically processed to give rise to a 35-kDa N-terminal fragment and a 20-kDa C-terminal fragment. This latter fragment is associated with the detergent-insoluble cellular fraction consistent with localization to the cytoskeletal protein pool (Kim et al., submitted). Likewise, for PS1, four species are observed by Western analysis, a 45–50-kDA full-length polypeptide, a high-mol-wt aggregate, and two proteolytic cleavage products, including a 28-kDa N-terminal fragment and a 19-kDa C-terminal fragment (unpublished data). Preliminary studies in our laboratory reveal that the high-mol-wt form of PS2 is polyubiquitinated and is normally degraded via the 26S proteosome complex (Kim et al., submitted). Interestingly, we have found that accumulation of the C-terminal, potentially cytoskeletal-associated 20-kDa PS2 fragment appears to be heightened in H4 human neuroglioma cells transfected with mutant PS2 (containing the Volga German N141I FAD mutation) as compared to H4 cells expressing wild-type PS2 (Kim et al., submitted). This enhanced accumulation of the 20-kDa fragment appears to be the result of inefficient degradation of PS2 via the ubiquitin-proteosome pathway. These data suggest that the mechanism by which the Volga German mutilation causes FAD may involve altered processing and degradation of PS2 (Kim et al., submitted).

The normal subcellular localization of FLAG-tagged PS1 and PS2 in transiently transfected mammalian cells has recently been reported *(85)*. PS1 and PS2 were both detected in the nuclear envelope, endoplasmic reticulum (ER), and the Golgi in COS cells and in H4 human neuroglioma cells. Interestingly, although the overall staining patterns for PS1 and PS2 are quite similar, clear differences are also evident. PS1 routinely exhibits a more defined perinuclear staining pattern than PS2, whereas PS2 staining exhibits a much clearer Golgi component. For both PS1 and PS2, the staining pattern is both reticular and punctate in nature, reminiscent of possible vesicular staining throughout the cytoplasm. Meanwhile, no staining for PS1 or PS2 has been observed on the plasma membrane. No gross abnormalities in subcellular localization have been observed for PS1 and PS2 containing FAD-associated mutations, although in COS cells transfected with PS1 carrying the A246E mutation, staining of the nuclear envelope has been reported to be somewhat more diffuse, irregular, and discontinuous in comparison to the consistently tight and uniform perinuclear staining observed with wild-type PS1 *(85)*. Cook et al. (submitted) have also demonstrated that PS1 is localized to the rough ER and in dendrites of NT2N human neuronal cell lines infected with human PS1.

The normal physiological roles of both of the presenilins remain unknown. However, clues about their function in mammalian cells can be derived from the interesting observation that both PS1 and PS2 share significant amino acid homology with two *C. elegans* proteins, *sel-12 (95)* and *spe-4 (96; see* Table 2). *Sel-12* was first isolated during a screen for suppressors of a *lin-12* hypermorphic gain-of-function mutation. The

Table 2
Percent Identity Between the Presenilins and the
***C. elegans* Gene Products**

	PS1	PS2	Sel-12	Spe-4
PS1	—	67	48	26
PS2	67	—	51	26
Sel-12	48	51	—	24
Spe-4	26	26	24	—

lin-12 gene is a member of the *lin-12*/Notch family of receptors for intracellular signals that specify cell fate in the nematode *(95)*. It produces a protein that has a single membrane-spanning domain. A hypermorphic mutation in the *lin-12* gene results in a multivulva phenotype that is characterized by the production of ectopic pseudovulvae. The fact that this phenotype can be corrected by specific loss-of-function mutations in *sel-12* indicates that there is an interaction between the SEL-12 and LIN-12 proteins, and that the function of SEL-12 may be to facilitate the LIN-12-mediated reception of intracellular signals. Although the exact details of the interaction remain unclear, the *sel-12* gene product may be directly involved in the LIN-12-mediated reception of signals by functioning as a coreceptor. Alternatively, SEL-12 may act as a downstream effector that is influenced by LIN-12 activation. Finally, SEL-12 may also play a role in receptor trafficking, localization, or recycling of LIN-12 *(95)*. This latter possibility, first raised by Levitan and Greenwald *(95)*, is most consistent with our recent observation that the human homologs of SEL-12, PS1 and PS2, are localized to the ER and Golgi, where they may play roles in protein processing and cellular trafficking.

Although the degree of identity of the presenilins with *spe-4* is not quite as striking as it is with *sel-12*, it is clear that the proteins are related. Mutations in *spe-4* disrupt the fibrous body membrane organelle (FB-MO), an unusual organelle that is involved in spermatogenesis in the nematode *(96)*. The function of the FB-MO is to package and deliver proteins to the spermatids during the unequal cytoplasmic partitioning that takes place during meiosis II. Unlike other organisms, the nematode spermatids do not contain ribosomes— they are discarded as the cells form. Thus, all of the proteins that are necessary for normal differentiation into functional sperm must be placed within the spermatid as it forms. Therefore, it is crucial for normal development of spermatids that the orderly segregation of components takes place during meiosis II. *Spe-4* mutations disrupt the coordination of cytokinesis with meiotic nuclear divisions during spermatogenesis and result in the production of a spermatocyte-like cell that contains four haploid nuclei instead of four spermatids. Thus, *spe-4* appears to play a role in cytoplasmic partitioning of proteins.

Overall, the display of homology between PS1 and PS2 with the two aforementioned *C. elegans* proteins suggests that the presenilins may play a role in the intracellular trafficking or localization/recycling of proteins. Interestingly, as described above, it has been demonstrated that mutations in APP lead to relative increases in the ratio of Aβ42:Aβ40 and it has been shown that this is most likely the result of altered intracellular trafficking and/or sorting of APP *(79,80)*. This hypothesis may ultimately gain further support from the recent observation that the levels of Aβx-42 are increased in the plasma and fibroblasts taken from patients with FAD-associated mutations in PS1 or PS2 *(14)*.

A second clue to the normal role of the presenilins may be provided by the observation that a truncated PS2 protein produced by a clone containing the nucleotides that encode the C-terminal 103 amino acids of PS2 appears to inhibit T-cell receptor- and Fas-induced apoptosis *(86)*. This study utilized a "death trap" system, which is based on the assumption that the expression transcripts derived from a transfected cDNA library constructed in a mammalian expression vector should protect some of the recipient cells from programmed cell death. A second cDNA clone isolated in this study encodes a Ca^{2+}-binding protein. Interestingly, the manner in which these two cDNA clones protect the cells from death appears to differ. The Ca^{2+}-binding protein cDNA is inserted in the expression vector in the antisense orientation, and presumably the antisense RNA that is produced on transfection reduces the steady-state amounts of the Ca^{2+}-binding protein. In contrast, the cDNA encoding the last 103 bp of PS2 is inserted in the vector in the sense orientation. Thus, the protection it provides against programmed cell death appears to be owing to an increase in the steady state of the truncated protein. An alternative explanation is that the truncated protein product competes for factors that normally interact with the C-terminus of PS2, suggesting that the cells are protected because the endogenous PS2 is unable to carry out its normal role efficiently.

SUMMARY

Genetic analyses of FAD kindreds have arguably led to the greatest advances in the quest to understand the etiology of this enigmatic and devastating neurodegenerative disorder. To date, four different genes have been discovered and confirmed to carry mutations associated with the onset of AD. Any of over 30 different pathogenic mutations discovered in the early onset FAD genes, APP, PS1, and PS2, can directly cause AD with 100% penetrance and are thus considered to be "deterministic" gene defects. Meanwhile, in a subset of AD cases with onset over the age of 60, a normal variant of the ApoE gene (ApoE-ε4) appears to confer increased risk for AD, but is not deterministic for the disease. A common and critical event resulting from the FAD-associated alterations in all four of these genes involves the excessive buildup of β-amyloid in the brains of affected individuals. This suggests a common pathogenic pathway for the mutations in these three genes centering around the abnormal cellular trafficking/processing of APP and the generation of Aβ. Given the demonstrated effects of FAD-associated mutations on the cellular trafficking of APP and subsequent changes in Aβ release (along with the potential role of the presenilins in intracellular transport in the ER and Golgi and the report that PS mutations lead to increased levels of Aβx-42), it is conceivable that, as a group, early onset FAD gene defects adversely affect the cellular sorting and processing of APP. In this scenario, mutations in APP as well as in the presenilins would most likely act as either "gain-of-function" or "negative dominant" gene defects, ultimately leading to the transport of APP into cellular compartments that are more conducive to the production of Aβ or specifically, Aβx-42.

AD patients who possess the allelic risk factor, ApoE-ε4, also manifest increased amyloid load in the brain. Thus, the mechanism by which this polymorphic allele confers increased susceptibility to AD most likely involves either the generation of Aβ, its aggregation in the brain parenchyma, or the clearance of β-amyloid deposits. It has been shown that APP must first undergo endocytosis before Aβ is generated and secreted by cell cultures *(64)*. APP can be internalized by clathrin-coated pits or by

LRP, the multifunctional neuronal receptor for ApoE in brain. We have recently shown that LRP is able to bind, internalize, and mediate the degradation of secreted forms of APP containing the KPI domain *(69)*. If LRP can also bind and internalize full-length transmembrane APP (Glabe, C., personal communication) in which the Aβ domain is intact, specific isoforms of ApoE could be envisioned to compete differentially with the internalization of APP concurrently affecting the production and release of Aβ. KPI-containing forms of APP are increased in the aging brain, suggesting that a potential internalization pathway utilizing LRP may become more critical in later stages of life. Thus, the degree to which specific ApoE isoforms interfere with a potential age-related demand on LRP to internalize KPI-containing forms of APP could serve as one possible explanation for the pathogenic role of ApoE 4 in its capacity as a risk factor for late-onset AD. Alternatively, different isoforms of ApoE could differentially affect the rate of aggregation of Aβ or the clearance of β-amyloid deposits in brain. The elucidation of the exact mechanism by which the four known FAD genes induce or accelerate AD-related neuropathology should continue to provide valuable new clues regarding the etiology of AD as well as vitally needed data to guide the development of effective new therapies.

REFERENCES

1. Tanzi, R., Gaston, S., Bush, A., Romano, D., Pettingell, W., Peppercorn, J., Paradis, M., Gurubhagavatula, S., Jenkins, B., and Wasco, W. (1994) Genetic heterogenity of gene defects responsible for familial Alzheimer disease, *Genetics* **91**, 255–263.
2. Glenner, G. G. and Wong, C. W. (1984) Alzheimer's disease: initial report of the purification and characterization of a novel cerebrovascular amyloid protein, *Biochem. Biophys. Res. Commun.* **120**, 885–890.
3. Goate, A., Chartier-Harlin, M., Mullan, M., Brown, J., Crawford, F., Fidani, L., Giuffra, L., Haynes, A., Irving, N., James, L., Mant, R., Newton, P., Rooke, K., Roques, P., Talbot, C., Pericak-Vance, M., Roses, A., Williamson, R., Rossor, M., Owen, M., and Hardy, J. (1991) Segregation of a missense mutation in the amyloid precursor protein gene with familial Alzheimer's disease, *Nature* **349**, 704–706.
4. Levy, E., Carman, M. D., Fernandez-Madrid, I. J., Power, M. D., Lieberburg, I., Van Duinen, S. G., Bots, G. T. A. M., Luyendijk, W., and Frangione, B. (1990) Mutation of the Alzheimer's disease amyloid gene in hereditary cerebral hemorrhage, Dutch type, *Science* **248**, 1124–1126.
5. Murrell, J., Farlow, M., Ghetti, B., and Benson, M. D. (1991) A mutation in the amyloid precursor protein associated with hereditary Alzheimer disease, *Science* **254**, 97–99.
6. Chartier-Harlin, M., Crawford, F., Hamandi, K., Mullan, M., Goate, A., Hardy, J., Backhovens, H., Martin, J., and van Broeckhoven, C. (1991) Screening for the β-amyloid precursor protein mutation (APP717: Val-Ile) in extended pedigrees with early onset Alzheimer's disease, *Neurosci. Lett.* **129**, 134,135.
7. Chartier-Harlin, M., Crawford, F., Houlden, H., Warren, A., Hughes, D., Fidani, L., Goate, A., Rossor, M., Roques, P., Hardy, J., and Mullan, M. (1991) Early-onset Alzheimer's disease caused by mutations at codon 717 of the β-amyloid precursor protein gene, *Nature* **353**, 844–846.
8. Hendriks, L., van Duijn, C. M., Cras, P., Cruts, M., van Hul, W., van Harskamp, F., Martin, J.-J., Hofman, A., and van Broeckhoven, C. (1992) Presenile dementia and cerebral haemorrhage caused by a mutation at codon 692 of the β-amyloid precursor protein gene, *Neurobiol. Aging* **13(Suppl. 1)**, S67.
9. Mullan, M., Crawford, F., Axelman, K., Houlden, H., Lilius, L., Winblad, W., and Lannfelt, L. (1992) A pathogenic mutation for probable Alzheimer's disease in the N-terminus of β-amyloid, *Nature Genet.* **1**, 345–347.

10. Tanzi, R. E., Vaula, G., Romano, D., Mortilla, M., Huang, T., Tupler, R., Wasco, W., Hyman, B., Gusella, J., and St. George-Hyslop, P. (1992) Assessment of APP gene mutations in a large set of familial and sporadic AD patients, *Neurobiol. Aging* **13(Suppl. 1),** S65.

11. Sherrington, R., Rogaev, E. I., Liang, Y., Rogaeva, E. A., Levesque, G., Ikeda, M., Chi, H., Lin, C., Li, G., Holman, K., Tsuda, T., Mar, L., Foncin, J.-F., Bruni, A. C., Montesi, M. P., Sorbi, S., Rainero, I., Pinessi, L., Nee, L., Chumakov, Y., Pollen, D., Wasco, W., Haines, J. L., Da Silva, R., Pericak-Vance, M., Tanzi, R. E., Roses, A. D., Fraser, P. E., Rommens, J. M., and St. George-Hyslop, P. H. (1995) Cloning of a novel gene bearing missense mutations in early onset familial Alzheimer disease, *Nature* **375,** 754–760.

12. Levy-Lahad, E.,* Wasco, W.,* Poorkaj, P., Romano, D. M., Oshima, J. M. Pettingell, W. H., Yu, C., Jondro, P. D., Schmidt, S. D., Wang, K., Crowley, A. C., Fu, Y.-H., Guenette, S. Y., Galas, D., Nemens, E., Wijsman, E. M., Bird, T. D., Schellenberg, G. D., and Tanzi, R. E. (1995) Candidate gene for the chromosome 1 familial Alzheimer's disease locus, *Science,* **269,** 973–977 (*shared first author*).

13. Rogaev, E. I., Sherrington, R., Rogaeva, E. A., Levesque, G., Ikeda, M., Liang, Y., Chi, H., Lin, C., Holman, K., Tsuda, T., Mar, L., Sorbi, S., Nacmias, B., Piacentini, S., Amaducci, L., Chumakov, I., Cohen, D., Lannfelt, L., Fraser, P. E., Rommens, J. M., and St. George-Hyslop, P. H. (1995) Familial Alzheimer's disease in kindreds with missense mutations in a gene on chomosome 1 related to the Alzheimer's disease type 3 gene, *Nature* **376(6543),** 775–778.

14. Scheuner, D., Eckman, C., Jensen, M., Song, X., Citron, M., Suzuki, N., Bird, T. D., Hardy, J., Hutton, M., Kukull, W., Larson, E., Levy-Lahad, E., Viitanen, M., Peskind, E., Poorkaj, P., Schellenberg, G., Tanzi, R. E., Wasco, W., Lannfelt, L., Selkoe, D., and Younkin, S. (1996) Aβ42(43) is increased *in vivo* by the *PS1/2* and *APP* mutations linked to familial Alzheimer's disease, *Nature Med.* **2,** 864–870.

15. Wasco, W. and Tanzi, R. E. (1995) Molecular Genetics of Amyloid and Apolipoprotein E in Alzheimer's Disease, in *Neurobiology of Alzheimer's Disease* (Dawbarn, D. and Allen, S. J., eds.), BIOS Scientific, Oxford, UK, pp. 51–76.

16. Goldgaber, D., Lerman, M. I., McBride, O. W., Saffiotti, U., and Gajdusek, D. C. (1987) Characterization and chromosomal localization of a cDNA encoding brain amyloid of Alzheimer's disease, *Science* **235,** 877–880.

17. Kang, J., Lemaire, H., Unterbeck, A., Salbaum, J. M., Masters, C. L., Grzeschik, K., Multhaup, G., Beyreuther, K., and Muller-Hill, B. (1987) The precursor of Alzheimer's disease amyloid A4 protein resembles a cell-surface receptor, *Nature* **325,** 733–736.

18. Robakis, N. K., Ramakrishna, N., Wolfe, G., and Wisniewski, H. M. (1987) Molecular cloning and characterization of a cDNA encoding the cerebrovascular and neuritic plaque amyloid peptides, *Proc. Natl. Acad. Sci. USA* **84,** 4190–4194.

19. Tanzi, R. E., Gusella, J. F., Watkins, P. C., Bruns, G. A. P., St George-Hyslop, P., van Keuren, M. L., Patterson, D., Pagan, S., Kurnit, D. M., and Neve, R. L. (1987) Amyloid β protein gene: cDNA, mRNA distribution and genetic linkage near the Alzheimer locus, *Science* **235,** 880–884.

20. Van Nostrand, W. E., Wagner, S. L., Shankle, W. R., Farrow, J. S., Dick, M., Rozemuller, J. M., Kuiper, M. A., Wolters, E. C., Zimmerman, J., Cotman, C. W., and Cunningham, D. D. (1992) Decreased levels of soluble amyloid beta-protein precursor in cerebrospinal fluid of live Alzheimer disease patients, *Proc. Natl. Acad. Sci. USA* **89,** 2551–2555.

21. Oltersdorf, T., Fritz, L. C., Schenk, D. B., Lieberburg, I., Johnson-Wood, K. L., Beattie, E. C., Ward, P. J., Blacher, R. W., Dovey, H. F., and Sinha, S. (1989) The secreted form of the Alzheimer's amyloid precursor protein with the Kunitz domain is protease nexin-II, *Nature* **341,** 144–147.

22. Weidemann, A., Konig, G., Bunke, D., Fischer, P., Salbaum, J. M., Masters, C. L., and Beyreuther, K. (1989) Identification, biogenesis and localization of precursors of Alzheimer's disease A4 amyloid protein, *Cell* **57,** 115–126.

23. Podlisny, M. B., Mammen, A. L., Schlossmacher, M. G., Palmert, M. R., Younkin, S. G., and Selkoe, D. J. (1990) Detection of soluble forms of the β-amyloid precursor protein in human plasma, *Biochem. Biophys. Res. Commun.* **167**, 1094–1101.

24. Kitaguchi, N., Takahashi, Y., Tokushima, Y., Shiojiri, S., and Ito, H. (1988) Novel precursor of Alzheimer's disease shows protease inhibitory activity, *Nature* **331**, 530–532.

25. Ponte, P., Gonzalez-DeWhitt, P., Schilling, J., Miller, J., Hsu, D., Greenberg, B., Davis, K., Wallace, W., Lieberburg, I., Fuller, F., and Cordell, B. (1988) A new A4 amyloid mRNA contains a domain homologous to serine proteinase inhibitors, *Nature* **331**, 525–527.

26. Tanzi, R. E., McClatchey, A. I., Lamperti, E. D., Villa-Komaroff, L., Gusella, J. F., and Neve, R. L. (1988) Protease inhibitor domain encoded by an amyloid protein precursor mRNA associated with Alzheimer's disease, *Nature* **331**, 528–530.

27. Konig, G., Monning, U., Czech, C., Prior, R., Baniti, R., Schreiter-Gasser, U., Bauer, J., Masters, C. L., and Beyreuther, K. (1992) Identification and expression of a novel alternative splice form of the βA4 amyloid precursor protein (APP) mRNA in leukocytes and brian microglial cells, *J. Biol. Chem.* **267**, 10,804–10,809.

28. Johnson, S. A., Pasinetti, G. M., May, P. C., Ponte, P. A., Cordell, B., and Finch, C. E. (1988) Selective reduction of mRNA for the β-amyloid precursor protein that lacks a Kunitz-type protease inhibitor motif in cortex from Alzheimer brains, *Exp. Neurol.* **102**, 264–268.

29. Koo, E. H., Sisodia, S. S., Cork, L. C., Unterbeck, A., Bayney, R. M., and Price, D. L. (1990) Differential expression of amyloid precursor protein mRNAs in cases of Alzheimer's disease and in aged nonhuman primates, *Neuron* **2**, 97–104.

30. Kovacs, D. M., Wasco, W., Witherby, J., Felsenstein, K. M., Brunel, F., Roeder, R. G., and Tanzi, R. E. (1995) The upstream stimulatory factor functionally interacts with the Alzheimer amyloid β-protein precursor gene, *Hum. Mol. Genet.* **9**, 1527–1533.

31. Wasco, W., Bupp, K., Magendantz, M., Gusella, J. F., Tanzi, R. E., and Solomon, F. (1992) Identification of a mouse brain cDNA that encodes a protein related to the Alzheimer disease-associated β precursor protein, *Proc. Natl. Acad. Sci. USA* **89**, 10,758–10,762.

32. Wasco, W., Gurubhagavatula, S., Paradis, M. D., Romano, D., Sisodia, S. S., Hyman, B. T., Neve, R. L., and Tanzi, R. E. (1993) Isolation and characterization of the human APLP2 gene encoding a homologue of the Alzheimer's associated amyloid β protein precursor, *Nature Genet.* **5**, 95–100.

33. Sprecher, C. A., Grant, F. J., Grimm, G., O'Hara, P. J., Norris, F., Norris, K., and Foster, D. C. (1993) Molecular cloning of the cDNA for a human amyloid precursor protein homolog: evidence for a multigene family, *Biochemistry* **32**, 4481–4486.

34. Slunt, H. H., Thinakaran, G., Von Koch, C., Lo, A. C., Tanzi, R. E., and Sisodia, S. S. (1994) Expression of a ubiquitous, cross-reactive homologue of the mouse β-amyloid precursor protein (APP), *J. Biol. Chem.* **269**, 2637–2644.

35. Rosen, D. R., Martin-Morris, L., Luo, L., and White, K. (1989) A drosophila gene encoding a protein resembling the human β-amyloid protein precursor, *Proc. Natl. Acad. Sci. USA* **86**, 2478–2482.

36. Daigle, I. and Li, C. (1993) apl-1, a Caenorhabditis elegans gene encoding a protein related to the human β-amyloid protein precursor, *Proc. Natl. Acad. Sci. USA* **90**, 12,045–12,049.

37. Saitoh, T., Sundsmo, M., Roch, J. M., Kumura, N., Cole, G., Schubert, D., Oltersdorf, T., and Schenk, D. B. (1989) Secreted form of amyloid-β protein is involved in the growth regulation of fibroblasts, *Cell* **58**, 615–622.

38. Mattson, M. P., Cheng, B., Culwell, A. R., Esch, F. S., Lieberberg, I., and Rydel, R. E. (1993) Evidence for excitoprotective and intraneuronal calcium-regulating roles for secreted forms of the beta-amyloid precursor protein, *Neuron* **10**, 243–254.

39. Smith, R. P., Higuchi, D. A., Broze, G. J., Jr. (1990) Platelet coagulation factor XIa-inhibitor, a form of Alzheimer amyloid precursor protein, *Science* **248**, 1126–1128.

40. Small, D. H., Nurcombe, V., Moir, R., Michaelson, S., Monad, D., Beyreuther, K., and Masters, C. L. (1992) Association and relase of amyloid protein precursor of Alzheimer's disease from chick brain extracellular matrix, *J. Neurosci.* **12**, 4143–4150.

41. Buee, L., Ding, W., Delacourte, A., and Flint, H. (1993) Binding of secreted human neuro-blastoma proteoglycans to the Alzheimer's amyloid A4 peptide, *Brain Res.* **601,** 154–163.
42. Breen, K. C. (1992) APP-collagen interaction is mediated by a heparin bridge mechanism, *Mol. Chem. Neuropathol.* **16,** 109–121.
43. Narindrasorasak, S., Lowery, D. E., Altman, R. A., Gonzalez-DeWhitt, P., Greenberg, B. D., and Kisilevsky, R. (1992) Characterization of high affinity binding between laminin and Alzheimer's disease amyloid precursor proteins, *Lab. Invest.* **67,** 643–652.
44. Kibbey, M. C., Jucker, M., Weeks, B. S., Neve, R. L., Van Nostrand, W. E., and Kleinman, H. K. (1993) β-amyloid precursor protein binds to the neurite-promoting IKVAV site of laminin, *Proc. Natl. Acad. Sci. USA* **90,** 10,150–10,153.
45. Bush, A. I., Pettingell, W. H., de Paradis, M., Tanzi, R. E., and Wasco, W. (1994) The amyloid beta-protein precursor and its mammalian homologues: evidence for a zinc-modu-lated heparin-binding superfamily, *J. Biol. Chem.* **269,** 26,618–26,621.
46. Jin, L. W., Ninomiya, H., Roch, J. M., Schubert, D., Masliah, E., Otero, D. A. C., and Saitoh, T. (1994) Peptides containing the RERMS sequence of amyloid b/A4 protein pre-cursor bind cell surface and promite neurite extension, *J. Neurosci.* **14,** 5461–5470.
47. Gandy, S. E. and Greengard, P. (1994) Processing of Aβ-amyloid precursor protein: Cell biology, regulation and role in Alzheimer's disease, *Int. Rev. Neurobiol.* **36,** 29–50.
48. Gandy, S., Caporaso, G., Buxbaum, J., Frangione, B., and Greengard, P. (1994) APP pro-cessing, Aβ amyloidogenesis, and the pathogenesis of Alzheimer's disease, *Neurobiol. Aging* **15,** 253–256.
49. Nitsch, R. M., Slack, B. E., Wurtman, R. J., and Growdon, R. H. (1992) Release of Alzheimer amyloid precursor derivatives stimulated by activation of muscarinic acetylcholine recep-tors, *Science* **358,** 304–307.
50. Sisodia, S. S., Koo, E. H., Beyreuther, K., Unterbeck, A., and Price, D. L. (1990) Evidence that β-amyloid protein in Alzheimer's disease is not derived by normal processing, *Science* **248,** 492–495.
51. Esch, F. S., Keim, P. S., Beattie, E. C., Blacher, R. W., Culwell, A. R., Oltersdorf, T., McClure, D., and Ward, P. J. (1990) Cleavage of amyloid b peptide during constitutive processing of its precursor, *Science* **248,** 1122–1124.
52. Nordstedt, C., Caporaso, G. L., Thyberg, J., Gandy, S. E., and Greengard, P. (1993) Iden-tification of the Alzheimer beta/A4-amyloid precursor protein in clathrin-coated vessicles purified from PC-12 cells. *J. Biol. Chem.* **268,** 608–612.
53. Golde, T. E., Estus, S., Younkin, L. H., Selkoe, D. J., and Younkin, S. G. (1992) Processing of the amyloid protein precursor to potentially amyloidogenic derivatives, *Science* **255,** 728–730.
54. Haass, C., Koo, E. H., Mellon, A., Hung, A. Y., and Selkoe, D. J. (1992) Targeting of cell-surface β-amyloid precursor protein to lysosomes: alternative processing into amyloid-bearing fragments, *Nature* **357,** 500–503.
55. Caporaso, G. L., Gandy, S. E., Buxbaum, J. D., Ramabhadran, T. V., and Greengard, P. (1992) Protein phosphorylation regulates secretion of Alzhiemer beta/A4 malyoid presursor protein, *Proc. Natl. Acad. Sci. USA* **89,** 3055–3059.
56. Seubert, P., Vigo-Pelfrey, C., Esch, F., Lee, M., Dovey, H., Davis, D., Sinha, S., Schlossmacher, M., Whaley, J., Swindlehurst, C., McCormack, R., Wolfert, R., Selkoe, D., Lieberberg, I., and Schenk, D. (1992) Isolation and quantification of soluble Alzheimer's β-peptide from biological fluids, *Nature* **359,** 325–327.
57. Gandy, S. E., Bhasin, R., Ramabhadran, T. V., Koo, E. L., Price, D. L., Goldgaber, D., and Greengard, P. (1992) Alzheimer β/A4 amyloid precursor protein: Evidence for putative amyloidogenic fragment, *J. Neurochem.* **58,** 383–386.
58. Estus, S. J., Golde, T. E., and Younkin, S. G. (1992) Normal processing of the Alzheimer's disease amyloid beta protein precursor generates potentially amyloidogenic carboxyl-ter-minal derivatives, *Ann. N.Y. Acad. Sci.* **674,** 138–148.

59. Tamaoka, A., Kalaria, R. N., Lieberberg, I., and Selkoe, D. (1992) Identification of a stable fragment of the Alzheimer amyloid precursor containing the β-protein in brain microvessels, *Proc. Natl. Acad. Sci. USA* **89,** 1345–1349.

60. Knops, J., Lieberberg, I., and Sinha, S. (1992) Evidence for a non-secretory acidic degradation pathway for amyloid precursor protein in 293 cells, *J. Biol. Chem.* **267,** 16,022–16,044.

61. Shoji, M., Golde, T. E., Ghiso, J., Cheung, T. T., Estus, S., Shaffer, L. M., Cai, X. -D., McKay, D. M., Tintner, R., Frangione, B., and Younkin, S. G. (1992) Production of the Alzheimer amyloid b protein by normal proteolytic processing, *Science* **258,** 126–129.

62. Haass, C., Schlossmacher, M. G., Hung, A. Y., Vigo-Pelfrey, C., Mellon, A., Ostaszewski, B. L., Lieberburg, I., Koo, E. H., Schenk, D., Teplow, D. B., and Selkoe, D. S. (1992) Amyloid β-peptide is produced by cultured cells during normal metabolism, *Nature* **359,** 322–325.

63. Jacobsen, S. J., Spruy, M. A., Brown, A. M., Sahasrabudhe, S. R., Blume, A. J., Vitek, M. P., Muenkel, H. A., Sonnenberg-Reines, J. (1994) The release of Alzheimer's disease beta amyloid peptide is reduced by phorbol treatment, *J. Biol. Chem.* **269,** 8376–8382.

64. Koo, E. H. and Squazzo, S. L. (1994) Evidence that production and release of amyloid β-protein involves the endocytic pathway, *J. Biol. Chem.* **269,** 17,386–17,389.

65. Chen, W., Goldstein, J. L., and Brown, M. S. (1990) NPXY, a sequence often found in cytoplasmic tails, is required for coated pit mediated internalization of the low density lipoprotein receptor, *J. Biol. Chem.* **265,** 3116–3123.

66. Lai, A., Sisiodia, S. S., and Trowbridge, I. S. (1995) Characterization of sorting signals in the beta-amyloid precursor protein cytoplamsic domain, *J. Biol. Chem.* **270,** 3565–3573.

67. Rebeck, G. W., Reiter, J. S., Strickland, D. K., and Hyman, B. T. (1993) Apolipoprotein E in sporadic Alzheimer's disease: allelic variation and receptor interactions, *Neuron* **11,** 575–580.

68. Kim, T. W., DiFiglia, M., Wasco, W., Rebeck, W. G., Hyman, B. T., Strickland, D. K., and Tanzi, R. E. (1995) Neuronal apolipoprotein E receptor, LRP, in the human central nervous system synaptic nerve terminal, *Soc. Neurosci.* abstract 21, p. 1008.

69. Kounnas, M. Z., Moir, R. D., Rebeck, G. W., Bush, A. I., Argaves, W. S., Hyman, B. T., Tanzi, R. E., and Strickland, D. K. (1995) LDL receptor-related protein, a multifunctional apolipoprotein E receptor, binds seceted beta-amyloid precursor protein and mediates its degradation, *Cell* **82,** 331–340.

70. Cai, X.-D., Golde, T. E., and Younkin, S. G. (1993) Release of excess amyloid β protein from a mutant amyloid b protein precursor, *Science* **259,** 514–516.

71. Suzuki, N., Cheung, T. T., Cai, X. D., Odaka, A., Otvos, L. Jr., Eckman, C., Golde, T. E., and Younkin, S. G. (1994) An increased percentage of long amyloid beta protein secreted by familial amyloid beta protein precursor (beta APP717) mutants, *Science* **264,** 1336–1340.

72. Citron, M., Oltersdorf, T., Haass, C., McConlogue, L., Hung, A. Y., Seubert, P., Vigo-Pelfrey, C., Lieberburg, I., and Selkoe, D. J. (1992) Mutation of the β-amyloid precursor protein in familial Alzheimer's disease increases β-protein production, *Nature* **360,** 672–674.

73. Yankner, B. A., Caceres, A., and Duffy, L. K. (1990a) Nerve growth factor potentiates the neurotoxicity of β-amyloid, *Proc. Natl. Acad. Sci. USA* **87,** 9020–9023.

74. Yankner, B. A., Duffy, L. K., and Kirschner, D. A. (1990b) Neurotrophic and neurotoxic effects of amyloid β protein: reversal by tachykinin neuropeptides, *Science* **250,** 279–282.

75. Frautschy, S. A., Baird, A., and Cole, G. M. (1991) Effects of injected Alzheimer β-amyloid cores in rat brain, *Proc. Natl. Acad. Sci. USA* **88,** 8362–8366.

76. Cotman, C. W., Bridges., R., Pike, C., Kesslak, P., Loo, D., and Copani, A. (1993) Mechanisms of neuronal cell death in Alzheimer's disease, in *Alzheimer's Disease: Advances in Clinical and Basic Research* (Corain, B., et al., eds.), Wiley, West Sussex, UK, pp. 281–290.

77. Pike, C. J., Burdick, D., Walencewicz, A. J., Glabe, C. G., and Cotman, C. W. (1993) Neurodegeneration induced by β-amyloid peptides in vitro: the role of peptide assembly state, *J. Neurosci.* **13,** 1676–1687.

78. Haass, C., Koo, E. H., Teplow, D. B., and Selkoe, D. J. (1994) Polarized secretion of beta-amyloid precursor protein and amyloid beta-peptide in MDCK cells, *Proc. Natl. Acad. Sci. USA* **91,** 1564–1568.

79. Mellman, I., Matter, K., Yamamoto, E., Pollack, N., Roome, J., Felsenstein, K., and Roberts, S. (1995) Mechanisms of molecular sorting in polarized cells: Relavance to Alzheimer's disease, in *Alzheimer's Disease: Lessons from Cell Biology* (Kosik, K. S., Christen, Y., and Selkoe, D. J., eds.), Springer-Verlag, Berlin, pp. 14–26.

80. Selkoe, D. J. (1995) Physiological roduction and polarized secretion of the amyloid, β-peptide in epithelial cells: a route to the mechanism of Alzheimer's disease, in *Alzheimer's Disease: Lessons from Cell Biology* (Kosik, K. S., Christen, Y., and Selkoe, D. J., eds.), Springer-Verlag, Berlin, pp. 70–77.

81. Games, D., Adams, D., Alessandrini, R., Barbour, R., Berthelette, P., Blackwell, C., Carr, T., Clemens, J., Donaldson, T., Gillespie, F., Guido, T., Hagopian, S., Johnson-Wood, K., Khan, K., Lee, M., Leibowitz, P., Lieberburg, I., Little, S., Masliah, E., McConlogue, L., Montoya-Zavala, M., Mucke, L., Paganini, L., Penniman, E., Power, M., Schenk, D., Seubert, P., Snyder, B., Soriano, F., Tan, H., Vitale, J., Wadsworth, S., Wolozin, B., and Zhao, J. (1995) Alzheimer-type neuropathology in transgenic mice overexpressing V717F β-amyloid precursor protein, *Nature* **373,** 523–527.

82. Levy-Lahad, E., Wijsman, E. M., Nemens, E., Anderson, L., Goddard, K. A. B., Weber, J. L., Bird, T. D., and Schellenberg, G. D. (1995) A familial Alzheimer's disease locus on chromosome 1, *Science* **269,** 970–972.

83. Schellenberg, G. D. (1992) Genetic linkage for a novel familial Alzheimer's disease locus on chromosome 14, *Science* **258,** 868–871.

84. Clark, R. F. and the Alzheimer's Disease Collaboration Group (1995) The structure of the presenilin 1 (S182) gene and identification of six novel mutations in early onset AD families, *Nature Genet.* **11,** 219–222.

85. Kovacs, D. M., Fausett, H. J., Page, K. J., Kim, T.-W., Mori, R. D., Merriam, D. E., Hoillister, R. D., Hallmark, O. G., Mancini, R., Felsenstein, K. M., Hyman, B. T., Tanzi, R. E., and Wasco, W. (1996) Alzheimer associated presenilins 1 and 2: Neuronal expression in brain and localization to intracellular membranes in mammalian cells, *Nature Med.* **2,** 224–229.

86. Vito., P., Lancana, E., and D'Adamio, L. (1996) Interfering with apoptosis: Ca^{2+}-binding protein ALG-2 and Alzhiemer's disease gene ALG-3, *Science* **271,** 521–525.

87. Wasco, W., Pettingell, W. P., Jondro, P. D., Schmidt, S. D., Gurubhagavatula, S., Rodes, L., DiBlasi, T., Romano, D. M., Guenette, S. Y., Kovacs, D. M., Growdon, J. H., and Tanzi, R. E. (1995) Familial Alzheimer's chromosome 14 mutations, *Nature Med.* **1,** 848.

88. Cruts, M., et al. (1995) Molecular genetic analysis of familial early-onset Alzheimer's disease linked to chromosome 14q24.3, *Hum. Mol. Genet.* **4,** 2363–2371.

89. Sorbi, S., et al. (1995) Missense mutation of S182 gene in Italian families with early-onset Alzheimer's disease, *Lancet* **346,** 439,440.

90. Campion, D., et al. (1995) Mutations of the presenilin 1 gene in families with early-onset Alzheimer's disease, *Hum. Mol. Genet.* **4,** 2373–2377.

91. Tanahashi, H., Tanahai, H., Mitsunaga, K., Takanshi, H., Tasaki, S., Watanabe, S., and Tabira, T. (1995) Missense mutation of S182 gene in Japanese familial Alzheimer's disease, *Lancet* **346,** 440.

92. Van Broeckhoven, C., et al. (1995) Presenilins and Alzheimer disease, *Nature Genet.* **11,** 230–232.

93. Wragg, M., Hutton, M., Talbot, C., and the Alzheimer's Disease Collaborative Group (ADCG) (1996) Genetic association between intronic polymorphism in presenilin 1 gene and late-onset Alzheimer's disease, *Lancet* **347,** 509–512.

94. Anwar, R., Moynihan, T. P., Ardley, H., Brindle, N., Coletta, L., Cairns, N., Markham, A. F., and Robinason, P. A. (1996) Molecular analysis of the presenilin 1 (S182) gene in "spo-

radic" case of Alzheimer's disease: Identification and characterization of unusual splice variants, *J. Neurochem.* **66,** 1774–1777.

95. Levitan, D. and Greenwald, I. (1995) Facilitation of lin-12-mediated signalling by sel-12, a *Caenorhabditis elegans* S182 Alzheimer's disease gene, *Nature* **377,** 351–354.

96. L'Hernault, S. W. and Arduengo, P. M. (1992) Mutation of a putative sperm membrane protein in *Caenorhabditis elegans* prevents sperm differentiation but not its associated meiotic divisions, *J. Cell Biol.* **119,** 55–68.

2

Potential Biological Mechanisms of ApoE in Alzheimer's Disease

G. William Rebeck

1. GENETIC PREDISPOSITIONS TO ALZHEIMER'S DISEASE (AD)

Other chapters in this book discuss the three genes involved in the development of early onset forms of AD: APP, presenilin-1, and presenilin-2. These genes share a number of features. First, mutations in these genes lead to early onset-forms of AD. Second, mutations in these genes invariably lead to AD; i.e., they are completely penetrant. Third, the functions of the APP, presenilin-1, and presenilin-2 gene products are unknown. In order to determine the functions of these genes, considerable research is being invested in examining the distribution of these proteins, the regulation of their expression, and the identification of proteins that interact with them.

The apolipoprotein E (ApoE) gene, in contrast, shares none of these features with APP or the presenilins. First, ApoE is associated primarily with late-onset forms of AD. Second, the ApoE variant associated with AD, the ApoE ε4 allele, can often be found in quite elderly, cognitively normal individuals *(1,2)*. That is, ApoE ε4 is incompletely penetrant and is therefore considered only a risk factor for AD. Third, at least some of the functions of the ApoE gene product are well known; ApoE has been studied as a protein involved in the transport of lipid particles in the plasma for over 20 yr *(3,4)*. Less well understood, however, are the functions of ApoE in the CNS, and how ApoE is involved in the development of AD.

2. ApoE STRUCTURE AND FUNCTION

The ApoE protein is composed of 299 amino acids cleaved from a signal peptide as it is secreted from the cell *(3,4)*. ApoE is composed of two large domains, an amino-terminal domain (aa 1–163) and a carboxy-terminal domain (aa 201–299), joined by a hinge region *(5)*. The amino-terminal domain interacts with ApoE receptors; the carboxy-terminal domain interacts with lipoprotein particles. The three isoforms of ApoE, ApoE2, E3, and E4 differ in the presence of cysteine/arginine residues in the receptor-binding domain: ApoE2, cys-112 cys-158; ApoE3, cys-112 arg-158; ApoE4, arg-112 arg-158. Only single ApoE isoforms have been found in the other animals examined *(6,7)*.

From: Molecular Mechanisms of Dementia *Edited by: W. Wasco and R. E. Tanzi Humana Press Inc., Totowa, NJ*

2.1. ApoE in the Periphery

Apolipoproteins are proteins complexed to lipid particles *(8)*. These lipid particles, lipoproteins, consist of phospholipids, free cholesterol, cholesterol esters, and triglycerides in addition to the apolipoproteins. In the plasma, ApoE is not present as a free protein; it is found complexed to three separate classes of lipoproteins, which differ in their composition, size, and density. These ApoE-containing lipoproteins are chylomicron remnants, very low-density lipoproteins (VLDL), and high-density lipoproteins (HDL). The largest of these are the chylomicron remnants, which are derived from lipoproteins made in the intestine using lipids absorbed from the diet. VLDL, generated by the liver using endogenous lipids, are smaller and denser than chylomicron remnants. These two types of large, lipid-rich particles are used to deliver lipids to cells; uptake is mediated by the interaction between ApoE and its receptors (*see* Table 1). ApoE is not found on another class of lipoprotein used for delivery of lipids to cells, the low-density lipoproteins (LDL). ApoE is found on a percentage of HDL, the smallest lipoproteins in the plasma. HDL are composed of 40–50% protein, most of which is ApoAI and ApoAII. In contrast to chylomicron remnants, VLDL and LDL, these small, lipid-poor particles are used primarily to remove lipids from cells, a process known as reverse cholesterol transport.

The binding of ApoE to lipoproteins occurs via the carboxy-terminal domain of ApoE. These 99 amino acids form amphipathic α helices, and the hydrophobic face of these helices interacts with the lipid particle *(9)*. Paradoxically, although the isoforms of ApoE differ in amino acids in the receptor-binding domain, they possess different lipid-binding characteristics *(10,11)*. ApoE3 preferentially binds to HDL particles, and ApoE4 preferentially binds to VLDL particles. Truncation studies of ApoE indicate that the amino acids 260–272 in the carboxy-terminal domain are important for the differences in lipoprotein binding seen for ApoE3 and ApoE4 *(12)*, presumably through an interaction with the receptor-binding domain of ApoE.

The binding of ApoE to receptors occurs via the amino-terminal domain of ApoE. These 163 amino acids form an antiparallel four-helix bundle *(13)* which interacts with a family of receptors, the LDL receptor family. Binding occurs via a highly charged region of ApoE from approximately amino acids 140–160 *(14–16)*. The amino acid substitution in ApoE2 at position 158 decreases binding of ApoE to the LDL receptor to only 2% of the binding observed in ApoE3; no differences have been found in ApoE3 and ApoE4 binding to receptors *(17,18)*. Binding of ApoE to specific receptors is altered by the type and composition of the lipoprotein on which the ApoE is present *(5)*, further evidence that the two domains of ApoE interact and influence each other's conformation. Recent X-ray crystallography showed that the ApoE3/4 residue (cys/arg-112) can affect the position of the arg-61 residue in human ApoE, and this residue interacts with the carboxy-terminal domain *(12)*. Interestingly, while the ApoE of most animals has an arginine at position 112 like human ApoE4, they do not have an arginine at position 61, and hence are structurally more related to human ApoE3 *(12)*.

ApoE can form dimers through the cysteine residues in the receptor-binding domain. ApoE3, with a single cysteine, can form ApoE3 homodimers *(19)* or ApoE3-ApoAII heterodimers (ApoAII is a 7-kDa protein with a single cysteine residue). ApoE2, with two cysteines, can form ApoE2 homodimers, ApoAII-ApoE2-ApoAII trimers, or other

Table 1
Members of LDL Receptor Family

		Types of repeats	
	EGF	Ligand binding	Spacer
LDL receptor	3	7	1
ApoE receptor 2	3	7	1
VLDL receptor	3	8	1
GP330/megalin	16	36	7
LRP	16	31	7

multimers *(20)*. ApoE4, without cysteines, is only monomeric. Formation of ApoE dimers affects both the lipoprotein and receptor-binding functions of ApoE: ApoE3 dimers have a higher affinity for HDL particles than for other lipoproteins *(21,22)*, and ApoE3 dimers interact less avidly with ApoE receptors than ApoE3 monomers *(23)*.

The receptors that bind ApoE-containing lipoproteins are the five members of the LDL receptor family cloned so far:

1. The LDL receptor *(24)*;
2. The LDL receptor-related protein, LRP *(25,26)*;
3. Glycoprotein 330, GP330 (also known as megalin and LRP-2) *(27)*;
4. The VLDL receptor *(28)*; and
5. The ApoE receptor 2 *(29)*.

These receptors share a number of features. Each is a cell-surface receptor that spans the plasma membrane once. Each has a short carboxy-terminal, intracellular domain, which contains at least one NPxY sequence for targeting receptor–ligand complexes to coated pits. Extracellularly, each possesses three types of sequence repeats: EGF repeats, cysteine-rich ligand-binding repeats, and spacer regions. The five members of the LDL receptor family differ mostly in the number and organization of these repeats (Table 1).

Binding of ApoE-containing lipoproteins to these receptors allows internalization of the lipoprotein. The receptor–lipoprotein complex is directed to the endosomal/lysosomal pathway *(30)*. In the internal, acidic compartments, ApoE is dissociated from the receptor, and the receptor is recycled to the plasma membrane. The protein component of the lipoproteins can be degraded in these compartments; the lipid components are absorbed into other cellular compartments.

2.2. ApoE in the CNS

Much less is known about the biochemistry of ApoE and the processes of lipid transport in the CNS. Although there are several classes of lipoproteins in the periphery, there is just one type of lipoprotein in the CNS, an HDL-like particle *(31–33)*. There seem to be several different types of CSF HDL particles: those containing primarily ApoE, those containing primarily ApoAI, and those containing a number of apolipoproteins, including ApoAIV, ApoD, and ApoJ *(31–33)*. ApoE2 and ApoE3 exist mostly as monomers in the CSF, but can form homo- and heterodimers like those seen

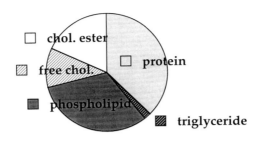

Fig. 1. Composition of CSF lipoproteins.

in the plasma (unpublished data). The CSF HDL are approximately one-third protein, one-third phospholipid, and one-third cholesterol and cholesterol esters (*31,33; see* Fig. 1). Coomassie staining of CSF HDL revealed that almost all the protein present in these lipoproteins is ApoE and ApoAI (unpublished data).

Some of the CSF apolipoproteins are synthesized in the CNS, whereas others seem to enter as plasma filtrate. Immunohistochemistry and *in situ* hybridization studies indicate that ApoE is synthesized in astrocytes *(32–35)*. Cell-culture experiments showed that ApoE is produced by astrocyte-like cells in culture, and is secreted associated with HDL-like particles (unpublished data; *36)*. These studies confirmed earlier suggestions that ApoE must be produced in the CNS because its levels were approx 5% of the levels found in the plasma *(33)*. Proteins that enter the CSF as plasma filtrate are present at levels <1% of their plasma concentration. Furthermore, the form of ApoE produced in the CNS differs from that in the periphery in that it is primarily glycosylated at Thr-194, whereas plasma ApoE is not *(37)*.

These HDL-like particles are the only lipoproteins present in the CNS; the larger lipoproteins responsible for the delivery of lipids to cells are not present. Thus, we speculated that CSF HDL may perform both of the transport functions of the many plasma lipoproteins, i.e. the removal of lipids from cells and the delivery of lipids to cells. Cholesterol found in the brain is synthesized locally *(38,39)* and probably not imported from the circulation. However, during neuronal degeneration, there is a need for the removal of lipids degenerating neurons and perhaps the need for delivery of lipids to sprouting neurites. For example, during synaptic remodeling after lesioning of rat brains, cholesterol sythesis was decreased and ApoE-binding sites were increased *(40)*, suggesting that excess cholesterol was being cleared from degenerating neurons, and being delivered to regenerating neurons. Astrocytic production of ApoE was induced in response to neuronal damage *(35)*. ApoE-containing lipoproteins produced around nerve lesions in the periphery act to clear cholesterol *(41)*. The ApoAI-containing particles that are found in the CSF are also likely to remove lipids from degenerating neurons; these particles are, after all, used in reverse cholesterol transport in the periphery. Using cultured fibroblasts, we have found that isolated CSF HDL (containing both ApoE and ApoAI) can act to remove cholesterol from fibroblast cells in culture, similar to plasma HDL (unpublished data). Whether ApoAI-containing CSF HDL function differently from ApoE-containing CSF HDL in the removal of lipids is as yet unknown.

Delivery of lipids to cells, on the other hand, is not the normal function of HDL particles. Pitas et al. *(33)* showed that CSF HDL can act to block interaction of LDL with receptors in culture. In order to examine more directly whether CSF HDL can deliver lipids to cells, we radiolabeled CSF HDL and showed that they can be taken up and degraded by fibroblasts in culture, but at levels much lower than observed for LDL particles (unpublished data). These data are supported by studies showing that dense ApoE-containing lipoproteins can interact with cells and promote neurite outgrowth in cell culture (*see* Section 3.1.1.; *42*).

Uptake of the CSF HDL into cells likely involves an interaction between ApoE and the ApoE receptors on the various types of CNS cells. We have been examing expression of the various ApoE receptors in the CNS. Immunohistochemical staining for the LDL receptor showed diffuse staining throughout the neuropil, in addition to weak astrocytic staining *(32,33,43)*. These observations are in agreement with *in situ* hybridization studies showing LDL receptor mRNA in neurons and glia (*44*; Liu et al., manuscript in preparation). LRP immunohistochemistry revealed strong expression on pyramidal neurons in hippocampal subfields, granule cells of the dentate gyrus, and activated astrocytes *(43,45–48)*. Strong LRP staining was also seen in choroid plexus *(49)*, and diffuse LRP staining was found throughout the neuropil. The VLDL receptor was found expressed on microglia as well as occasional pyramidal neurons in cortical layers III and V *(50,52)*. GP330 expression is seen in ependymal cells *(49)*. Finally, *in situ* hybridization indicated that the ApoE receptor 2 was present in cerebellar cortex, choroid plexus, ependyma, hippocampus, and olfactory bulb *(29)*. Thus, each of the ApoE receptors is found on a distinct subset of cells in the CNS.

In addition, there is another class of receptor that is involved with the clearance of lipoproteins, the scavenger receptors *(53)*. These receptors in the periphery bind oxidized or acetylated LDL particles. In the CNS, the macrophage scavenger receptor has been localized to microglia *(51)* where it may also play a role in clearing lipoproteins.

3. ApoE IN AD

With this background of ApoE structure and function, we can begin to evaluate the models of the involvement of ApoE in AD. There are three basic models put forth so far:

1. ApoE-containing lipoproteins are important for prevention of neurodegeneration, and ApoE4 is less capable of supporting neuronal survival under toxic conditions;
2. ApoE interacts with τ and microtubules and ApoE4 does not protect τ from aggregation into neurofibrillary tangles (NFT); and
3. ApoE interacts with Aβ or APP and either promotes the formation of Aβ aggregates or is involved in Aβ clearance.

Again, an ApoE isoform-specific effect must be hypothesized.

3.1. ApoE in Neurodegeneration

Expression of ApoE is induced in lesion models of both peripheral *(54)* and CNS *(35)* neurons, suggesting that ApoE plays a role in removal of membrane lipids from degenerating neurons *(41)*. A role for ApoE in synaptic regeneration is also implied from studies of ApoE knockout mice *(55)*, which showed an increased loss of synapses with age. In vitro analyses have shown that treatment of dorsal root ganglion neurons in culture with ApoE-containing lipoproteins stimulates neurite outgrowth *(56)*. Together these studies strongly support a role for ApoE in neuronal repair and regeneration. Perhaps ApoE4 is less able to support neuron survival during neurodegeneration than ApoE3 or ApoE2. This hypothesis has so far been tested two ways: by analysis of neurite outgrowth promoted by ApoE4- vs ApoE3-containing lipoproteins; and by analysis of ApoE genotype effects on other neurodegenerative diseases.

3.1.1. Neurite Outgrowth

Both ApoE3- and ApoE4-containing lipoproteins deliver lipids to neurons in culture, apparently via LRP *(57)*. However, although ApoE3-containing lipoproteins stimulate neurite outgrowth, ApoE4-containing lipoproteins do not *(57–59)*. This observation has been made for ApoE on the surface of large lipoproteins as well as for more relevant HDL-like lipoproteins *(42)*. ApoE3 and ApoE4 are both competent to deliver lipoproteins to these cultured neurons *(57)*, in accord with previous studies showing no difference in ApoE3 and ApoE4 binding to LRP *(17)*. Thus, ApoE, in addition to acting to deliver lipids to cells, could activate an intracellular signaling pathway that affects the growth of neurites. This observed difference in the biology of ApoE3 and ApoE4 is exactly the type of effect that could explain the genetic risk associated with ApoE ε4. ApoE4-positive individuals would be impaired in the sprouting of neurites after neuronal damage, perhaps leading to decreased synaptic plasticity and poorer survival of surrounding neurons. However, there is as yet no direct evidence for a signaling pathway stimulated by ApoE.

3.1.2. Other Neurodegenerative Diseases

Many studies have now been conducted examining the influence of ApoE ε4 on onset and progression of neurodegenerative diseases other than AD. Although not all studies agree, there are convincing data that ApoE ε4 is not overrepresented in Parkinson's disease *(60–62)*, amyolateral sclerosis (ALS) *(63)*, Creutzfeld-Jacob disease *(64–68)*, Pick's disease *(69)*, or progressive supranuclear palsy *(69)*. Together, these data imply that ApoE isoforms do not affect the neuropathological processes found in other neurodegenerative diseases. It is possible that inheritance of ApoE ε4 affects the age of onset or the severity of neuropathological changes in these other neurodegenerative diseases. So far, only a few studies have examined these factors. Inheritance of ApoE ε4 had no effect on age of onset of ALS *(63,70)*, although there may be differences in bulbar-onset and limb-onset forms of the disease *(70)*. Inheritance of ApoE ε4 also had no effect on the number of cortical Lewy bodies in patients with Parkinson's disease and AD *(71)*. Thus, there are few data supporting a role for ApoE in neurodegenerative processes other than those seen in AD.

3.2. ApoE in the development of NFT

Several reports *(69,72)* showed that AD patients who were positive for the ApoE ε4 allele did not show increased numbers of NFTs. (Several other reports linking ApoE ε4 to higher levels of NFT formation did not control for strong confounding factor of disease duration *[73–75]*). A role for ApoE in NFT development was first suggested by in vitro assays showing that ApoE bound to the microtubule-associated protein τ *(76)*. However, ApoE is a protein associated with soluble lipoproteins, and *in situ* hybridization studies have shown that ApoE is not synthesized in neurons *(35;* Page, et al., manuscript in preparation). Thus, an interaction between τ and ApoE would require uptake of ApoE from the extracellular space into intracellular vesicles, and transfer of ApoE from these vesicles into the cytoplasm. Electromicrographic studies of human neurons *(77)* and rat hepatocytes *(79)* suggest that ApoE may indeed be found in cytoplasm, although the mechanism of its transfer is still undefined. In addition, there are now several reports of ApoE immunoreactivity in NFT and apparently healthy neurons in postmortem human brain *(78,80)*. Evidence for the mechanism of transfer of ApoE into the neuronal cytoplasm of neurons would greatly support the plausibility of the hypothesis that ApoE affects development of NFTs in AD.

The hypothesis that ApoE can affect tangle formation is based on the in vitro data showing that ApoE3 bound unphosphorylated τ, whereas ApoE4 did not *(76)*. Neither isoform of ApoE bound to phosphorylated forms of τ. These observations gave rise to the model that ApoE3 binds to unphosphorylated τ and protects it from the phosphorylation that occurs in AD. ApoE4, in contrast, is unable to protect τ from phosphorylation. This hypothesis has recently been supported by studies of ApoE-deficient mice showing increased levels of τ phosphorylation *(81)*. Furthermore, neurite outgrowth experiments of cells treated with ApoE3- and ApoE4-containing lipoproteins showed that ApoE4-treated cells had higher levels of depolymerized microtubules *(82)*. Thus, ApoE may affect microtubule assembly, either directly or indirectly.

3.3. ApoE in the Deposition of Amyloid

There are several reasons to favor the hypothesis that ApoE affects the development of AD by affecting the deposition of amyloid. First, ApoE is consistently found asssociated with Aβ deposits in the brain parenchyma and in amyloid angiopathy *(58,83)*. Second, the levels of amyloid deposited in the brains of individuals with AD and with Down's syndrome vary with ApoE genotype *(43,69,72,73,75,84)* (Fig. 2). Third, ApoE genotype affects the level of amyloid deposition associated with head injury *(85)*, with ApoE ε4 associated with higher levels of amyloid deposition. Finally, ApoE genotype affects the age of onset of AD *(69,86,87)*, and amyloid deposition appears to be the earliest neuropathological change that occurs in AD *(88,89)*.

There are at least three processes affecting amyloid deposition that could be influenced by ApoE:

1. The clearance of Aβ;
2. The deposition of Aβ; and
3. The generation of Aβ.

3.3.1. Clearance of Aβ

ApoE binds hydrophobic and amphipathic molecules for clearance by cells, and Aβ is an amphipathic molecule. The connection between ApoE and Aβ first depended on two observations, the binding of ApoE to senile plaques *(58)* and the binding of ApoE to soluble Aβ *(90)*. We hypothesized that ApoE could prevent Aβ aggregation, or even target for removal microaggregates of Aβ molecules and thus prevent accumulation of amyloid *(43)*. An early in vitro study with purified ApoE (not complexed to lipoproteins) showed that Aβ bound to ApoE4 more quickly than to ApoE3, but there were no differences in avidity of binding *(91)*. Studies with ApoE on lipoproteins, however, showed that Aβ bound to ApoE3, to both ApoE monomers and dimers, with greater

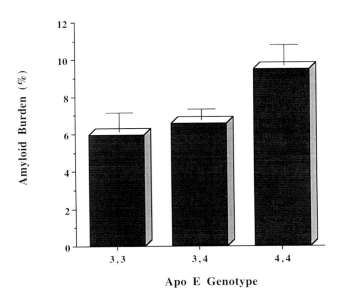

Fig. 2. Amyloid burden in AD patients separated by ApoE genotype *(69)*.

affinity than to ApoE4 *(92–94)*. These studies suggested that ApoE on lipoproteins could bind and clear Aβ, and that ApoE3-containing lipoproteins were more efficient at this clearance. Indeed, in the plasma, Aβ was found associated with HDL *(95)*, and in the brain, Aβ was found associated with lipids *(96)*, supporting an association between lipoproteins and Aβ.

We also hypothesized that Aβ clearance might be impaired in ApoE ε4 individuals based on the presence of the ApoE receptor LRP on amyloid deposits *(43,97)*. This hypothesis received further support when we found that other LRP ligands were also found on amyloid deposits *(2)*. LRP is a multifunctional receptor, acting to clear protease–protease inhibitor complexes, lipoprotein-associated proteins, and other molecules (Table 2). Since most of the LRP ligands have already been found associated with senile plaques in AD *(2,110–114)*, we hypothesized that LRP may not be clearing its ligands normally in AD brain. Impaired clearance of ApoE–Aβ complexes may be part of a larger problem of impaired cellular uptake of many molecules in AD brain. Indeed, impaired metabolism of lipoproteins may underlie the lipid deficits seen in AD brains *(115–117)*.

3.3.2. Deposition of Aβ

A second hypothesis concerning interactions between ApoE and Aβ suggests that ApoE alters assembly of Aβ into insoluble aggregates. This hypothesis builds on the observations outlined above showing that ApoE and Aβ proteins interact in vitro. Several studies reported that ApoE facilitated the aggregation of Aβ into fibrils in cell-free systems, and that ApoE2, E 3, and E 4 differed in their ability to aid in this process *(118–121)*. Another study, however, reported that ApoE3 and ApoE4 inhibited the formation of Aβ fibrils *(122)*. Again, these studies were conducted with purified ApoE, rather than with ApoE-containing lipoproteins. In the hydrophobic environment of

Table 2
Functions of LRP Ligands

LRP ligand	Function
Lipid-associated molecules	
ApoE-containing lipoproteins	Lipoprotein transport *(97a,98)*
Lipoprotein lipase	Cleave triglycerides and phospholipids *(99)*
Hepatic lipase	Cleave triglycerides and phospholipids *(100)*
Proteases/inhibitors	
α2-macroglobulin	Multi-functional proteinase inhibitor *(26)*
Tissue plasminogen activator	Cleaves plasminogen to plasmin *(102)*
Urokinase plasminogen activator	Cleaves plasminogen to plasmin *(103)*
Plasminogen activator inhibitor-1	Inhibits tPA and uPA *(104,105)*
Tissue factor pathway inhibitor-1	Inhibits factors VIIa and Xa *(106)*
Protease nexin II (APP-770)	Inhibits factors IXa and XIa *(101)*
Other	
Lactoferrin	Iron transport *(107)*
Thrombospondin	Cellular attachment *(108)*
Exotoxin A	Pseudomonas toxin *(109)*

lipoproteins, the assembly of Aβ into fibrils could be altered dramatically. Terzi et al. *(123)* reported that lipid vesicles affected the secondary structure of Aβ, favoring the formation of β-structure, suggesting that Aβ aggregation may be altered in the presence of lipoproteins or cell membranes. It is possible that aggegation of Aβ in lipoproteins may compete with clearance of Aβ in lipoproteins, and a change in the kinetics of either aggregation or clearance could lead to amyloid deposition.

3.3.3. Generation of Aβ

A third mechanism by which ApoE could influence amyloid formation is through an effect on APP metabolism. Recently two interesting connections between ApoE metabolism and APP metabolism found. First, the ApoE receptor LRP was found also to be a receptor for soluble APP containing the Kunitz protease inhibitor domain *(101)*. Thus, two genetic risk factors for AD, APP, and ApoE share a single cell-surface receptor, LRP. Second, the processing of APP was found to be altered by the level of cholesterol in the cell *(124)*. Thus, cell cholesterol levels, which are modulated by ApoE-containing lipoproteins, affect APP metabolism. However, there is as yet no direct evidence that ApoE affects the production of Aβ: CSF Aβ levels were found not to differ in AD patients of the various ApoE genotypes *(125)*.

SUMMARY

Despite a large amount of information concerning the form and function of the ApoE isoforms, we do not how these molecules affect the AD neuropathological processes. With the large number of DNA databases assembled in labs around the world, there will be more and more genetic risk factors identified for many diseases. These experiences, over the last three years of research into ApoE and AD, suggest that converting genetic risks into concrete pathways of biological mechanisms will be a difficult task.

REFERENCES

1. Louhija, J., Miettinen, H. E., Kontula, K., Tikkanen, M. J., Mietinen, T. A., and Tilvis, R. S. (1994) Aging and genetic variation of plasma apolipoproteins: relative loss of the apolipoprotein E4 phenotype in centenarians, *Arteriosclerosis Thrombosis* **14**, 1084–1089.
2. Rebeck, G. W., Perls, T. T., West, H. L., Sodhi, P., Lipsitz, L. A., and Hyman, B. T. (1994) Reduced apolipoprotein E4 allele frequency in the oldest old Alzheimer's patients and cognitively normal individuals, *Neurology* **44**, 1513–1516.
3. Davignon, J., Gregg, R. E., and Sing, C. F. (1988) Apolipoprotein E polymorphism and atherosclerosis, *Arteriosclerosis* **8**, 1–21.
4. Mahley, R. W. (1988) Apolipoprotein E: cholesterol transport protein with expanding role in cell biology, *Science* **240**, 622–630.
5. Weisgraber, K. H. (1994) Apolipoprotein E:structure-function relationships, *Advances in Protein Chemistry* **45**, 249–302.
6. Poduri, A., Gearing, M., Rebeck, G. W., Mirra, S. S., Tigges, J., and Hyman, B. T. (1994) Apolipoprotein E4 and beta amyloid in senile plaques and cerebral blood vessels of aged rhesus monkeys, *Am. J. Pathol.* **144**, 1183–1187.
7. Zannis, V. I., Nicolosi, R. J., Jensen, E., Breslow, J. L., and Hayes, K. C. (1985) Plasma and hepatic ApoE isoproteins of nonhuman primates. Differences in apoE among humans, apes, and new and old world monkeys, *J. Lipid Res.* **26**, 1421–1430.
8. Assmann, G. (1982) *Lipid Metabolism and Atherosclerosis*, F. K. Schattauer, Stuttgart, Germany.
9. Segrest, J. P., Jones, M. K., De Loof, H., Brouillette, C. G., Venkatachalapathi, Y. V., and Anantharamaiah, G. M. (1992) The amphipathic helix in the exchangeable apolipoproteins: a review of secondary structure and function, *J. Lipid Res.* **33**, 141–166.
10. Gregg, R. E., Zech, L. A., Schaefer, E. J., Stark, D., Wilson, D., and Brewer, H. B., Jr. (1986) Abnormal in vivo metabolism of apolipoprotein E4 in humans, *J. Clin. Invest.* **78**, 815–821.
11. Weisgraber, K. H. (1990) Apolipoprotein E distribution among human plasma lipoproteins: role of the cysteine-arginine interchange at residue 112, *J. Lipid Res.* **31**, 1503–1511.
12. Dong, L.-M., Wilson, C., Wardell, M. R., Simmons, T., Mahley, R. W., Weisgraber, K. H., and Agard, D. A. (1994) Human apolipoprotein E: role of arginine 61 in mediating the lipoprotein preferences of the E3 and E4 isoforms, *J. Biol. Chem.* **269**, 22,358–22,365.
13. Wilson, C., Wardell, M. R., Weisgraber, K. H., Mahley, R. W., and Agard, D. A. (1991) Three-dimensional structure of the LDL receptor binding domain of human apolipoprotein E, *Science* **252**, 1817–1822.
14. Innerarity, T. L., Friedlander, E. J., Rall, S. C., Jr, Weisgraber, K. H., and Mahley, R. (1983) The receptor-binding domain of human apolipoprotein E, *J. Biol. Chem.* **258**, 12,341-12,347.
15. Lalazar, A., Weisgraber, K. H., Rall, S. C., Jr., Giladi, H., Innerarity, T. L., Levanon, A. Z., Boyles, J. K., Amit, B., Gorecki, M., Mahley, R. W., and Vogel, T. (1988) Site-specific mutagenesis of human apolipoprotein E: recptor binding activity of variants with single amino acid substitutions, *J. Biol. Chem.* **263**, 3542–3545.
16. Weisgraber, K. H., Innerarity, T. L., Harder, K. J., Mahley, R. W., Milne, R. W., Marcel, Y. L., and Sparrow, J. T. (1983) The receptor-binding domain of human apolipoprotein E, *J. Biol. Chem.* **258**, 12,348–12,354.
17. Kowal, R. C., Herz, J., Weisgraber, K. H., Mahley, R. W., Brown, M. S., and Goldstein, J. L. (1990) Opposing effects of apolipoproteins E and C on lipoprotein binding to low density lipoprotein receptor-related protein, *J. Biol. Chem.* **265**, 10,771–10,779.
18. Weisgraber, K. H., Innerarity, T. L., and Mahley, R. W. (1982) Abnormal lipoprotein receptor-binding activity of the human E apoprotein due to cysteine-arginine interchange at a single site, *J. Biol. Chem.* **257**, 2518–2521.
19. Weisgraber, K. H., and Mahley, R. W. (1978) Apoprotein (E-AII) complex of human plasma lipoproteins. I. Characterization of this mixed disulfide and its identification in a high density lipoprotein subfraction, *J. Biol. Chem.* **253**, 6281–6288.

20. Tozuka, M., Hidaka, H., Miyachi, M., Furihata, K., Katsuyama, T., and Kanai, M. (1992) Identification and characterization of apolipoprotein (AII-E2-AII) complex in human plasma lipoprotein, *Biochim. Biophys. Acta* **1165**, 61–67.

21. Borghini, I., James, R. W., Blatter, M.-C., and Pometta, D. (1991) Distribution of apolipoprotein E between free and A-II complexed forms in very-low- and high-density lipoproteins: functional implications, *Biochim. Biophys. Acta.* **1083**, 139–146.

22. Innerarity, T. L., Mahley, R. W., Weisgraber, K. H., and Bersot, T. P. (1978) Apoprotein (E-AII) complex of human plasma lipoproteins. II. Receptor binding activity of a high density lipoprotein subfraction modulated by the apo(E-AII) complex, *J. Biol. Chem.* **253**, 6289–6295.

23. Weisgraber, K. H. and Shinto, L. H. (1991) Identification of the disulfide-linked homodimer of apolipoprotein E3 in plasma. Impact on receptor binding activity, *J. Biol. Chem.* **266**, 12,029–12,034.

24. Yamamoto, T., Davis, C. G., Brown, M. S., Schneider, W. J., Casey, M. L., Goldstein, J. L., and Russell, D. W. (1984) The human LDL receptor: a cysteine-rich protein with multiple Alu sequences in its mRNA, *Cell* **39**, 27–38.

25. Herz, J., Hamann, U., Rogne, S., Myklebost, O., Gausepohl, H., and Stanley, K. K. (1988) Surface location and high affinity for calcium of a 500-kd liver membrane protein closely related to the LDL-receptor suggest a physiological role as lipoprotein receptor, *EMBO J.* **7**, 4119–4127.

26. Strickland, D. K., Ashcom, J. D., Williams, S., Burgess, W. H., Migliorini, M., and Argraves, W. S. (1990) Sequence identity between the α_2-macroglobulin receptor and low density lipoprotein receptor-related protein suggests that this molecule is a multifunctional receptor, *J. Biol. Chem.* **265**, 17,401–17,404.

27. Saito, A., Pietromonaco, S., Loo, A. K.-C., and Farquhar, M. G. (1994) Complete cloning and sequencing of rat gp330/"megalin," a distinctive member of the low density lipoprotein receptor gene family, *Proc. Natl. Acad. Sci. USA* **91**, 9725–9729.

28. Sakai, J., Hoshino, A., Takahashi, S., Miura, Y., Ishii, H., Suzuki, H., Kawarabayasi, Y., and Yamamoto, T. (1994) Structure, chromosome location, and expression of the human very low density lipoprotein receptor gene, *J. Biol. Chem.* **269**, 2173–2182.

29. Kim, D.-H., Iijima, H., Goto, K., Sakai, J., Ishii, H., Kim, H.-J., Suzuki, H., Kondo, H., Saeki, S., and Yamamoto, T. (1996) Human apolipoprotein E receptor 2, *J. Biol. Chem.* **271**, 8373–8380.

30. Brown, M. S. and Goldstein, J. L. (1986) A receptor-mediated pathway for cholesterol homeostasis, *Science* **232**, 34–47.

31. Borghini, I., Barja, F., Pometta, D., and James, R. W. (1995) Characterization of subpopulations of lipoprotein particles isolated from human cerebrospinal fluid, *Biochim. Biophys. Acta.* **1255**, 192–200.

32. Pitas, R. E., Boyles, J. K., Lee, S. H., Foss, D., and Mahley, R. W. (1987) Astrocytes synthesize apolipoprotein E and metabolize apolipoprotein E-containing lipoproteins, *Biochim. Biophys. Acta* **917**, 148–161.

33. Pitas, R. E., Boyles, J. K., Lee, S. H., Hui, D., and Weisgraber, K. H. (1987) Lipoproteins and their receptors in the central nervous system, *J. Biol. Chem.* **262**, 14,352–14,360.

34. Boyles, J. K., Pitas, R. E., Wilson, E., Mahley, R. W., and Taylor, J. M. (1985) Apolipoprotein E associated with astrocytic glia of the central nervous system and with nonmyelinating glia of the peripheral nervous system, *J. Clin. Invest.* **76**, 1501–1513.

35. Poirier, J., Hess, M., May, P. C., and Finch, C. E. (1991) Astrocytic apolipoprotein E mRNA and GFAP mRNA in hippocampus after entorhinal cortex lesioning, *Mol. Brain Res.* **11**, 97–106.

36. Dyer, C. and Philibotte, T. (1995) A clone of the MOCH-1 glial tumor in culture: multiple phenotypes expressed under different environmental consitions, *J. Neuropathol. Exp. Neurol.* **54**, 852–863.

37. Warnette-Hammond, M. E., Lauer, S. J., Corsini, A., Walker, D., Taylor, J. M., and Rall, Jr., S. C. (1989) Glycosylation of human apolipoprotein E. *J. Biol. Chem.* **264**, 9094–9101.

38. Edmond, J., Korsak, R. A., Morrow, J. W., Torok-Both, G., and Catlin, D. H. (1991) Dietary cholesterol and the origin of cholesterol in the brain of developing rats, *J. Nutr.* **121,** 1323–1330.
39. Jurevics, H. and Morell, P. (1995) Cholesterol for synthesis of myelin is made locally, not imported into the brain, *J. Neurochem.* **64,** 895–901.
40. Poirier, J., Baccichet, A., Dea, D., and Gauthier, S. (1993) Cholesterol synthesis and lipoprotein reuptake during synaptic remodelling in hippocampus in adult rats, *Neuroscience* **55,** 81–90.
41. Goodrum, J. F. (1991) Cholesterol from degenerating nerve myelin becomes associated with lipoproteins containing apolipoprotein E, *J. Neurochem.* **56,** 2082–2086.
42. Bellosta, S., Nathan, B. P., Orth, M., Dong, L.-M., Mahley, R. W., and Pitas, R. E. (1995) Stable expression and secretion of apolipoproteins E3 and E4 in mouse neuroblastoma cells produces differential effects on neurite outgrowth, *J. Biol. Chem.* **270,** 27,063–27,071.
43. Rebeck, G. W., Reiter, J. S., Strickland, D. K., and Hyman, B. T. (1993) Apolipoprotein E in sporadic Alzheimer's disease: allelic variation and receptor interactions, *Neuron* **11,** 575–580.
44. Swanson, L. W., Simmons, D. M., Hofmann, S. L., Goldstein, J. L., and Brown, M. S. (1988) Localization of mRNA for low density lipoprotein receptor and a cholesterol synthetic enzyme in rabbit nervous system by in situ hybridization, *Proc. Natl. Acad. Sci. USA* **85,** 9821–9825.
45. Bu, G., Maksymovitch, E. A., Nerbonne, J. M., and Schwartz, A. L. (1994) Expression and function of the low density lipoprotein receptor-related protein (LRP) in mammalian central neurons, *J. Biol. Chem.* **269,** 18,521–18,528.
46. Moestrup, S. K., Gliemann, J., and Pallensen, G. (1992) Distribution of the α_2-macroglobulin receptor/low density lipoprotein receptor-related protein in human tissues, *Cell Tissue Res.* **269,** 375–382.
47. Tooyama, I., Kawamata, T., Akiyama, H., Kimura, H., Moestrup, S. K., Gliemann, J., Matsuo, A., and McGeer, P. L. (1995) Subcellular localization of the low density lipoprotein receptor-related protein (α_2-macroglobulin receptor) in human brain, *Brain Res.* **691,** 235–238.
48. Wolf, B. B., Lopes, M. B. S., VandenBerg, S. R., and Gonias, S. L. (1992) Characterization and immunohistochemical localization of α_2-macroglobulin receptor (low-density lipoprotein receptor-related protein) in human brain, *Am. J. Pathol.* **141,** 37–42.
49. Zheng, G., Bachinsky, D. R., Stamenkovic, I., Strickland, D. K., Brown, D., Andres, G., and McCluskey, R. T. (1994) Organ distribution in rats of two members of the low-density lipoprotein receptor gene family, gp330 and LRP/a2MR, and the receptor-associated protein (RAP), *J. Histochem. Cytochem.* **42,** 531–542.
50. Christie, R. H., Chung, H., Rebeck, G. W., Strickland, D., and Hyman, B. T. (1996) Expression of the very low density lipoprotein receptor (VLDL-r), an apolipoprotein E receptor, in the central nervous system and in Alzheimer disease, *J. Neuropath. Exp. Neurol.* **55,** 491–498.
51. Christie, R. H., Freeman, M., and Hyman, B. T. (1996) Expression of the macrophage scavenger receptor, a multifunctional lipoprotein receptor, in microglia associated with senile plaques in Alzheimer's disease, *Am. J. Pathol.* **148,** 399–403.
52. Okuizumi, K., Onodera, O., Namba, Y., Ikeda, K., Yamamoto, T., Seki, K., Ueki, A., Nanko, S., Tanaka, H., Takahashi, H., Oyanagi, K., Mizusawa, H., Kanazawa, I., and Tsuji, S. (1995) Genetic association of the very low density lipoprotein (VLDL) receptor with sporadic Alzheimer's disease, *Nature Genet.* **11,** 207–209.
53. Krieger, M. and Herz, J. (1994) Structures and functions of multiligand lipoprotein receptors: macrophage scavenger receptors and LDL receptor-related protein (LRP), *Ann. Rev. Biochem.* **63,** 601–37.
54. Snipes, G. J., McGuire, C. B., Norden, J. J., and Freeman, J. A. (1986) Nerve injury stimulates the secretion of apolipoprotein E by nonneuronal cells, *Proc. Natl. Acad. Sci. USA* **83,** 1130–1134.
55. Masliah, E., Mallory, M., Ge, N., Alford, M., Veinbergs, I., and Roses, A. D. (1995) Neurodegeneration in the central nervous system of apoE-deficient mice, *Exp. Neurol.* **136,** 107–122.

56. Handelmann, G. E., Boyles, J. K., Weisgraber, K. H., Mahley, R. W., and Pitas, R. E. (1992) Effects of apolipoprotein E, β-very low density lipoproteins, and cholesterol on the extensions of neurites by rabbit dorsal root ganglion neurons in vitro, *J. Lipid Res.* **33**, 1677–1688.

57. Holtzman, D. M., Pitas, R. E., Kilbridge, J., Nathan, B., Mahley, R. W., Bu, G., and Schwartz, A. L. (1995) Low density lipoprotein receptor-related protein mediates apolipoprotein E-dependent neurite outgrowth in a central nervous system-derived neuronal cell line, *Proc. Natl. Acad. Sci. USA* **92**, 9480–9484.

58. Namba, Y., Tomonaga, M., Kawasaki, H., Otomo, E., and Ikeda, K. (1991) Apolipoprotein E immunoreactivity in cerebral amyloid deposits and neurofibrillary tangles in Alzheimer's disease and kuru plaque amyloid in Creutzfeldt-Jakob disease, *Brain Res.* **541**, 163–166.

59. Nathan, B. P., Bellosta, S., Sanan, D. A., Weisgraber, K. H., Mahley, R. W., and Pitas, R. E. (1994) Differential effects of apolipoproteins E3 and E4 on neuronal growth in vitro, *Science* **264**, 850–852.

60. Arai, H., Muramatsu, T., Higuchi, S., Sasaki, H., and Trojanowski, J. Q. (1994) Apolipoprotein E gene in Parkinson's disease with or without dementia, *Lancet* **344**, 889.

61. Benjamin, R., Leake, A., Edwardson, J. A., McKeith, I. G., Ince, P. G., Perry, R. H., and Morris, C. M. (1994) Apolipoprotein E genes in Lewy body and Parkinson's disease, *Lancet* **343**, 1565.

62. Koller, W. C., Glatt, S. L., Hubble, J. P., Paolo, A., Troster, A. I., Handler, M. S., Horvat, R. T., Martin, C., Schmidt, K., Karst, A., Wijsman, E. M., Yu, C.-E., and Schellenberg, G. D. (1995) Apolipoprotein E genotypes in Parkinson's disease with and without dementia, *Ann. Neurol.* **37**, 242–245.

63. Mui, S., Rebeck, G. W., McKenna-Yasek, D., Hyman, B. T., and Brown, R. H. (1995) Apolipoprotein E ε4 allele is not associated with earlier age at onset in amyotrophic lateral sclerosis, *Ann. Neurol.* **380**, 460–463.

64. Nakagawa, Y., Kitamoto, T., Furukawa, H., Ogomori, K., and Tateishi, J. (1995) Apolipoprotein E in Creutzfeldt-Jakob disease, *Lancet* **345**, 68.

65. Pickering-Brown, S. M., Mann, D. M. A., Owen, F., Ironside, J. W., de Silva, R., Roberts, D. A., Balderson, D. J., and Cooper, P. N. (1995) Allelic variation in apolipoprotein E and prion protein genotype related to plaque formation and age of onset in sporadic Creutzfeld-Jakob disease, *Neurosci. Lett.* **187**, 127–129.

66. Roses, A. D., Saunders, A. M., Strittmatter, W. J., Schmechel, D. E., Pericak-Vance, M. A., and Hyman, B. (1995) Apolipoprotein E in Creutzfeldt-Jakob disease, *Lancet* **345**, 69.

67. Saunders, A. M., Schmader, K., Breitner, J. C. S., Benson, M. D., Brown, W. T., Goldfarb, L., Goldgaber, D., Manworing, M. G., Szymanski, M. H., McCown, N., Dole, K. C., Schmechel, D. E., Strittmatter, W. J., Pericak-Vance, M. A., and Roses, A. D. (1993) Apolipoprotein E e4 allele distributions in late-onset Alzheimer's disease and in other amyloid-forming diseases, *Lancet* **342**, 710–711.

68. Zerr, I., Helmhold, M., and Weber, T. (1995) Apolipoprotein E in Creutzfeldt-Jakob disease, *Lancet* **345**, 68,69.

69. Gomez-Isla, T., West, H. L., Rebeck, G. W., Harr, S. D., Growdon, J. H., Locasio, J. J., Perls, T. T., Lipsitz, L. A., and Hyman, B. T. (1996) Clinical and pathological correlates of apolipoprotein E e4 in Alzheimer disease, *Ann. Neurol.* **39**, 62–70.

70. Al-Chalabi, A., Enayat, Z. E., Bakker, M. C., Sham, P. C., Ball, D. M., Shaw, C. E., Lloyd, C. M., Powell, J. F., and Leigh, P. N. (1996) Association of apolipoprotein E e4 with bulbar onset motor neuron disease, *Lancet* **347**, 159,160.

71. Gearing, M., Schneider, J. A., Rebeck, G. W., Hyman, B. T., and Mirra, S. S. (1995) Alzheimer's disease with and without coexisting Parkinson's disease changes: apolipoprotein E genotype and neuropathological correlates, *Neurology* **45**, 1985–1990.

72. Schmechel, D. E., Saunders, A. M., Strittmatter, W. J., Crain, B., Hulette, C., Joo, S. H., Pericak-Vance, M. A., Goldgaber, D., and Roses, A. D. (1993) Increased amyloid β-peptide deposition in cerebral cortex as a consequence of apolipoprotein E genotype in late-onset Alzheimers disease, *Proc. Natl. Acad. Sci. USA* **90**, 9649–9653.

73. Nagy, Z. S., Esiri, M. M., Jobst, K. A., Johnston, C., Litchfield, S., Sim, E., and Smith, A. D. (1995) Influence of the apolipoprotein E genotype on amyloid deposition and neurofibrillary tangle formation in Alzheimer's disease, *Neuroscience* **69**, 757–761.

74. Ohm, T. G., Kirca, M., Bohl, J., Scharnagl, H., Gross, W., and Marz, W. (1995) Apolipoprotein E polymorphism influences not only cerebral senile plaque load but also Alzheimer-type neurofibrillary tangle formation, *Neuroscience* **66**, 583–587.

75. Polvikoski, T., Sulkava, R., Haltia, M., Kainulainen, K., Vuorio, A., Verkkoniemi, A., Niinisto, L., Halonen, P., and Kontula, K. (1995) Apolipoprotein E, dementia, and cortical deposition of β-amyloid protein, *N. Engl. J. Med.* **333**, 1242–1247.

76. Strittmatter, W. J., Saunders, A. M., Goedert, M., Weisgraber, K. H., Dong, L.-M., Jakes, R., Huang, D. Y., Pericak-Vance, M., Schmechel, D., and Roses, A. D. (1994) Isoform-specific interactions of apolipoprotein E with microtubule-associated protein tau: implications for Alzheimer disease, *Proc. Natl. Acad. Sci. USA* **91**, 11,183–11,186.

77. Han, S.-H., Einstein, G., Weisgraber, K. H., Strittmatter, W. J., Saunders, A. M., Pericak-Vance, M., Roses, A. D., and Schmechel, D. E. (1994) Apolipoprotein E is localized to the cytoplasm of human cortical neurons: a light and electron microscopic study, *J. Neuropathol. Exp. Neurol.* **53**, 535–544.

78. Han, S.-H., Hulette, C., Saunders, A. M., Einstein, G., Pericak-Vance, M., Strittmatter, W. J., Roses, A. D., and Schmechel, A. E. (1994) Apolipoprotein E is present in hippocampal neurons without neurofibrillary tangles in Alzheimer's disease and in age-matched controls, *Exp. Neurol.* **128**, 13–26.

79. Hamilton, R. L., Wong, J. S., Guo, L. S. S., Krisans, S., and Havel, R. J. (1990) Apolipoprotein E localization in rat hepatocytes by immunogold labeling of cyrothin sections, *J. Lipid Res.* **31**, 1589–1603.

80. Metzger, R. E., LaDu, M. J., Pan, J. B., Getz, G. S., Frail, D. E., and Falduto, M. T. (1996) Neurons of the human frontal cortex display apolipoprotein E immunoreactivity: implications for Alzheimer's disease, *J. Neuropathol. Exp. Neurol.* **55**, 372–380.

81. Genis, I., Gordon, I., Sehayek, E., and Michaelson, D. M. (1995) Phosphorylation of tau in apolipoprotein E-deficient mice, *Neurosci. Lett.* **199**, 5–8.

82. Nathan, B. P., Chang, K.-C., Bellosta, S., Brisch, E., Ge, N., Mahley, R. W., and Pitas, R. E. (1995) The inhibitory effect of apolipoprotein E4 on neurite outgrowth is associated with microtubule depolymerization, *J. Biol. Chem.* **370**, 19,791–19,799.

83. Wisniewski, T., and Frangione, B. (1992) Apolipoprotein E: a pathological chaperone protein in patients with cerebral and systemic amyloid, *Neurosci. Lett.* **135**, 235–238.

84. Greenberg, S. M., Rebeck, G. W., Vonsattel, J. P. G., Gomez-Isla, T., and Hyman, B. (1995) Apolipoprotein E e4 and cerebral hemorrhage associated with amyloid angiopathy, *Ann. Neurol.* **38**, 254–259.

85. Nicoll, J. A. R., Roberts, G. W., and Graham, D. I. (1995) Apolipoprotein ε4 allele is associated with deposition of amyloid β-protein following head injury, *Nature Med.* **1**, 135–137.

86. Corder, E. H., Saunders, A. M., Strittmatter, W. J., Schmechel, D. E., Gaskell, P. C., Small, G. W., Roses, A. D., Haines, J. L., and Pericak-Vance, M. A. (1993) Gene dose of apolipoprotein E type 4 allele and the risk of Alzheimer's disease in late onset families, *Science* **261**, 921–923.

87. Tsai, M.-S., Tangalos, E. G., Petersen, R. C., Smith, G. E., Schaid, D. J., Kokmen, E., Ivnek, R. J., and Thibodeau, N. (1994) Apoliprotein E: risk factor for Alzheimer's disease, *Am. J. Hum. Genet.* **54**, 643–649.

88. Hardy, J. and Allsop, D. (1991) Amyloid deposition as the central event in the aetiology of Alzheimer's disease, *Trends Pharmacol. Sci.* **12**, 383–388.

89. Mann, D. M. A., Marcyniuk, B., Yates, P. O., Neary, D., and Snowden, J. S. (1988) The progression of the pathological changes of Alzheimer's disease in frontal and temporal neocortex examined at both biopsy and autopsy, *Neuropathol. Appl. Neurobiol.* **14**, 177–195.

90. Strittmatter, W. J., Saunders, A. M., Schmechel, D., Pericak-Vance, M., Enghild, J., Salvesen, G. S., and Roses, A. D. (1993) Apolipoprotein E: high-avidity binding to β-amyloid and increased frequence of type 4 allele in late-onset familial Alzheimer disease, *Proc. Natl. Acad. Sci. USA* **90,** 1977–1981.

91. Strittmatter, W. J., Weisgraber, K. H., Huang, D., Dong, L. M., Salvesen, G. S., Pericak-Vance, M., Schmechel, D., Saunders, A. M., Goldgaber, D., and Roses, A. D. (1993) Binding of human apolipoprotein E to βA4 peptide: isoform specific effects and impications for late onset Alzheimer disease, *Proc. Natl. Acad. Sci. USA* **90,** 8098–8102.

92. LaDu, M. J., Falduto, M. T., Manelli, A. M., Reardon, C. A., Getz, G. S., and Frail, D. E. (1994) Isoform-specific binding of apolipoprotein E to β-amyloid, *J. Biol. Chem.* **269,** 23,403–23,406.

93. LaDu, M. J., Pederson, T. M., Frail, D. E., Reardon, C. A., Getz, G., and Falduto, M. T. (1995) Purification of apolipoprotein E attenuates isoform-specific binding to β-amyloid, *J. Biol. Chem.* **270,** 9039–9042.

94. Zhou, Z., Smith, J. D., Greengard, P., and Gandy, S. (1996) Alzheimer amyloid-β peptide forms denaturant-resistant complex with type E3 but not type E4 isoform of apolipoprotein E, *Mol. Med.* **2,** 175–180.

95. Koudinov, A., Matsubara, E., Frangione, B., and Ghiso, J. (1994) The soluble form of Alzheimer's amyloid beta protein is complexed to high density lipoprotein 3 and very high density lipoprotein in normal human plasma, *Biochem. Biophys. Res. Commun.* **205,** 1164–1171.

96. Yanagisawa, K., Odaka, A., Suzuki, N., and Ihara, Y. (1995) GM1 ganglioside-bound amyloid β-protein (Aβ): a possible form of preamyloid in Alzheimer's disease, *Nature Med.* **1,** 1062–1066.

97. Tooyama, I., Kawamata, T., Akiyama, H., Moestrup, S. K., Gliemann, J., and McGeer, P. L. (1993) Immunohistochemical study of α_2 macroglobulin receptor in Alzheimer and control postmortem human brain, *Mol. Chem. Neuropathol.* **18,** 153–160.

97a. Kowal, R. C., Herz, J., Goldstein, J. L., Esser, V., and Brown, M. S. (1989) Low density lipoprotein receptor-related protein mediates uptake of cholesteryl esters derived from apoprotein E-enriched lipoproteins, *Proc. Natl. Acad. Sci. USA* **86,** 5810–5814.

98. Beisiegel, U., Weber, W., Ihrke, G., Herz, J., and Stanley, K. K. (1989) The LDL-receptor-related protein, LRP, is an apolipoprotein E-binding protein, *Nature* **341,** 162–164.

99. Beisiegel, U., Weber, W., and Bengtsson-Olivecrona, G. (1991) Lipoprotein lipase enhances the binding of chylomicrons to low density lipoprotein receptor-related protein, *Proc. Natl. Acad. Sci. USA* **88,** 8342–8346.

100. Kounnas, M. Z., Chappell, D. A., Wong, H., Argraves, W. S., and Strickland, D. K. (1995) The cellular internalization and degradation of hepatic lipase is mediated by low density lipoprotein receptor-related protein and requires cell surface proteoglycans, *J. Biol. Chem.* **270,** 9307–9312.

101. Kounnas, M. Z., Moir, R. D., Rebeck, G. W., Bush, A. I., Argraves, W. S., Tanzi, R. E., Hyman, B. T., and Strickland, D. K. (1995) LDL receptor-related protein, a multifunctional apoE receptor, binds secreted β-amyloid precursor protein and mediates its degradation, *Cell* **82,** 331–340.

102. Bu, G., Williams, S., Strickland, D. K., and Schwartz, A. L. (1992) Low density lipoprotein receptor-related protein/α_2-macroglobulin receptor is a hepatic receptor for tissue-type plasminogen activator, *Proc. Natl. Acad. Sci. USA* **89,** 7427–7431.

103. Kounnas, M. Z., Henkin, J., Argraves, W. S., and Strickland, D. K. (1993) Low density lipoprotein receptor-related protein/α_2-macroglobulin receptor mediates cellular uptake of pro-urokinase, *J. Biol. Chem.* **268,** 21,862–21,867.

104. Nykjaer, A., Petersen, C. M., Moeller, B., Jensen, P. H., Moestrup, S., Holtet, T. L., Etzerodt, M., Thorgersen, H. C., Munch, M., Andreasen, P. A., and Gliemann, J. (1992) Purified α_2-macroglobulin receptor/LDL receptor-related protein binds urokinase-plasminogen activator inhibitor type-1 complex, *J. Biol. Chem.* **267,** 14,543–14,546.

105. Orth, K., Madison, E. L., Gething, M.-J., Sambrook, J. F., and Herz, J. (1992) Complexes of tissue-type plasminogen activator and its serpin inhibitor plasminogen activator inhibitor type 1 are internalized by means of the low density lipoprotein receptor-related protein/α_2-macroglobulin receptor, *Proc. Natl. Acad. Sci. USA* **89,** 7422–7426.

106. Warshawsky, I., Broze, G. J., Jr, and Schwartz, A. L. (1994) The low density lipoprotein receptor-related protein mediates the cellular degradation of tissue factor pathway inhibitor, *Proc. Natl. Acad. Sci. USA* **91,** 6664–6668.

107. Willnow, T. E., Goldstein, J. L., Orth, K., Brown, M. S., and Herz, J. (1992) Low density lipoprotein receptor-related protein and gp330 bind similar ligands, including plasminogen activator-inhibitor complexes and lactoferrin, an inhibitor of chylomicron remnant clearance, *J. Biol. Chem.* **267,** 26,172–26,180.

108. Mikhailenko, I., Kounnas, M. Z., and Strickland, D. K. (1995) Low density lipoprotein receptor-related protein/α_2-macroglobulin receptor mediates the cellular internalization and degradation of thrombospondin, *J. Biol. Chem.* **270,** 9543–9549.

109. Kounnas, M. Z., Morris, R. E., Thompson, M. R., FitzGerald, D. J., Strickland, D. K., and Saelinger, C. B. (1992) The α_2-macroglobulin receptor/low density lipoprotein receptor-related protein binds and internalizes Pseudomonas exotoxin A, *J. Biol. Chem.* **267,** 12,420–12,423.

110. Bauer, J., Strauss, S., Schreiter-Gasser, U., Ganter, U., Schlegel, P., Witt, I., Yolk, B., and Berger, M. (1991) Interleukin-6 and α_2-macroglobulin indicate an acute-phase state in ALzheimer's disease cortices, *FEBS Lett.* **285,** 111–114.

111. Buee, L., Hof, P. R., Roberts, D. D., Delacourte, A., Morrison, J. H., and Fillit, H. M. (1992) Immunohistochemical identification of thrombospondin in normal human brain and in Alzheimer's disease, *Am. J. Pathol.* **141,** 783–788.

112. Hollister, R. D., Kisiel, W., and Hyman, B. T. (1996) Immunohistochemical localization of tissue factor pathway inhibitor-1 (TFPI-1), a kunitz proteinase inhibitor, in Alzheimer's disease, *Brain Res.* in press.

113. Kawamata, T., Tooyama, I., Yamada, T., Walker, D. G., and McGeer, P. L. (1993) Lactotransferrin immunocytochemistry in Alzheimer and normal human brain, *Am. J. Pathol.* **142,** 1574–1585.

114. van Gool, D., de Strooper, B., van Leuven, F., Triau, E., and Dom, R. (1993) α_2-Macroglobulin expression in neuritic-type plaques in patients with Alzheimer's disease, *Neurobiol. Aging* **14,** 233–237.

115. Nitsch, R. M., Blusztajn, J. K., Pittas, A. G., Slack, B. E., Growdon, J. H., and Wurtman, R. J. (1992) Evidence for a membrane defect in Alzheimer disease brain, *Proc. Natl. Acad. Sci. USA* **89,** 1671–1675.

116. Soderberg, M., Edlund, C., Alafuzoff, I., Kristensson, K., and Dallner, G. (1992) Lipid composition in different regions of the brain in Alzheimer's disease/senile dementia of Alzheimer's type, *J. Neurochem.* **59,** 1646–1653.

117. Svennerholm, L., and Gottfries, C.-G. (1994) Membrane lipids, selectively diminished in Alzheimer brains, suggest synapse loss as a primary event in early-onset form (type I) and demyelination in late onset form (type II), *J. Neurochem.* **62,** 1039–1047.

118. Castano, E. M., Prelli, F., Wisniewski, T., Golabek, A., Kumar, R. A., Soto, C., and Frangione, B. (1995) Fibrillogenesis in Alzheimer's disease of amyloid β peptides and apolipoprotein E, *Biochem. J.* **306,** 599–604.

119. Ma, J., Yee, A., Brewer, A. Y. H., Jr., Das, S., and Potter, H. (1994) Amyloid-associated proteins α_1-antichymotrypsin and apolipoprotein E promote assembly of Alzheimer β-protein into filaments, *Nature* **372,** 92–94.

120. Sanan, D. A., Weisgraber, K. H., Russell, S. J., Mahley, R. W., Huang, D., Saunders, A., Schmechel, D., Wisniewski, T., Frangione, B., Roses, A., and Strittmatter, W. J. (1994) Apolipoprotein E associates with β-amyloid peptide of Alzheimer's disease to form novel monofibrils, *J. Clin. Invest.* **94,** 860–869.

121. Wisniewski, T., Castano, E. M., Golabek, A., Vogel, T., and Frangione, B. (1994) Acceleration of Alzheimer's disease fibril formation by apolipoprotein E in vitro, *Am. J. Pathol.* **145,** 1030–1035.
122. Evans, K. C., Berger, E. P., Cho, C.-G., Weisgraber, K. H., and Lansbury, P. T. (1995) Apolipoprotein E is a kinetic but not a thermodynamic inhibitor of amyloid formation: implications for the pathogenesis and treatment of Alzheimer disease, *Proc. Natl. Acad. Sci. USA* **92,** 763–767.
123. Terzi, E., Holzemann, G., and Seelig, J. (1995) Self-association of β-amyloid peptide (1-40) in solution and binding to lipid membranes, *J. Mol. Biol.* **252,** 633–642.
124. Bodovitz, S. and Klein, W. L. (1996) Cholesterol modulates a-secretase cleavage of amyloid precursor protein, *J. Biol. Chem.* **271,** 4436–4440.
125. Nitsch, R. M., Rebeck, G. W., Deng, M., Richardson, U. I., Tennis, M., Schenk, D. B., Vigo-Pelfrey, C., Lieberburg, I., Wurtman, R. J., Hyman, B. T., and Growdon, J. H. (1995) Cerebrospinal fluid levels of amyloid β-protein in Alzheimer's disease: inverse correlation with severity of dementia and effect of apoE genotype, *Ann. Neurol.* **37,** 512–518.

3

Understanding the Biology and Molecular Pathogenesis of Alzheimer's Disease in Transgenic Mice Expressing Amyloid Precursor Proteins

Karen K. Hsiao

1. INTRODUCTION

Recent developments in transgenic mice expressing Alzheimer amyloid precursor proteins (APP) have provided a powerful new means for testing hypotheses about the biology and molecular pathogenesis of Alzheimer's disease (AD). This chapter will delineate some key features of experimental design that are known to influence transgenic phenotypes. Knowledgeable application of these parameters in experimental design and interpretation may facilitate the production of reproducible and reliable results. The use of these parameters in designing experiments to test hypotheses about the pathogenesis of AD will be illustrated.

2. KEY FEATURES OF EXPERIMENTAL DESIGN AND INTERPRETATION

2.1. Primary Structure of APP

The primary structure of the APP transgene can influence the temporal presentation of neurologic signs in transgenic mice *(1)*. Human APP transgenes containing mutations associated with familial AD, induced death and neophobia earlier than wild-type mouse APP expressed at similar levels, indicating an effect of the APP species, APP mutations, or both. Further experiments are required to determine the relative contributions that APP species and mutations make to differences in the timing of neurologic manifestations.

Whether different APP isoforms affect the transgenic phenotype is unknown, since comparisons of different APP isoforms that control for host strain and precise transgenic APP expression levels are lacking. It is noteworthy that transgenic mice overexpressing predominantly KPI-containing APP isoforms develop significant numbers of amyloid plaques that are virtually identical in appearance to human AD plaques *(2,3)*. In contrast, transgenic mice overexpressing APP lacking the KPI domain develop central nervous system (CNS) dysfunction in specific regions of the brain that are virtually identical to the regions affected in AD, yet lack amyloid plaques *(1)*. This observation suggests the possibility that KPI-containing APP isoforms facilitate the

From: Molecular Mechanisms of Dementia *Edited by: W. Wasco and R. E. Tanzi Humana Press Inc., Totowa, NJ*

generation of amyloid plaques, but not the induction of CNS dysfunction. This hypothesis can be tested in carefully quantified and controlled experiments using transgenic mice (*see* Section 3). Alternatively, amyloid formation may depend on specific mutations or properties of the expression vector or host strain.

2.2. Host Strain and Outcome Measures

The mouse host strain can influence the transgenic phenotype *(1,4)*. FVB/N mice overexpressing human or mouse APP die early, and develop a CNS disorder that includes neophobia and impaired spatial alternation, with diminished glucose utilization and astrogliosis mainly in the cerebrum. In contrast, human APP overexpressed in C57B6/SJL transgenic mice backcrossed to C57B6 mice do not exhibit early death or neophobia, but do exhibit impaired spatial alternation and spatial reference memory.

Both FVB/N mice and C57B6 hybrid mice exhibit hippocampal dysfunction in behavioral tests, and FVB/N mice show a significant decrease in hippocampal glucose utilization that corroborates the behavioral tests. These results indicate that there are both strain-dependent and strain-invariant features associated with expression of APP transgenes. It is possible that the strain-dependent features associated with transgenic APP expression involve particular genes, which may be possible to identify through genetic analysis, and some of these genes could potentially influence the expression of Alzheimer's disease in humans. The strain-dependent features can serve as invaluable outcome measures for assaying the biological activity of APP within a given strain. The strain-invariant features are more likely to be relevant in other species, including humans, and may provide important clues about fundamental pathogenic mechanisms in AD.

Dichotomous outcome measures are often useful for assaying effects of transgenic APP expression, so that Kaplan-Meier and other nonparametric statistics can be used in data analysis. FVB/N transgenic mice overexpressing APP exhibit three easily measurable dichotomous clinical outcomes: death, neophobia, and thigmotaxis. Histopathologic outcomes, such as gliosis, plaque formation, and neuronal loss, may also be scored dichotomously under some circumstances.

Some measurements of behavior, such as learning and memory, cannot easily be scored for nonparametric analysis, because the behavioral instruments for measuring learning and memory in this fashion are not readily available for mice. In these circumstances, it is useful to apply parametric tests at different ages to ascertain whether any observed deficits are age-related, as would be expected for a degenerative disorder like AD. C57B6/SJL mice overexpressing human APP with the K670N/M671L mutation exhibit no deficits in spatial reference memory in the Morris water maze *(5)* or in spatial alternation in a Y-maze at 2 mo of age, but are seriously impaired by 9 mo of age *(5a)*, and JU mice expressing wild-type human APP exhibit no deficits in these same tests at 6 mo of age, but are significantly impaired by 12 mo of age *(6)*.

The clinical abnormalities in transgenic FVB/N mice overexpressing human or mouse APP closely resemble those occurring in a subset of older nontransgenic FVB/N mice, indicating that overexpression of APP accelerates a naturally occurring, age-related CNS disorder in this strain of mouse *(1)*. The pattern of diminished regional brain glucose utilization in aged, impaired nontransgenic FVB/N mice overlaps strikingly with that observed in patients with AD. Regions associated with cognitive and emotional learning and memory, such as the association areas of the cerebral cortex, the hippocampus, entorhinal cortex, and amygdala, are the regions most affected in both aged, impaired nontransgenic FVB/N mice and AD patients. Since APP overexpression accelerates a senescent CNS disorder in FVB/N mice that is functionally similar to AD, it is possible that aberrant APP expression in each species or strain would give rise to age-dependent CNS dysfunction characteristic for each type of animal. Therefore, in certain instances, it may be helpful to evaluate the phenotypes of transgenic mice expressing APP and other AD-associated genes, e.g., PS1 or S182 *(7)* and PS2 or STM2 *(8)*, in the context of specific senescent CNS syndromes known to occur naturally in the host.

2.3. Levels and Sites of Expression

Experience to date suggests that transgenic APP levels exceeding 1 U (1 U representing the amount of endogenous mouse APP present in the brain) are more likely to induce abnormal behavioral or pathological phenotypes. By precisely quantitating transgenic APP levels in multiple lines of mice expressing a particular APP transgene, it becomes possible to transform transgenic mice from a qualitative tool into a quantitative one. For instance, lines harboring APP transgenes driven by the hamster prion protein gene cosmid vector have been created expressing brain APP levels ranging from <1 U to approx 5 U *(1)*. This enables APP dose–response curves to be generated where each data point represents a single transgenic line. This is easily feasible when dichotomous outcome measures can be employed to score the percentage of animals at a given age exhibiting the biological effects of the APP transgenes. In host strains where dichotomous outcome measures are not available, an inverse relationship between onset of abnormalities and APP dosage would be expected.

The site of APP expression may also influence the transgenic phenotype. Cell type, regional brain and body tissue distribution, and intracellular localization would all be expected to play a role. The observation that transgenic FVB/N mice expressing intracellular, but not secreted Aβ exhibited early death, and seizures may be an illustration of this phenomenon *(9)*. It is also possible that the distinct phenotypes in this case were owing to different levels of Aβ expression, since respective levels of Aβ expression for the intracellular and secreted forms were not reported.

3. USING TRANSGENIC MICE TO TEST TWO HYPOTHESES ABOUT THE PATHOGENESIS OF AD

Two central questions about the pathogenesis of AD can be answered using transgenic mice in experimental paradigms where the parameters discussed above are carefully applied. The first question pertains to whether the primary structure of APP determines whether amyloid plaques form in transgenic mice and, if they do form, whether the plaques exert any effect on the behavioral phenotype. The second question pertains to whether Aβ has pathogenic activity that can be dissociated from amyloid plaque deposition, and is therefore the pathogenic moiety in transgenic mice that have behavioral abnormalities, but no amyloid plaques. The methods by which each of these questions can be answered will be briefly outlined.

Hypothesis 1a: The presence of the KPI domain favors amyloid plaque formation in transgenic mice overexpressing APP.

Hypothesis 1b: Amyloid plaque formation influences the behavioral abnormalities observed in transgenic mice overexpressing APP.

To test Hypothesis 1, the following parameters must be selected:

1. Primary structures of APP transgenes;
2. Host strain;
3. Transgenic APP expression levels; and
4. Outcome measures.

The primary structures of the APP transgenes required to perform this experiment include APP695 and APP770 or APP751 transgenes with and without AD-associated mutations. The host strain should **not** be one like the FVB/N strain with early death induced by APP overexpression. Early death appears to preclude extracellular Aβ or Aβ-like deposits from forming spontaneously *(10)*. Amyloid plaques found to date in transgenic mice have all occurred in animals >5 mo of age *(2,11)*. Ideally, transgenic APP expression levels should exceed 2–4 U. Outcome measures should include plaque formation in transgenic mice over a range of ages from 4 to 24 mo. If plaques are found in some transgenic mice, then assays of memory and learning in lines with and without plaques possessing similar levels of transgenic APP expression should be compared.

Hypothesis 2: Aβ is the pathogenic domain of APP in transgenic mice with behavioral abnormalities but no amyloid plaques.

To test Hypothesis 2, the following parameters must be selected:

1. Primary structure of APP transgenes;
2. Host strain;
3. Transgenic APP expression levels; and
4. Outcome measures.

The primary structures of the APP transgenes required to perform this experiment include APP695 transgenes with mutations that raise the levels of Aβ as well as APP695 transgenes that are unable to produce Aβ (i.e., transgenes in which the Aβ region has been substituted). The ideal host strain for this experiment is FVB/N, because two nonparametric outcome measures, death and neophobia, can be completed in the relatively short period of 100 d from birth. Creating lines with a range of transgenic APP expression from <1–4 U would be required to titrate the effects of the different transgenes optimally.

4. CONCLUSION

It is clear that the recent development of a transgenic mouse with authentic amyloid plaques and several other AD-related pathologies *(2)* is a boon to the pharmaceutical industry wishing to test drugs that will inhibit amyloid plaque formation. However, many questions remain about the cause or causes of CNS dysfunction in AD. It is possible that discoveries of novel mechanisms of CNS dysfunction in AD will lead to other therapies that are as effective or more effective than inhibitors of Aβ deposition. Transgenic mice expressing APP and other AD-related genes now enable scientists to pose and test hypotheses about the pathogenesis of AD, both with respect to its molecular pathology and its molecular pathophysiology. This can be done most successfully and reproducibly if the parameters outlined in this chapter are carefully established, thus transforming APP transgenesis from a qualitative into a quantitative science.

Note Added in Proof

We have recently created transgenic mice overexpressing the 695-amino acid isoform of human K670N-M671L APP exhibiting the correlative appearance of learning and memory abnormalities, elevations in Aβ levels, and classic amyloid plaques *(5a)*. These results mitigate against Hypothesis 1a, that the KPI domain is required for the formation of amyloid plaques in transgenic mice. These mice can be used to test Hypothesis 1b by performing careful temporal studies of the relationship between the onset of behavioral abnormalities and the appearance of amyloid plaques.

REFERENCES

1. Hsiao, K. K., Borchelt, D. R., Olson, K., Johannsdottir, R., Kitt, C., Yunis, W., Xu, S., Eckman, C., Younkin, S., Price, D., Iadecola, C., Clark, H. B., and Carlson, G. (1995) Age-related CNS disorder and early death in transgenic FVB/N mice overexpressing Alzheimer amyloid precursor proteins, *Neuron* **15**, 1–16.
2. Games, D., Adams, D., Alessandrini, R., Barbour, R., Berthelotte, P., Blackwell, C., Carr, T., Clemens, J., Donaldson, T., Gillespie, F., Guido, T., Hagoplan, S., Johnson-Wood, K., Khan, K., Lee, M., Leibowitz, P., Lieberburh, I., Little, S., Masliah, E., McConlogue, L., Montoya-Zavaia, M., Mucke, L., Paganini, L., Penalman, E., Power, M., Schenk, D., Peubert, P., Snyder, B., Soriano, F., Tan, H., Vitale, J., Wadsworth, S., Wolozin, B., and Zhao, J. (1995) Alzheimer-type neuropathology in transgenic mice overexpressing V717F β-amyloid precursor protein, *Nature* **373**, 523–527.
3. Mucke, L., Rockenstein, E., Tan, H., Gordon, M., Power, M., Masliah, E., and McConlogue, L. (1995) Levels and alternative splicing of amyloid precursor protein (APP) transcripts in brains of transgenic mice and humans with Alzheimer's disease (AD), *Soc. Neurosci. Abstracts* **21**, 258 (109.8).
4. Hsiao, K. K., Loh, J., Nilsen, S., and Johannsdottir, R. (1995) Strain dependence of longevity and behavior in transgenic mice expressing mutant Alzheimer amyloid precursor protein, *Soc. Neurosci. Abstracts* **21**, 257 (109.6).
5. Morris, R. G. M. (1984) Development of a water-maze procedure for studying spatial learning in the rat, *J. Neurosci. Methods* **11**, 47–60.
5a. Hsiao, K., Chapman, P., Nilsen, S., Eckman, C., Harigaya, Y., Younkin, S., Yong, F., and Cole, G. Correlative memory deficits, Aβ elevation and amyloid plaques in transgenic mice, *Science* (in press).
6. Moran, P. M., Higgins, L. S., Cordell, B., and Moser, P. C. (1995) Age-related learning deficits in transgenic mice expressing the 751-amino acid isoform of human β-amyloid precursor protein, *Proc. Natl. Acad. Sci. USA* **92**, 5341–5345.
7. Sherrington, R., Rogaev, E. I., Liang, Y., Rogaeva, E. A., Levesque, G., Ikeda, M., Chi, H., Lin, C., Li, G., Holman, K., Tsuda, T., Mar, L., Foncin, J. -F., Bruni, A. C., Montesi, M. P., Sorbi, S., Rainero, I., Pinessi, L., Nee, L., Chumakov, I., Pollen, D., Brookes, A., Sanseau, P., Polinsky, R. J., Wasco, W., DaSilva, H. A. R., Haines, J. L., Pericak-Vance, M. A., Tanzi, R. E., Roses, A. D., Fraser, P. E., Rommens, J. M., and George-Hyslop, P. H. S. (1995) Cloning of a gene bearing missense mutations in early-onset familial Alzheimer's disease, *Nature* **375**, 754–760.
8. Levy-Lehad, E., Wasco, W., Poorkaj, P., Romano, D. M., Oshima, J., Pettingell, W. H., Yu, C., Jondro, P. D., Schmidt, S. D., Wang, K., Crowley, A. C., Fu, Y., Guenette, S. Y., Galas, D., Nemens, E., Wijsman, E. M., Bird, T., Schellenberg, G. D., and Tanzi, R. E. (1995) Candidate gene for the chromosome 1 familial Alzheimer's disease locus, *Science* **269**, 973–977.
9. LaFerla, F. M., Tinkle, B. T., Bieberich, C. J., Haudenschild, C. C., and Jay, G. (1995) The Alzheimer's Aβ peptide induces neurodegeneration and apoptotic cell death in transgenic mice, *Nature Genet.* **9**, 21–30.
10. Cole, G. M., Frautschy, S. A., Saido, T. C., and Hsiao, K. (1995) Age-related β-amyloid immunoreactivity in APP transgenic mice, *Neurosci. Abstracts* **21**, 258 (109. 7).
11. Higgins, L. S., Holtzman, D. M., Rabin, J., Mobley, W. C., and Cordell, B. (1994) Transgenic mouse brain histopathology resembles early Alzheimer's disease, *Ann. Neurol.* **35**, 598–607.

4

Mechanism for β-amyloid Overproduction in Alzheimer Disease

Possible Antisense RNA-mediated Generation of a 5'-truncated βAPP MRNA Encoding 12-kDa C-terminal Fragment of βAPP, the Immediate Precursor of Aβ

Vladimir Volloch

1. INTRODUCTION

The overproduction of β-amyloid (Aβ) is associated with and appears to be a primary cause of Alzheimer's disease (AD). Aβ can be generated by proteolysis of β-amyloid precursor protein (βAPP) in both AD-affected and normal cells. There is no evidence, however, that proteolytic cleavage leading to the production of Aβ in sporadic AD-affected and in normal tissues differs qualitatively or quantitatively to account for the overproduction of Aβ in AD. Therefore, an additional pathway for the enhanced production of Aβ may be involved in sporadic AD. A mechanism is proposed that may be responsible for the overproduction of Aβ in sporadic AD, which constitutes the majority of all AD cases. The proposed mechanism, which may be activated or enhanced in sporadic AD-affected tissues, is based on a model for cellular mRNA replication developed in the author's laboratory and proposes the antisense RNA-mediated generation of a 5'-truncated βAPP mRNA encoding 12-kDa C-terminal fragment of βAPP, the immediate precursor of Aβ, followed by initiation of translation at met_{596} contiguously preceding Aβ. The proposed model makes several verifiable predictions and suggests new directions of experimentation that may lead to a better understanding of the mechanisms involved in AD. It also sheds a new light on some previously unexplained results in the field of AD.

2. Aβ AND AD

The overproduction of Aβ, a small, 4-kDa segment in the C-terminal portion of βAPP, is associated with and considered by many to be the primary cause of AD *(1)*. Several types of results argue strongly for the causative role of Aβ in AD. First, Down's syndrome, associated with trisomy 21 and, consequently, increased dosage of the βAPP gene, which is located on chromosome 21, is characterized by a fivefold increase in βAPP expression over normal levels and by the early cerebral deposition of Aβ in

From: Molecular Mechanisms of Dementia *Edited by: W. Wasco and R. E. Tanzi Humana Press Inc., Totowa, NJ*

affected subjects *(2,3)*. Second, presence of the ε4 allele of apolipoprotein E , the major genetic factor in the late-onset AD, correlates with an increase in cerebral deposits of Aβ *(4,5)*. Third, cells from patients with a defect in the S182 gene, associated with the most common form of the early onset AD, make abnormally high amounts of Aβ *(6)*. Fourth, many mutations in the βAPP gene that underlie some forms of familial AD were found to increase the production of Aβ *(7–9)*. Finally, and probably most convincingly, transgenic mice overexpressing full-length human βAPP generate high levels of Aβ and develop AD-like neuropathology *(10)*, consistent with the notion that overproduction of Aβ is sufficient for AD.

3. Aβ CAN BE PRODUCED BY PROTEOLYSIS OF βAPP IN BOTH AD-AFFECTED AND NORMAL CELLS

Proteolytic processing of βAPP is a well-known phenomenon that occurs constitutively in both normal and AD-affected tissues as well as in cultured cells. It is affected by yet-to-be-identified enzymes designated α-, β-, and γ-secretases and occurs at met_{596}/asp_{597} (β-secretase; $βAPP_{695}$ numbering), at lys_{612}/leu_{613} (α-secretase) and between val_{635} and thr_{639} (γ-secretase). Cleavage by β-secretase generates an ectodomain fragment ending at met_{596} and a 12-kDa C-terminal βAPP fragment containing Aβ at its N-terminus (beginning with asp_{597}). The production of Aβ by proteolysis of βAPP requires cleavage by both β- and γ-secretases. Cleavage by α-secretase generates an ectodomain fragment ending at lys_{612} and precludes formation of Aβ because it occurs within the Aβ sequence. Evidence that proteolysis in the Aβ region of βAPP occurs in AD-affected tissues as well as in normal cells includes the demonstration of soluble ectodomain fragments generated proteolytically from βAPP in human cerebrospinal fluid *(11,12)* and of the 12-kDa C-terminal βAPP fragment in both normal and AD brains as well as in cells transfected with βAPP transgenes *(13,14)*. In addition, transgenic mice expressing human βAPP generate both free Aβ and the complementary ectodomain fragment *(10)*. Are there differences in the βAPP proteolytic pathway in normal and affected cells sufficient to explain the overproduction of Aβ in AD?

4. MOLECULAR MECHANISMS UNDERLYING SOME TYPES OF FAMILIAL, BUT NOT SPORADIC, AD ARE WELL UNDERSTOOD

In some types of familial AD, generation of Aβ deposits is caused by mutations within the βAPP gene that affect either βAPP proteolytic pathway or the functional properties of Aβ. In such familial AD cases, mutation-mediated alteration of proteolytic cleavage of βAPP or enhancement of Aβ's amyloidogenicity is sufficient for an accelerated cerebral deposition of Aβ and there is no need to invoke an additional mechanism except for the mutations. For example, in patients with the Dutch mutation (glu_{617} to gln_{617}), altered functional properties of mutated Aβ *(15)* may contribute to the early and often severe cerebrovascular Aβ deposition. The naturally occuring Flemish mutation (ala_{616} to gly_{616}) and the genetically engineered mutation phe_{614} to pro_{614} interfere with the cleavage at the α-secretase site and consequently increase the production of Aβ *(9,16)*. Probably the best example is proteolytic processing of βAPP containing the mutation lys_{595}-met_{596} to asp_{595}-leu_{596}, seen in Swedish familial AD, where the enhanced production of Aβ is owing to the increased efficiency of cleavage at the mutated β-secretase site *(17)* and the consequent unsusceptibility (*see* Section 6.) of the resulting 12-kDa fragment to α-secretase cleavage *(18,19)*. The Aβ production pathway in Swedish familial AD, however, is qualitatively different from that responsible for the production of Aβ from wild-type βAPP in that leu_{596}/asp_{597} cleavage occurs in a different cellular compartment *(17,19)* and possibly by a different enzyme *(19)*, and therefore is not relevant to Aβ production in sporadic, i.e., involving wild-type βAPP, AD.

On the other hand, there is no evidence that proteolytic cleavage leading to the production of Aβ in sporadic AD-affected and in normal tissues differ qualitatively or quantitatively so as to account for the overproduction of Aβ in AD involving wild-type βAPP. Therefore, since proteolytic processing alone cannot account for the increased production of Aβ in sporadic AD, an additional Aβ production pathway may be employed in this type of AD, which constitutes the majority of all AD cases. How could this new mechanism operate? To answer this question, it would be instructive to define the rate-limiting step in production of Aβ.

5. GENERATION OF 12-kDa C-TERMINAL FRAGMENT OF βAPP, THE IMMEDIATE PRECURSOR OF Aβ, IS THE RATE-LIMITING STEP IN PRODUCTION OF Aβ

The amount of the 12-kDa C-terminal βAPP fragment correlates with the amount of released Aβ *(20,21)*, indicative of the precursor–product relationship. Direct evidence that the 12-kDa C-terminal βAPP fragment is the immediate pecursor of Aβ and can be further cleaved by γ-secretase, thus generating Aβ, comes from the work of Dyrks and coworkers, who transfected cells with a 5'-truncated βAPP gene *(22,23)*. RNA transcribed from transfected DNA was translated starting at met_{596} and resulting in an extensive overproduction of the 12-kDa C-terminal βAPP fragment with *(23)* or without *(22)* signal sequence. In both cases, this fragment was rapidly cleaved by γ-secretase to generate Aβ, which was subsequently secreted. This observation indicates that generation of the 12-kDa fragment, and not cleavage at the γ-secretase site, is the rate-limiting step in the production of Aβ. This conclusion is consistent with the results of experiments involving βAPP gene containing the Swedish mutation where the increased efficiency of proteolytic cleavage at the β-secretase site, i.e., the increased production of the 12-kDa C-terminal fragment, leads to the increased generation and secretion of Aβ *(19)*.

6. THE 12-kDa C-TERMINAL βAPP FRAGMENT IS NOT SUSCEPTIBLE TO THE α-SECRETASE CLEAVAGE

Cleavage of βAPP at the α-secretase site precludes the production of Aβ. Unlike intact βAPP, however, the 12-kDa C-terminal βAPP fragment expressed in transfected cells independently of βAPP is not cleaved at the α-secretase site *(22,24)*. This observation is consistent with results obtained by Haass and coworkers, who demonstrated that cleavage of βAPP at the β-secretase site appears to prevent cleavage at the α-secretase site *(19)*. The facts that the 12-kDa C-terminal βAPP fragment is not susceptible to cleavage at the α-secretase site and that cleavage at the γ-secretase site is not a rate-limiting step in the generation of Aβ suggest that the increase in production of the 12-kDa C-terminal βAPP fragment may be an efficient way to overproduce Aβ. The most effective manner to achieve this would be generation of the 12-kDa fragment independently of βAPP.

7. TRANSLATION OF βAPP MRNA FROM AUG$_{1786}$ MAY GENERATE A 12-kDa C-TERMINAL βAPP FRAGMENT INDEPENDENTLY OF βAPP

In βAPP mRNA, the Aβ-coding segment is preceded immediately by the in-frame AUG codon at position 1786 (nucleotide residues are numbered from the start of the βAPP coding region as in ref. *25*) corresponding to the met$_{596}$. The initiation of translation at this position would produce the 12-kDa C-terminal βAPP fragment independently of βAPP. It is noteworthy that the AUG$_{1786}$ is situated within a nucleotide context optimal for initiation of translation, i.e., an A in position −3 and a G in position +4 relative to the A of the AUG codon *(26)*. In fact, AUG$_{1786}$ is one of only two AUG codons within the entire βAPP mRNA that are located within an optimal translation initiation context. Such favorable location of AUG$_{1786}$ was the basis for an earlier proposal that the 12-kDa C-terminal fragment may be generated independently from βAPP by internal initiation of translation of the βAPP mRNA at the AUG$_{1786}$ *(27)*, but this has been subsequently ruled out by the elegant experiments of Citron and coworkers *(28)*. There is, however, another possibility of utilization of the AUG$_{1786}$ as a translation initiation codon, namely the generation of a 5'-truncated βAPP mRNA in which the AUG$_{1786}$ becomes the first AUG codon. A possible mechanism for the generation of such a truncated βAPP mRNA is suggested by recent results from the author's laboratory.

8. ANTISENSE RNA-MEDIATED RNA-DEPENDENT RNA SYNTHESIS RESULTS IN GENERATION OF A 5'-TRUNCATED mRNA

Recently, we obtained evidence that, in erythroid cells, globin mRNA can be produced by RNA-dependent RNA synthesis via antisense RNA intermediates and that this process may also occur in other cell types with other mRNA species. Elucidation of the structure of antisense globin RNA suggested a possible mechanism *(29)* (Fig. 1). Antisense RNA contains a poly(U) stretch at the 5'-end, indicating that its synthesis starts within the poly(A) region of mRNA, presumably by a mechanism similar to that employed in viral systems *(30)*. At the 3'-end, antisense RNA contains two strongly complementary elements within the segment corresponding to the 5'-untranslated region of globin mRNA. This complementarity within the antisense strand is highly conserved during evolution of mammalian globins from marsupials to human *(31)*. It is important to note that it is the complementary relationship and not the nucleotide sequence that is conserved; although nucleotide sequences in this region have diverged during mammalian evolution, the complementarity between the two elements has been preserved. The conservation extends not only to the presence of complementary elements but also to their position, the complementary elements being always located within the segment of the antisense strand corresponding to the 5'-untranslated region of globin mRNA, one always being strictly 3'-terminal *(31)*.

This strong evolutionary conservation suggested an underlying function, namely the priming of the synthesis of a sense RNA strand by the 3'-terminal element of an antisense strand. The strict 3'-terminal location of one of the complementary elements appears to be an absolute requirement, the addition of only one "noncomplementary" nucleotide to the 3'-terminus of the antisense globin strand strongly inhibiting its self-priming capacity *(31)*. The initial product of such a self-priming process is a chimeric antisense–sense molecule in the form of a hairpin loop (Fig. 1). The separation of strands appears to involve cleavage at the 3'-end of the loop that generates 5'-truncated

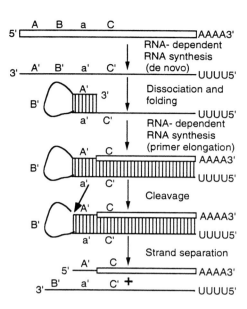

Fig. 1. Postulated mechanism of mRNA replication. Box, sense strand; line, antisense strand. A' and a', complementary elements within 3'-terminal segment of an antisense strand.

mRNA molecules. Since a full-size mRNA molecule can be repeatedly used as a template in such a process, it can direct the synthesis of many truncated mRNA molecules; the subsequent translation of this RNA would result in enhanced production of a polypeptide. Potentially, this process, which may have evolved to enhance expression of specific genes, may be involved in diseases, such as AD, associated with the overproduction of specific proteins.

Because self-priming by globin antisense RNA occurs within the segment corresponding to the 5'-untranslated region of mRNA, the resulting sense strand is truncated within its 5'-untranslated region, but retains an intact coding capacity. Recently, we identified antisense counterparts, putative intermediates in RNA-dependent RNA synthesis, for a number of spliced mRNA species in mammalian cells, an indication that this phenomenon may be quite widespread. Principally, in a nonglobin system, self-priming might occur within a portion of an antisense molecule corresponding to the coding region of an mRNA, thus generating sense strand with 5'-truncated coding region. In such a case, provided the first available AUG is in-frame, translation would result in the C-terminal portion of an original polypeptide. If the βAPP mRNA were subject to such a replication process and if truncation occurred so that the first available AUG is the AUG_{1786}, translation would result in the 12-kDa C-terminal fragment of βAPP.

9. COMPLEMENT OF βAPP mRNA IS CAPABLE OF SELF-PRIMING SYNTHESIS OF A SENSE βAPP STRAND WITH THE FIRST AUG CODON IN POSITION 1786

For a 5'-truncated βAPP mRNA with the first AUG codon in position 1786 to be produced by the mechanism described in Section 8., the antisense βAPP RNA should be able to self-prime the synthesis of a sense-strand in the manner illustrated in Fig. 1, starting upstream from and in the vicinity of the AUG_{1786}. For this to occur, the antisense strand would have to contain two topologicaly compatible complementary elements, one strictly 3'-terminal and another corresponding to a segment of βAPP mRNA upstream of the AUG_{1786}. Is this requirement satisfied in a complement of βAPP mRNA? An answer to this question could be obtained in a model experiment of a type carried out with globin mRNA *(31)*. In such an experiment, an mRNA of interest serves as a template for synthesis of cDNA (the antisense strand) and is subsequently removed by RNase H activity usually present in preparations of reverse transcriptase. If complementary elements were present within the antisense strand, if one of them were 3'-terminal, and if they were topologicaly compatible, self-priming of sense strand synthesis would occur. The result would be an antisense strand (cDNA) extended at the 3'-end by a segment of a sense strand in a hairpin-like structure. Moreover, provided that the 5'-terminus of an mRNA were defined, the junction between the antisense and sense components would indicate the site of self-priming.

In fact, such an experiment was actually carried out with βAPP mRNA. In 1988, when several βAPP cDNAs had already been obtained, but the sequence of the gene and its flanking regions were not yet known, a new βAPP cDNA was reported *(32)*. It differed from the others in that it contained, in addition to a known complement of βAPP mRNA, an over 70-nucleotide-long segment at the 3'-end. When the 5'-end of the βAPP gene and its flanking regions were sequenced *(33)*, no genomic sequence corresponding to the additional 3'-segment of the new cDNA could be seen. On the other hand, it was found that the noncoded segment of the new cDNA was identical to a segment of βAPP mRNA within the coding region of the molecule about 2 kb downstream from its 5'-terminus, which overlaps in part with the Aβ coding region *(34)*. This unusual βAPP cDNA can be analyzed in terms of our model for RNA-dependent RNA synthesis (Fig. 1). It consists of an antisense molecule (cDNA), extended by a sense-strand fragment identical to the segment of βAPP mRNA immediately downstream from residue 1728. It can thus be viewed as a chimeric antisense–sense molecule in which a hairpin loop connects a segment of the antisense portion with a complementary sense extension, which corresponds to a segment of the coding region of βAPP mRNA. Such an extension could have been triggered on completion of cDNA synthesis *(31)*, by complementarity of the 3'-terminal segment of βAPP antisense strand with a topologically compatible internal fragment of the same molecule corresponding to a segment of βAPP mRNA immediately upstream of nucleotide 1728.

As shown in Fig. 2A, such complementary elements are indeed present within the antisense βAPP strand. Because one of the elements must be strictly 3'-terminal to initiate the extension *(31)*, the self-priming ability of the antisense strand depends critically on the 5'-terminal sequence of βAPP mRNA. There are at least five known 5'-ends of βAPP mRNA in normal brain *(33)*. The corresponding 3'-ends of antisense strands are marked by dots in Fig. 2A. Only one of these, i.e., −149 in Fig. 2, would allow effective self-priming to yield the chimeric antisense–sense molecule; with other ends, the 3'-complementary element would be either nonterminal or form an unstable hybrid. In normal subjects, the predominant transcription start site is at residue −146, and whether it shifts in AD patients to residue −149 or elsewhere remains to be determined. Cleavage at the 3'-end of a hairpin loop (Fig. 2B) of the chimeric antisense–sense βAPP molecule would generate a severely 5'-truncated sense βAPP RNA

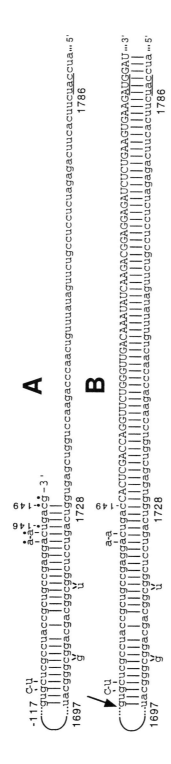

Fig. 2. 3'-Terminal and internal complementary elements of the βAPP antisense strand. **(A)** Folded antisense βAPP RNA strand; **(B)** self-primed synthesis of a 5'-truncated βAPP mRNA. Numbers indicate positions of corresponding residues in βAPP mRNA. Nucleotide residues are numbered as in ref. 25; the nucleotide sequence upstream from residue −146 is from ref. 33. Positions corresponding to transcription start sites of βAPP mRNA are marked by dots. Lower-case letters, antisense strand; upper-case letters, sense strand; arrow indicates postulated cleavage site at the 3'-end of a hairpin loop; underlined, translation initiation codon AUG_{1786} and its complement.

molecule in which the first AUG codon, AUG_{1786} corresponding to met_{596}, is in frame with and immediately precedes the Aβ coding region. Translation of the 5'-truncated βAPP mRNA would result, therefore, in the 12-kDa C-terminal portion of βAPP containing met_{596} followed by Aβ at its N-terminus. This polypeptide could be processed further by two known enzymes to generate Aβ: N-terminal methionine aminopeptidase *(35)*, which removes N-terminal methionine from a majority of newly synthesized eukaryotic proteins, and γ-secretase. Indeed, as was mentioned above, the 12-kDa C-terminal βAPP fragment, translated in transfected cells from the met_{596} without a leader sequence, is cleaved proteolytically at the γ-secretase site to generate Aβ, which is subsequently secreted *(22)*.

10. PREDICTIONS OF THE PROPOSED MODEL

The model for antisense RNA-mediated generation of a 5'-truncated βAPP mRNA encoding the 12-kDa C-terminal βAPP fragment, a process postulated to be activated or enhanced in AD-affected tissues, allows several verifiable predictions. These include the following for sporadic AD-affected brain tissues:

1. The presence of the antisense βAPP RNA, some of it specifically truncated at the 3' terminus;
2. Shift of the transcriptional start site for βAPP mRNA to position −149 or downstream from position −143;
3. The occurrence of a 5'-truncated βAPP mRNA encoding the 12-kDa C-terminal fragment of βAPP; and
4. The presence of RNA-dependent RNA polymerase activity.

The proposed model also predicts that mutations affecting the two complementary elements within the βAPP antisense RNA, and the 3'-terminal location of one of them would either increase the predisposition to AD or confer resistance to it. AD-promoting mutations could be detected by studying the βAPP gene of affected subjects. AD-inhibiting mutations, such as the deletion of one of the complementary elements, could be detected through search for what might be called a "familial resistance" to AD. Such a search would include analyzing the βAPP gene of subjects from long-lived families whose members are not susceptible to AD. It should be noted that, in terms of the proposed model, promotion or inhibition of AD could be achieved not only through mutations, but also through changes in the expression of the βAPP gene. For example, an early shift of the transcriptional start site establishing the 3'-terminal location of one of the complementary elements would increase the predisposition to AD. On the other hand, elimination of one of the complementary elements would confer resistance to sporadic AD. The 3'-terminal complementary element could be eliminated by a shift of the transcriptional start site of βAPP mRNA to a position downstream from a segment corresponding to this element, whereas the removal of the internal complementary element could be effected through alternative splicing leading to βAPP mRNA lacking exon 15, the location of a segment corresponding to the internal complementary element. Such splicing pattern, resulting in ubiquitously expressed βAPP mRNA isoforms lacking exon 15, was observed in rat tissues *(36)*.

Another prediction of the proposed model is the extensive synthesis of the 12-kDa C-terminal βAPP fragment as a primary translational product in Aβ-overproducing cells, a phenomenon that should be seen in pulse–chase experiments. Currently, however, this prediction cannot be verified for lack of an experimental model system.

The proposed model suggests an approach for establishing a genuine mouse model for sporadic AD. In the existing transgenic mouse model *(10)*, the pathology is owing to overexpression of the human βAPP transgene. Earlier attempts, where transgene was expressed at lower, relatively normal levels, did not result in AD neuropathology. Normally, mice develop neither amyloid plaques when aging nor AD pathology *(37,38)*. The rate of cleavage of mouse βAPP at the β-secretase site is much lower than that of human βAPP, but "humanization" of the Aβ segment of mouse βAPP by the substitution of three residues increases this rate to "human" levels *(39)*. On the basis of these findings, it was suggested that, in such "humanized" transgenic mice, the rate of sporadic AD would be comparable with that of human *(39)*. However, segments of the mouse βAPP antisense strand corresponding to two complementary elements of human βAPP antisense strand exibit much weaker complementarity. Therefore, in terms of the proposed model, "humanization" of mouse βAPP gene by increase in the extent of complementarity of the two elements in question, but not "humanization" of mouse Aβ segment alone, should generate rates of sporadic AD comparable with those of humans provided, of course, that the amyloidogenicity of mouse Aβ is similar to that of its human counterpart.

It should be noted that two technical aspects could complicate the investigation of the proposed mechanism. First, Aβ-overproducing cells are likely to be the first victims of AD neuropathology triggered by increased deposition of Aβ. Therefore, in postmortem samples from patients with advanced AD, Aβ-overproducing cells may be poorly represented. A possible solution to this potential problem is to analyze a sufficient number of samples from "normal" subjects old enough to have relatively high probability of developing AD. Second, by analogy with globin mRNA replication in erythroid precursor cells *(29,40)*, 5'-truncated βAPP mRNA encoding the 12-kDa βAPP fragment may be heavily modified and consequently hybridize poorly with specific probes at high-stringency conditions. In such a case, the analytical procedures used to study globin mRNA replication *(40)* can be employed.

11. CONCLUSIONS

The overproduction of Aβ is associated with and considered by many to be the primary cause of AD. In some cases, it can be caused by mutations within the βAPP gene that affect βAPP proteolytic pathway. In such familial AD cases, mutation-mediated enhancement or alteration of proteolytic cleavage is sufficient for the increased production of Aβ, and there is no need to invoke additional mechanisms other than the mutations. The best example to illustrate this point is the Swedish mutation, in which the mechanism proposed here cannot operate because met_{596} is replaced by leu, but neither the proposed nor any other additional mechanism is needed in this case; the mutation alone is sufficient. Indeed, the enhanced production of Aβ in Swedish familial AD is owing to the increased efficiency of cleavage at the mutated β-secretase site *(17)* and the consequent unsusceptibility of the resulting 12-kDa fragment to the α-secretase cleavage *(18,19)*. The Aβ production pathway in Swedish familial AD, however, is qualitatively different from and therefore not relevant to Aβ production in sporadic AD *(19)*.

On the other hand, there is no evidence that proteolytic cleavage leading to the production of Aβ in sporadic AD-affected and in normal tissues differ qualitatively or quantitatively so as to account for the overproduction of Aβ in AD involving wild-type βAPP. Therefore, since proteolytic processing alone cannot account for the increased production of Aβ in sporadic AD, an additional Aβ production pathway may be employed in this type of AD, which constitutes the majority of all AD cases. A mechanism is described in this chapter for the generation and overproduction of the 12-kDa C-terminal fragment of βAPP, the immediate precursor of the Aβ, not involving βAPP. It proposes the occurrence of antisense RNA-mediated generation of 5'-truncated βAPP mRNA followed by initiation of translation at the AUG_{1786} immediately preceding the Aβ coding region. It requires a shift of the transcriptional start site of βAPP mRNA and induction of RNA-dependent RNA synthesis machinery in response to an undefined stimulus, and is postulated to be activated or enhanced in the sporadic AD-affected tissues. In this model, two factors contribute to the increased production of Aβ: (1) the proposed mechanism for generation of 5'-truncated βAPP mRNA leads to its overproduction, and (2) in contrast to the intact βAPP, where cleavage at the the α-secretase site precludes formation of Aβ, the resulting 12-kDa C-terminal fragment of βAPP is not a subject to α-secretase cleavage, but is cleaved by γ-secretase. This cleavage generates Aβ, which is subsequently secreted.

The proposed model makes several verifiable predictions and suggests new directions of experimentation that may lead to a better understanding of the mechanisms involved in AD.

REFERENCES

1. Selkoe, D. J. (1995) Alzheimer's amyloid of another flavor, *Nature Medicine* **1**, 998,999.
2. Beyreuther, K., Pollwein, P., Multhaup, G., Monning, U., Konig, G., Dyrks, T., Schubert, W., and Masters, C. (1993) Regulation and expression of the Alzheimer's β/A4 amyloid protein precursor in health, disease, and Down syndrome, *Annals New York Acad. Sci.* **695**, 91–102.
3. Neve, R., Finch, E., and Dawes, L. (1988) Expression of the Alzheimer amyloid precursor gene transcripts in the human brain, *Neuron* **1**, 669–677.
4. Schmechel, D., Saunders, A., Strittmatter, W., Crain, B., Hulette, C., Joo, S., Pericak-Vance, M., Goldgaber, D. and Roses, A. (1993) Increased amyloid β-peptide deposition in cerebral cortex as a consequence of apolipoprotein E genotype in late-onset Alzheimer disease, *Proc. Natl. Acad. Sci. USA* **90**, 9649–9653.
5. Hyman, B., West, H., Budyrev, S., Mantgna, R., Ukleja, M., Havlin, S., and Stanley, H. (1995) Quantitative analysis of senile plaques in Alzheimer disease: observation of log-normal size distribution and molecular epidemiology of differences associated with apolipoprotein E genotype and trisomy 21 (Down syndrome), *Proc. Natl. Acad. Sci. USA* **92**, 3586–3590.
6. Querfurth, H., Wijsman, E., St. George-Hyslop, P., and Selkoe, D. (1995) βAPP mRNA transcription is increased in cultured fibroblasts from the familial Alzheimer's disease-1 family, *Molec. Brain Res.* **28**, 319–337.
7. Suzuki, N., Cheung, T., Cai, X-D., Odaka, A., Otvos, L., Eckman, C., Golde, T., and Younkin, S. (1994) An increased percentage of long amyloid β protein secreted by familial amyloid β precursor ($βAPP_{717}$) mutants, *Science* **264**, 1336–1340.
8. Citron, M., Vigo-Pelfrey, C., Teplow, D., Miller, C., Schenk, D., Jonston, J., Winblat, B., Venizelos, N., Lannfelt, L., and Selkoe, D. (1994) Excessive production of amyloid β-protein by peripheral cells of symptomatic and presymptomatic patients carrying the Swedish familial Alzheimer disease mutation, *Proc. Natl. Acad. Sci. USA* **91**, 11,993–11,997.
9. Haass, C., Hung, A., Selkoe, D., and Teplow, D. (1994) Mutations associated with a locus for familial Alzheimer's disease result in alternative processing of amyloid β-protein precursor, *J. Biol. Chem.* **269**, 17,741–17,748.

10. Games, D., Adams, D., Alessandrini, R., Barbour, R., Berthelette, P., Blackwell, C., Carr, T., Clemens, J., and Donaldson, T. (1995) Alzheimer-type neuropathology in transgenic mice overexpressing V717F β-amyloid precursor protein, *Nature* **373,** 523–527.

11. Palmert, M., Usiak, M., Mayeux, R., Raskind, R., Tourtelotte, W., and Younkin, S. (1990) Soluble derivatives of the β amyloid protein precursor in cerebrospinal fluid: alterations in normal aging and in Alzheimer's disease, *Neurology* **40,** 1028–1034.

12. Weidemann, A., Konig, G., Bunke, D., Fischer, P., Salbaum, J. M., Masters, C., and Beyreuther, K. (1989) Identification, biogenesis, and localization of precursors of Alzheimer's disease A4 amyloid protein, *Cell* **57,** 115–124.

13. Estus, S., Golde, T., Kunishita, T., Blades, D., Lowery, D., Eisen, M., Usiak, M., Qu, X., Tabira, T., Greenberg, B., and Younkin, S. (1992) Potentially amyloidogenic, carboxyl-terminal derivatives of the β-amyloid protein precursor, *Science* **255,** 726–728.

14. Golde, T. E., Estus, S., Younkin, I., Selkoe, D., and Younkin, S. (1992) Processing of the β-amyloid protein precursor to potentially amyloidogenic derivatives, *Science* **255,** 728–730.

15. Davis, J. and Van Nostrand, W. (1996) Enhanced pathologic properties of Dutch-type mutant amyloid-β protein, *Proc. Natl. Acad. Sci. USA* **93,** 2996–3000.

16. Hendriks, L., van Duijn, C., Cras, P., Cruts, M., Van Hul, W., van Harskamp, F., Warren, A., McInnis, M., Antonarakis, S., and Martin, J. (1992) Presenile dementia and cerebral haemorrhage linked to a mutation at codon 692 of the β-amyloid precursor protein gene, *Nature Genet.* **1,** 218–222.

17. Citron, M., Teplow, D., and Selkoe, D. (1995) Generation of amyloid-β protein from its precursor is sequence-specific, *Neuron* **14,** 661–670.

18. Dyrks, T., Dyrks, E., Monning, U., Urmoneit, B., Turner, J., and Beyreuther, K. (1993) Generation of βA4 from the amyloid protein precursor and fragments thereof, *FEBS Lett.* **335,** 89–93.

19. Haass, C., Lemere, C., Capell, A., Citron, M., Seubert, P., Schenk, D., Lannfelt, L., and Selkoe, D. (1995) The Swedish mutation causes early-onset Alzheimer's disease by β-secretase cleavage within the secretory pathway, *Nature Medicine* **1,** 1291–1296.

20. Cai, X-D., Golde, T. E., and Younkin, S. G. (1993) Release of excess amyloid-β protein from a mutant amyloid-β protein precursor, *Science* **259,** 514–516.

21. Higaki, J., Quon, D., Zhong, Z., and Cordell, B. (1995) Inhibition of β-amyloid formation identifies proteolytic precursors and subcellular site of catabolism, *Neuron* **14,** 651–659.

22. Dyrks, T., Dyrks, E., Monning, U., Urmoneit, B., Turner, J., and Beyreuther, K. (1993) Generation of βA4 from the amyloid protein precursor and fragments thereof, *FEBS Lett.* **335,** 89–93.

23. Dyrks, T., Monning, U., Beyreuther, K., and Turner, J. (1994) Amyloid precursor protein secretion and βA4 amyloid generation are not mutually exclusive, *FEBS Lett.* **349,** 210–214.

24. Iizuka, T., Shoji, M., Kawarabayashi, T., Sato, M., Kobayashi, T., Tada, N., Kasai, K., Matsubara, E., Watanabe, M., Tomidokoro,Y., and Hirai, S. (1996) Intracellular generation of amyloid β-protein from amyloid β-protein precursor fragment by direct cleavage with β- and γ-secretase, *Biochem. Biophys. Res Comm.* **218,** 238–242.

25. Kang, J., Lemaire, H-G., Unterbeck, A., Salbaum, J. M., Masters, C., Grzeschik, K-H., Multhaup, G., Beyreuther, K., and Muller-Hill, B. (1987) The precursor of Alzheimer's disease amyloid A4 protein resembles a cell-surface receptor, *Nature* **325,** 733–736.

26. Kozak, M. (1991) Structural features in eukaryotic mRNAs that modulate the initiation of translation, *J. Biol. Chem.* **266,** 19,867–19,870.

27. Breimer, L. H. and Denny, P. (1987) Alzheimer amyloid aspects, *Nature* **326,** 749,750.

28. Citron, M., Haass, C., and Selkoe, D. J. (1993) Production of amyloid-β-peptide by cultured cells: no evidence for internal initiation of translation at met_{596}, *Neurobiol. of Aging* **14,** 571–573.

29. Volloch, V., Schweitzer, B., and Rits, S. (1996) Antisense globin RNA in mouse erythroid tissues: structure, origin and possible function, *Proc. Natl. Acad. Sci. USA* **93,** 2476–2481.

30. Richards, O. and Ehrenfeld, E. (1990) Poliovirus RNA replication, *Curr. Topics Microbiol. Immunol.* **161,** 90–115.
31. Volloch, V., Schweitzer, B., and Rits, S. (1994) Evolutionarily conserved elements in the 5' untranslated region of globin mRNA mediate site-specific priming of a unique hairpin structure during cDNA synthesis, *Nucl. Ac. Res.* **22,** 5302–5309.
32. Mita, S., Sadlock, J., Herbert, J., and Schon, E. A. (1988) A cDNA specifying the human amyloid precursor protein (ABPP) encodes a 95-kDa polypeptide, *Nucl. Ac. Res.* **16,** 9351.
33. Salbaum, J. M., Weidemann, A., Lemaire, H-G., Masters, C., and Beyreuther, K. (1988) The promoter of Alzheimer's disease amyloid A4 precursor gene, *EMBO J.* **7,** 2807–2813.
34. Mita, S., Sadlock, J., Herbert, J., and Schon, E. A. (1988) A cDNA specifying the human amyloid precursor protein (ABPP) encodes a 95-kDa polypeptide (addendum), *Nucl. Ac. Res.* **16,** 11,402.
35. Rubenstein, P. and Martin, D. (1983) NH_2-terminal processing of actin in mouse L-cells *in vivo*, *J. Biol. Chem.* **258,** 3961–3966.
36. Sandbrink, R., Masters, C., and Beyreuther, K. (1994) βA4 amyloid protein precursor mRNA isoforms without exon 15 are ubiquitously expressed in rat tissues including brain, but not in neurons, *J. Biol. Chem.* **269,** 1510–1517.
37. Joachim, C. and Selkoe, D. (1992) The seminal role of beta-amyloid in the pathogenesis of Alzheimer disease, *Alzheimer Disease Association Discords* **6,** 7–34.
38. Chernak, J. (1993) Structural features of the 5' upstream regulatory region of the gene encoding rat amyloid-β precursor protein, *Gene* **133,** 255–260.
39. De Strooper, B., Simons, M., Multhoup, G., Van Leuven, F., Beyreuther, K., and Dotti, C. (1995) Production of intracellular amyloid-containing fragments in hippocampal neurons expressing human β-amyloid precursor protein and protection against amyloidogenesis by subtle amino acid substitutions in the rodent sequence, *EMBO J.* **14,** 4932–4938.
40. Volloch, V., Schweitzer, B., and Rits, S. (1996) Unusual hyperabundant globin RNA in erythroid precursor cells: possible end-product of globin mRNA replication. Submitted for publication.

5

Apoptosis and Alzheimer's Disease

Andréa LeBlanc

1. INTRODUCTION

The evolution of a tissue during aging requires a noninflammatory mechanism for the removal of cells that are no longer necessary. This task is accomplished by physiological cell death called programmed cell death or apoptosis. Programmed cell death is defined as an active mechanism often requiring novel transcription and translation of specific genes, which leads to distinct morphological alterations of the cell, such as DNA condensation, cell shrinkage, and membrane blebbing. The apoptotic cell retains membrane integrity, avoiding spillage of its intracellular milieu into the extracellular space. Consequently, the apoptotic cell debris are removed by a noninflammatory process *(1)*. In contrast, necrotic cell death is a response to an acute cellular insult that promotes membrane damage and extracellular release of the cell content, resulting in an inflammatory response of the organism.

Programmed cell death may be activated during aging by a genetically timed mechanism that prevents a senescent cell from becoming harmful to its environment, allows a response to environmental stress produced by altered trophic support *(2,3)*, or prevents cellular proliferation in terminally differentiated long-lived cells submitted to malignant transformation (*4*; reviewed in ref. *5*). Apoptosis in the nervous system would be a convenient mechanism to remove old cells without causing an inflammatory response, which would be deleterious to the organism. Therefore, apoptosis is a popular hypothesis to explain many neurodegenerative diseases, such as Alzheimer's disease (AD) *(6)*, Huntington's disease *(7,8)*, spinal muscular atrophy *(9,10)*, cerebellar degeneration, prion diseases, amyotropic lateral sclerosis, and Parkinson's disease (reviewed in ref. *11*). Although programmed cell death is well defined in the developing nervous system (reviewed in ref. *12*), very little is known about the aging nervous system. This chapter reviews molecular mechanisms of neuronal apoptosis identified in cell culture systems and mammalian models, and summarizes the evidence for the presence of apoptotic mechanisms in the brain of individuals with AD.

2. STAGES OF PROGRAMMED CELL DEATH

Most cells undergoing programmed cell death go through a series of temporally conserved regulated steps ultimately leading to cellular demise. These steps can be classified as:

From: Molecular Mechanisms of Dementia *Edited by: W. Wasco and R. E. Tanzi Humana Press Inc., Totowa, NJ*

1. Apoptosis activation signal;
2. Initiation;
3. Commitment;
4. Execution; and
5. Elimination.

The apoptosis activating signal is cell-type-dependent, but can be grossly catego-rized as either the absence of a factor required for cellular survival or the presence of a factor that triggers cell death *(1,13)*. Generally, cultured cells can be induced to undergo apoptosis by serum deprivation, which will deprive the cells from essential factors. The initiation of apoptosis can be observed as early as within 3 h within signaling. The time required to induce this phase is also cell-type- and signal-dependent. In response to the apoptotic signal, the cell undergoes morphological changes, which have been clearly described by Arends and Wyllie *(14)*.

Initiation of apoptosis includes the shrinkage of the nucleus, condensation of the chromatin, nucleolar disintegration, cytoplasmic volume reduction, and compaction of cytoplasmic organelles. The endoplasmic reticulum is dilated, and vesicular forma-tions fuse to the plasma membrane, cytoskeletal filaments are reorganized, and riboso-mal particles cluster *(14)*. In contrast to necrotic cell death, mitochondria remain intact and do not swell. In this phase, the cellular membrane is not permeable to vital dyes. Biochemically, a number of genes are actively expressed during the initiation of apop-tosis. However, in many cases, active gene expression is not required for a cell to undergo morphological changes resembling apoptosis. In fact, it has been shown that a cell can undergo apoptosis in the absence of a nuclei *(15)*. The activation of immediate early genes, *fos*, *myc*, and *jun*, has been confirmed in many apoptotic systems *(16–18)*.The expression of oncogenes, especially *fos* and *jun*, leads to the induction of the expression of a number of secondary genes, which probably function in the later stages of apoptosis. Other biochemical changes during the initiation of apoptosis include moderately increased calcium levels and alteration of protein kinase activity *(14,19)*.

Commitment of a cell to apoptosis is denoted as the time where the cell will not be saved on removal of the apoptosis activating signal. During this phase, plasma mem-brane blebbing and nuclear crenation are observed *(14)*. The cellular content is reorga-nized to form apoptotic bodies. Certain proteins are known to protect against the induction of apoptosis, the most universal being *bcl*-2 and related proteins. Others pre-cipitate or induce apoptosis, and are known as death proteins. The *bcl*-2-related protein family consists of proteins that protect against cell death, such as *bcl*-2 and *bcl*-x$_L$ *(20)*, and those that promote cell death, such as bax *(21)*, Bad *(22)*, Bak *(23–25)*, and *bcl*-x$_S$ *(20)*. Two highly conserved amino acid motifs, the *bcl*-2 homology domain 1 (BH1) and 2 (BH2), exist in *bcl*-2-related proteins *(26)*. Site-specific mutagenesis of a single amino acid within each of these domains is sufficient to abrogate *bcl*-2's protective function against programmed cell death as well as heterodimerization to bax. Overexpression of bax in a cell induces programmed cell death *(21)*. Therefore, it is hypothesized that one of the roles of *bcl*-2 is to prevent monomeric forms or homodimers of bax *(21,26)*. Thus, protein–protein interaction may be an important mechanism in cell survival or inhibition of apoptosis. Proteins, like Bag-1, share no homology to *bcl*-2-related proteins, but interact with *bcl*-2 to synergistically protect against cell death induced by a variety of stimuli *(27)*. It is very possible that a number of these proteins have yet to be discovered. Other functions have been attributed to *bcl-2*. There is evidence that it may act as an antioxidant *(28,29)*. In addition, *bcl-2*'s ability to regulate nuclear trafficking *(30)* suggests that it may mediate communications between the cytoplasmic and the nuclear compartments. However, *bcl-2* targets are also cytoplasmic, since *bcl-2* protects enucleated cells from apoptosis *(15)*. Other than the *bcl-2*-related proteins, one of the cytoplasmic proteins that interacts with *bcl-2* is R-*ras (31)*.

On commitment, a number of proteases and nucleases are activated to execute cellular degeneration. Some of the specific proteases known to be activated have been identified *(32)*. Of these, interleukin-1β-converting enzyme (ICE) and ICE-like proteases, prICE, Icht-1, Icht-2 (TX), apopain, Yama, or CPP32β probably play a critical role in apoptosis *(33–39)*. TX can proteolyze ICE and its own precursor, but not ICE substrates *(40)*. These proteases may mediate proteolytic cleavage of a wide range of substrates. One of these is poly (ADP-ribose) polymerase, which protects against the fragmentation of DNA *(36)*. Cytoskeletal structures, such as lamin B and actin, are proteolytically degraded or modified during apoptosis *(41,42)*. Changes in the actin cytoskeleton organization during apoptosis implicate ICE activity through proteolyzed Gas-2, an upregulated gene during growth arrest, which is part of the microfilament system *(42)*. Actin is also by itself a possible substrate of ICE *(43)*. In addition, it has been shown that apoptosis not only triggers disruption of microtubules, but microtubule-disrupting agents trigger massive apoptosis in human leukemia cells *(44)*. ICE gene expression and activation are regulated through integrins in the extracellular matrix *(45)* in tumor necrosis factor/FAS-mediated apoptosis pathway *(46,47)*.

Endonucleases are responsible for the fragmentation of DNA (reviewed in refs. *48–50*). Typically, the separation of a DNA ladder of 180 nucleotides or multiples thereof on an agarose gel is accepted as the confirmation of an apoptotic mechanism. However, recent evidence indicates that this process is either very slow or nonexistent in certain cell types, and larger DNA fragments only can be observed *(51)*. With degeneration of nuclear and cytoplasmic structures, cultured cells become permeable to vital dyes *(14)*.

Elimination of the apoptotic cells in a tissue is usually carried out by phagocytosis (reviewed in ref. *48*). In cell cultures, attached cells will round up and lift off the culture dish.

3. PROGRAMMED CELL DEATH IN NEURONS

An invaluable abundance of new information on apoptotic mechanisms has populated the research journals in the last year. Most of the work is on the study of apoptosis in dividing cells, and many of the identified mechanisms are cell-type-dependent. Since neurons are long-lived, irreversibly and terminally differentiated cells, it is crucial to clearly define the expression of possible mediators of neuronal programmed cell death. Many recent papers review the novel discoveries and the molecular mechanisms of apoptosis in neurons *(43,52–54)*. The following section describes some of the observed events in apoptosis of neuronal experimental models.

A number of cell-culture models, such as PC12 cells, are presently being used to study apoptosis as well as primary neuron cultures *(55–58)*. Continuous cell lines provide the advantage of unlimited cell numbers and synchronicity often required to clearly identify genes involved in cell death, whereas primary cultures have the advantage of truly being irreversibly differentiated similar to the in vivo neuronal state. It is of great interest to study the apoptotic mechanism in neurons, since, upon demise, these cells cannot be replaced. Whereas necrotic neuronal cell death can only be inhibited by preventing the acute insult, apoptotic neuronal cell death may be prevented by inhibiting neuronal degeneration before commitment to apoptosis.

3.1. Apoptotic Signals of Neurons

Neurons are known to undergo programmed cell death in the absence of target tissue or growth factors, source of metabolic energy, motor activity, or the presence of anabolic steroids, and glucocorticoids, especially when elevated by stress *(12,59)*. Neuronal cell death as a result of target deprivation appears to be developmentally regulated. In early development, cell death may eliminate aberrant cells from the environment, allowing for the healthy neurons to extend axons and dendrites and become functional. Neuronal cell death, after connections have been achieved, may eliminate neurons with a transient function. Recent evidence suggests that a neuron may undergo either apoptosis or necrosis in response to an identical signal *(60,61)*. Exposure of cerebellar granule neurons to toxic levels of glutamate results in necrosis and apoptosis of two subpopulations of neurons depending on the integrity of the cell's mitochondrial function *(62)*. Therefore, the intensity of a "death" signal and the state of the recipient cell can decide whether a neuron dies by apoptosis or necrosis.

3.2. Initiation of Apoptosis in Neurons

Mechanisms of neuronal cell death have been well characterized in peripheral neuron models. For example, nerve growth factor (NGF)-differentiated PC12 cells initially undergo transcription- and translation-dependent neuritic alterations, such as beading and thinning, culminating in massive neuritic degeneration with time of NGF deprivation. Cell lysis appears to follow neuritic alterations. Other cells show membrane blebbing from the cell body *(55)*. Membrane blebbing, neuritic degeneration, DNA fragmentation, nuclear compaction, and cell shrinkage have been observed in serum, or growth factor deprivation induced cell death in primary sympathetic cervical ganglia neurons *(57,58)*. Neuritic alterations, DNA fragmentation, and nuclear compaction characteristic of apoptosis also occur in serum deprived human primary CNS neurons *(63)*.

As stated, apoptosis is often accompanied by active gene expression. One group of genes that has been under intense scrutiny are the cellular oncogene families of *myc*, *fos*, and *jun*. Immediate early genes c-*fos*, c-*jun*, and *jun* B are increased on neuronal stimulation and possibly play a role in the regulation of expression of a number of genes required for neuronal activity (reviewed in ref. *64*). Characterization of the molecular mechanisms of programmed cell death in rat neurons shows that the level of *fos* is also elevated during developmental cell death *(65)*. Similarly, sympathetic cervical ganglion cells deprived of NGF show increased c-*jun*, *fos* B, and c-*fos* expression before morphological signs of apoptosis *(66)*. Intracellular injection of antibodies to either *fos* proteins (*fos* and *fos*-like proteins) or c-*jun* inhibits programmed cell death induction by NGF deprivation, whereas *jun* B or *jun* D had no effect *(66,67)*. c-*jun* expression increases before neurons are committed to cell death. In addition, c-*jun* overexpression in sympathetic cervical ganglia is in itself sufficient to induce apoptosis

(67). Increased expression may not be the only modification to c-*jun* during apoptosis. c-*jun* phosphorylation also occurs in NGF-deprived neurons undergoing apoptosis *(67)*. Therefore, c-*jun* appears to be a key element in the neuronal apoptotic pathway.

bcl-2 is developmentally regulated in the nervous system. Although *bcl*-2 is expressed in substantial amounts in the peripheral nervous system throughout life, it decreases to very low levels during aging in the rodent central nervous system *(53,68)*. However, *bcl*-x is expressed in the developing and aging CNS neuron, and appears to be more abundant than *bcl*-2 *(20,69–72)*. Although the elimination of *bcl*-2 expression has little effect on the central or peripheral nervous system in *bcl*-2 knockout mice *(73)*, elimination of *bcl*-x expression causes massive neuronal cell death *(20,22,70,74)*, which is independent of immature hematopoietic cell death also observed *(75)*.

Interestingly, *bcl*-2 prevents survival factor deprivation-induced neuronal apoptosis in the PC12 model cell line *(76,77)*, in sympathetic cervical ganglia primary neuron cultures *(78)*, and in sensory neurons *(79–80)*. *bcl*-2 and its counterpart, *bcl*-xL, also prevent hypoxia and axotomy-induced death in vivo *(74,79,81)*. Little is known about the regulation of *bcl*-2 expression in the nervous system. NGF-deprived sympathetic cervival ganglia cells show decreased levels of *bcl*-2 expression, suggesting that NGF deprivation not only activates a number of genes necessary to execute the demise of the neuron, but also removes protective mechanisms against apoptosis by downregulation of antideath proteins *(82)*. Regulation of *bcl*-2 activity also occurs through phosphorylation *(83)*. However, this mechanism has not yet been observed in neurons.

3.3. Commitment of Neurons to Apoptosis

In the sympathetic cervical ganglia primary neuron cultures, neurons can be rescued from NGF deprivation-induced apoptosis by adding NGF after 16–18 h *(57)*. As discussed, the commitment to apoptosis can also be prevented with high levels of expression of *bcl*-2, and ICE inhibitors also prevent apoptosis of motor neurons in vivo and in vitro *(84)*.

3.4. Execution of Apoptosis

This aspect of neuronal apoptosis is still not clear. Since the cytoskeleton of neurons is highly specialized, it is likely that neuritic beading and degeneration observed during apoptosis are mediated through proteolytic activities or through the activation of kinases that alter the phosphorylation state of neurofilaments, such as τ.

3.5. Elimination of Apoptosis

Cultured cells undergoing apoptosis usually round up and lift from the culture dish. In neuron cultures, this process is not obvious, because neuronal cultures require high-density plating and elaborate an extensive network of neurites, which prevent apoptotic cells from lifting until a large number of cells have undergone apoptosis. Therefore, it is common to see dead neurons interspersed with the surviving cells. Elimination of apoptotic bodies from the central nervous system is likely the responsibility of microglia.

4. APOPTOSIS AND AD

AD is characterized by neuronal degeneration. Neurons undergo cytoskeletal rearrangement and develop neurofibrillary tangles *(85,86)* and loss of synapse *(87)*; cell death is observed especially in cholinergic neurons *(88–90).* The progressive nature of neuronal cell dysfunction and death in AD individuals is consistent with an apoptotic mechanism of neuronal cell death, and there is growing support for neuronal apoptosis in AD *(11,91,92).* However, apoptosis in a tissue, such as the brain, will be very difficult if not impossible to test conclusively. First, apoptosis of a neuron is expected to occur within a defined time period, probably not exceeding 48–96 h. Thereafter, the apoptotic cell is phagocytosed. Therefore, progressive neuronal apoptosis will unlikely yield high numbers of detectable apoptotic neurons at any time after the onset of disease. Second, the brain cannot be invaded for study during the disease. Examination of postmortem brain gives a very limited view of a process that has developed over the years, and, probably, erased important clues to the initial mechanisms of cellular demise. Consequently, with the present technology, it may be difficult to identify apoptosis as a major component of AD or any other neurodegenerative diseases. The ideal situation would be to observe ongoing cell death in an AD patient. Since invasive methods are not yet available, we must rely on cellular models and postmortem material. However, it is still important to pursue the characterization of neuronal cell dysfunction and death in AD, since apoptotic cell death implies potential treatment to stop cellular demise in the aging brain of individuals with AD. Keeping in mind these caveats, the following paragraphs describe evidence for apoptosis in AD.

4.1. Signals of Apoptosis

There are at least two possible signals of apoptosis in AD: neurotrophin or target deprivation, and induction of apoptosis by amyloid β peptide.

Various mechanisms of neurotrophin deprivation are possible in the brain.

1. It has been proposed that the loss of cholinergic basal forebrain neurons in AD occurs as a result of depreciating neurotrophic factor levels, such as NGF *(59).* Since not all cholinergic neurons are NGF-dependent, other growth factors may be implicated in this disease. Glia may play an important role in maintaining the neurotrophic levels required for neuronal survival. Defective glia in *Drosophila* induce the apoptosis of neurons of the visual system *(93).* Therefore, although most of the research concentrates on the dysfunctional or dying neurons, one must keep in mind that the study of supporting glia may be as relevant as the study of the neuron itself.
2. Senescent cells in culture become resistant to apoptosis *(2,3).* Similarly, target dependency decreases or disappears in rat cholinergic neurons with aging *(94),* indicating a common mechanism to preserve the final aged population of cells. It is possible that cholinergic loss in AD is the result of the inability of neurons to acquire resistance to target-deprived apoptosis during aging. Consequently, normally decreasing levels of neurotrophic factors in aging could lead to neuron-specific cell death and result in neurodegeneration.
3. Loss of synapse in AD *(87)* also implies that the neuron is deprived of its target and target deprivation is well established as one of the signals initiating apoptosis. Therefore, synaptic loss may in some situations precede neuronal apoptosis.

Overproduction of the amyloid precursor protein (APP) metabolic product, amyloid β peptide (Aβ), is a fairly well supported hypothesis to explain the pathogenesis of AD. Aβ is increased in cells harboring various APP mutants in chromosome 21-linked familial AD (FAD) (reviewed in ref. *95),* and in cells of mutant presenillin 1 (S182) in chromosome 14-linked FAD *(96,97).* At high concentrations, the fibrillar form of Aβ is neurotoxic *(98)* and the cell death mechanism of Aβ toxicity under these conditions is apoptosis *(99,100)*. However, there are at least two possibilities that should be explored. First, overproduction of Aβ likely results in less metabolism of APP through the nonamyloidogenic pathway, leading to less sAPP, which is a known neuroprotector *(101)*. Therefore, it is possible that decreased sAPP renders the neurons vulnerable to a number of insults, which normally would be harmless. Second, the mutations of APP, presenillin I and II *(102)*, may also create a gain of function as observed in both Huntington's disease and Amyotropic lateral sclerosis. It is hypothesized that the mutant huntingtin and superoxide dismutase may interact abnormally with other proteins and induce cell death *(7,103)*. In view of the family of *bcl*-2-related proteins, which mediate cell survival and cell death by protein–protein interactions, this hypothesis is highly plausible.

4.2. Signs of Apoptosis in Brains Affected by AD

Senile plaques, neurofibrillary tangles, and neuronal loss are characteristic pathological manifestations in AD brains. Senile plaques represent extracellular deposits of a number of proteins of which the Aβ peptide is most abundant. The plaques are surrounded by reactive astrocytes and microglia, and are interspersed with dystrophic neurites. Therefore, neuritic alterations observed in cultured neurons undergoing apoptosis are also evident in vivo in AD individuals. Terminal deoxynucleotidyl transferase dUTP end labeling (TUNEL) staining, which identifies 3'-ends of DNA strands, a phenomena resulting from DNA fragmentation, is increased in AD brains *(104,105)*. TUNEL staining of some neurofibrillary tangle-containing neurons indicates that apoptosis is part of AD pathology *(105)*. However, there is contradictory evidence. Some studies fail to see fragmented DNA *(106)*. In one study, the majority of cells with fragmented DNA showed swelling of the cytoplasm, which is more typical of necrosis than apoptosis *(104)*. Surprisingly, according to this study, neurons are not the only cells containing fragmented DNA in AD. Glial cells, such as oligodendrocytes and microglia, also showed fragmented DNA *(104)*. On the other hand, 41% of neurons with fragmented DNA contained neurofibrillary tangles *(104)*, indicating a link between apoptosis and neurofibrillary tangles.

There is evidence for increased *fos* expression in the hippocampus of AD brains *(107,108)*. Both *jun* and *fos* colocalize with neurofibrillary tangle marker, PHF-1, in some neurons. Increased levels of SGP-2 (clusterin, apo J) in AD brains *(109)* indicate an apoptotic mechanism, since this gene is highly expressed in cells undergoing apoptosis *(5,110)*. *bcl*-2 levels are generally increased in AD brains except in the neurofibrillary tangle-containing neuron *(111)*. Finally, the presence of microglia in close proximity to the senile plaque *(112)* indicates active phagocytosis of the cellular remnants similar to removal of apoptotic bodies in tissues.

With the growing interest in this field, more molecular markers of apoptosis are likely to be studied in AD brains and should populate the literature soon.

4.3. Aβ and Apoptosis

Aβ, through a short 10 amino acid region extending from amino acids 25–35 of the Aβ, causes rat hippocampal and cortical neuronal death in culture *(98)*. The neurotoxic effect of Aβ appears to be dependent on its aggregation and conformation state *(113)*. Chronic treatment of neurons with Aβ induces neuritic dystrophy, neuronal membrane blebbing, condensed chromatin, and DNA fragmentation, which are typical features of apoptosis *(99,100,114)*. c-*jun* expression is increased and sustained in cultured rat hippocampal neurons treated with Aβ *(115)*. τ Protein kinase I is activated by Aβ, and Aβ-induced neuronal cell death can be inhibited by suppression of τ protein kinase I with antisense oligonucleotides *(116)*. The mechanism by which Aβ induces cell death or apoptosis is not yet clearly defined. Thus far, Aβ toxicity has been attributed to altered calcium levels, thereby promoting susceptibility to excitotoxic damage *(117)*, free radical formation *(118–123)*, and a possible competition for NGF low-affinity receptor *(124)*. It is suggested that the differential expression of the low-affinity NGF receptor in various neuronal types would explain the variable in vivo susceptibility of neurons to Aβ toxicity. Much evidence indicates that fibrillar Aβ peptide initiates apoptosis. However, in these studies, apoptosis occurs using 20–100 μ*M* of Aβ. Since the level of Aβ is approx 4 n*M* in the aging and AD cerebrospinal fluid *(125)*, the effect of physiological or pathological concentration that neurons are likely to encounter should be studied to clearly define a role for Aβ in neuronal apoptosis of AD.

Other negative effects of Aβ include hyperphosphorylation of τ, which may promote neurofibrillary tangle formation *(126)*; formation of calcium channels when incorporated in membrane lipid bilayer *(127,128)*; promotion of potassium channel dysfunction *(129)*; and induction of cytokines, tumor necrosis factor, or reactive nitrogen intermediates in glial cells *(130,131)*. Each of these effects of Aβ could in some way be related to an apoptotic mechanism in neuronal cells.

5. CONCLUSIONS

Although not yet conclusive, there is evidence to suggest that neuronal apoptosis is one of the main mechanisms of neuronal cell death in aging diseases. Protection against neuronal apoptosis induced by a variety of signals, such as *bcl*-2 overexpression or with inhibitors of ICE, indicates possible future treatment against in vivo neuronal apoptosis in the aging brain. Attacking the disease through apoptotic inhibitors may provide the well-sought goal of postponing the effects of neuronal death in aging individuals by 10–20 yr. Therefore, individuals predisposed to neurodegenerative diseases, such as AD, could truly benefit from the extended life provided by improved health care in the 20th century. This notion alone warrants further extensive research on neuronal apoptosis.

REFERENCES

1. Kerr, J. F. R. and Harmon, B. V. (1991) Definition and incidence of apoptosis: an historical perspective, in *Apoptosis: The Molecular Basis of Cell Death. Current Communications in Cell and Molecular Biology*, vol. 3 (Tomei, L. D. and Cope, F. O., eds.), Cold Spring Harbor Laboratory, Cold Spring Harbor, NY, pp. 5–29.
2. Peacocke, M. and Campisi, J. (1991) Cellular senescence: a reflection of normal growth control, differentiation, and aging? *J. Cell Biochem.* **45,** 147–155.
3. Wang, E. (1995) Senescent human fibroblasts resist programmed cell death, and failure to suppress *bcl*2 is involved, *Cancer Res.* **55,** 2284–2292.
4. Heintz, N. (1993) Cell death and the cell cycle: a relationship between transformation and neurodegeneration? *Trends Biol. Sci.* **18,** 157–159.
5. Lockshin, R. A. and Zakeri, Z. F. (1990) Programmed cell death: new thoughts and relevance to aging, *J. Gerontol. Biol. Sci.* **45,** B135–140.

6. Johnson, E. M. (1994) Possible role of neuronal apoptosis in Alzheimer's disease, *Neurobiol. Aging* **15(2),** 5187–5189.
7. Zeitlin, S., Liu, J.-P., Chapman, D. L., Papaioannou, V. E., and Efstratiadis, A. (1995) Increased apoptosis and early embryonic lethality in mice nullizygous for the Huntington's disease gene homologue, *Nature Genet.* **11,** 155–163.
8. Portera-Caillau, C., Hedreen, J. C., Price, D. L., and Koliatsos, V. E. (1995) Evidence for apoptotic cell death in Huntington Disease and excitotoxic animal models, *J. Neurosci.* **15(5),** 3775–3787.
9. Roy, N., Mahadevan, M. S., McLean, M., Farahani, R., Baird, S., BesnerJohnston, A., Lefebvre, C., Kang, X., Salih, M., Aubry, H., Tamai, K., Guan, X., Ioannou, P., Crawford, T. O., de Jong, P. J., Surh, L., Ikeda, J., Korneluk, R. G., and MacKenzie, A. (1995) The gene for neuronal apoptosis inhibitory protein is partially deleted in individuals with spinal muscular atrophy, *Cell* **80,** 167–178.
10. Lefebvre, S., Burglen, L., Reboullet, S., Clermont, O., Burlet, P., Viollet, L., Benichou, B., Cruaud, C., Millasseau, P., Zeviani, M., Le Paslier, D., Frezal, J., Cohen, D., Weissenbach, J., Munnich, A., and Melki, J. (1995) Identification and characterization of a spinal muscular Atrophy-determining gene, *Cell* **80,** 155–165.
11. Thompson, C. (1994) Apoptosis in the pathogenesis and treatment of disease, *Science* **267,** 1456–1462.
12. Oppenheim, R. W. (1991) Cell death during development of the nervous system, *Ann. Rev. Neurosci.* **14,** 453–501.
13. Tomei, L. D. and Cope, F. O. (eds.) (1994) *Apoptosis II: The Molecular Basis of Apoptosis in Disease: Current Communications in Cell and Molecular Biology*, vol. 8, Cold Spring Harbor Laboratory, Cold Spring Harbor, NY, p. 430.
14. Arends, M. J. and Wyllie, A. H. (1991) Apoptosis: mechanisms and roles in pathology, *Int. Rev. Exp. Pathol.* **32,** 223–254.
15. Jacobson, M. D., Burne, J. F., and Raff, M. C. (1994) Programmed cell death and *bcl*-2 protection in the absence of a nucleus, *EMBO J.* **13(8),** 1899–1910.
16. Evans, G. I., Wyllie, A. H., Gilbert, C. S., Littlewood, T. D., Land, H., Brooks, M., Waters, M., Waters, C. M., Penn, L. Z., and Hancock, D. C. (1992) Induction of apoptosis in fibroblasts by c-*myc* protein, *Cell* **69,** 119–128.
17. Collota, F., Polentarutti, N., Sironi, M., and Mantovani, A. (1992) Expression and involvement of c-*fos* and c-*jun* protooncogenes in programmed cell death induced by growth factor deprivation in lymphoid cell lines, *J. Biol. Chem.* **267(26),** 18,278–18,283.
18. Barrett, J. C. and Preston, G. (1994) Apoptosis and cellular senescence: forms of irreversible growth arrest, in *Current Communications in Cell and Molecular Biology: Apoptosis II: The Molecular Basis of Apoptosis in Disease* (Tomei, L. D. and Cope, F. O., eds.), Cold Spring Harbor Laboratory, Cold Spring Harbor, NY, pp. 253–281.
19. Xia, Z., Dickens, M., Raingeaud, J., Davis, R. J., and Greenberg, M. E. (1995) Opposing effects of ERK and JNK-p38 MAP kinases on apoptosis, *Science* **270,** 1326–1331.
20. Boise, L. H., Gonzalez-Garcia, M., Postema, C. E., Ding, L., Lindsten, T., Turka, L. A., Mao, X., Nunez, G., and Thompson, C. B. (1993) *bcl*-x, a *bcl*-2-related gene that functions as a dominant regulator of apoptotic cell death, *Cell* **74,** 597–608.
21. Oltvai, Z. N., Milliman, C. L., and Korsmeyer, S. J. (1993) *bcl*-2 heterodimerizes in vivo with a conserved homolog, bax, that accelerates programmed cell death, *Cell* **74,** 609–619.
22. Yang, E., Zha, J., Jockel, J., Boise, L. H., Thompson, C. B., and Korsmeyer, S. J. (1995) Bad, a heterodimeric partner for *bcl*-x_L and *bcl*-2 displaces Bax and promotes cell death, *Cell* **80,** 285–291.
23. Chittenden, T., Harrington, E. A., O'Connor, R., Flemington, C., Lutz, R. J., Evan, G. I., and Guild, B. C. (1995) Induction of apoptosis by the *bcl*-2 homologue bak, *Nature* **374,** 733–736.
24. Kiefer, M. C., Brauer, M. J., Powers, V. C., Wu, J. J., Umansky, S. R., Tomei, D., and Barr, P. J. (1995) Modulation of apoptosis by the widely distributed *bcl*-2 homologue Bak, *Nature* **374,** 736–739.

25. Farrow, S. N., White, J. H. M., Martinou, I., Aven, T., Pun, K., Grinham, C. J., Martinou, J. C., and Brown, R. (1995) Cloning of a *bcl-2* homologue by interaction with adenovirus E1B 19K, *Nature* **374,** 731–733.

26. Yin, X.-M., Oltval, Z. N., and Korsmeyer, S. J. (1994) BH1 and BH2 domains of *bcl-2* are required for inhibition and heterodimerization with bax, *Nature* **369,** 321–323.

27. Takayama, S., Sato, T., Krajewski, S., Kochel, K., Irie, S., Millan, J. A., and Reed, J. C. (1995) Cloning and functional analysis of Bag-1: a novel *bcl-2* Binding protein with anticell death activity, *Cell* **80,** 279–284.

28. Hockenberry, D., Nunez, G., Milliman, C., Schreiber, R. D., and Korsmeyer, S. J. (1990) *bcl-2* is an inner mitochondrial membrane protein that blocks programmed cell death, *Nature* **348,** 334–336.

29. Kane, D. J., Sarafian, T. A., Anton, R., Hahn, H., Gralla, E., Valentine, J. S., Ord, T., and Bredesen, D. E. (1993) *bcl-2* inhibition of neural cell death: Decreased generation of reactive oxygen species, *Science* **262,** 1274–1277.

30. Reed, J. C. (1994) *bcl-2* and the regulation of programmed cell death, *J. Cell. Biol.* **124,** 1–6.

31. Fernandez-Sarabia, M. J. and Bischoff, J. R. (1993) *bcl-2* associates with the *ras*-related protein R-*ras* p23, *Nature* **366,** 274,275.

32. Martin, S. J. and Green, D. R. (1995) Protease activation during apoptosis: death by a thousand cuts? *Cell* **82,** 349–352.

33. Miura, M., Zhu, H., Rotello, R., Hartwieg, E. A., and Yuan, J. (1993) Induction of apoptosis in fibroblasts by IL-1β-converting enzyme, a mammalian homolog of the *C. elegans* cell death gene ced-3, *Cell* **75,** 653–660.

34. Yuan, J., Shaham, S., Ledoux, S., Ellis, H., and Horvitz, R. H. (1993) The *C. elegans* cell death gene ced-3 encodes a protein similar to mammalian interleukin-1β-converting enzyme, *Cell* **75,** 641–652.

35. Kumar, S., Kinoshita, M., Noda, M., Copeland, N. G., and Jenkins, N. A. (1994) Induction of apoptosis by the mouse Nedd2 gene, which encodes a protein similar to the product of the *Caenorhabditis elegans* cell death gene ced-3 and the mammalian IL-1β-converting enzyme, *Genes Dev.* **8,** 1613–1626.

36. Lazebnik, Y. A., Kaufmann, S. H., Desnoyers, S., Poirier, G. G., and Earnshaw, W. C. (1994) Cleavage of poly(ADP-ribose) polymerase by a proteinase with properties like ICE, *Nature* **371,** 346,347.

37. Wang, L., Miura, M., Bergeron, L., Zhu, H., and Yuan, J. (1994) Ich-1, an Ice/ced-3-related gene, encodes both positive and negative regulators of programmed cell death, *Cell* **78,** 739–750.

38. Nicholson, D. W., Ali, A., Thornberry, N. A., Vaillancourt, J. P., Ding, C. K., Gallant, M., Gareau, Y., Griffin, P. R., Labelle, M., Lazebnik, Y. A., Munday, N. A., Raju, S. M., Smulson, M. E., Yamin, T.-T., Yu, V. L., and Miller, D. K. (1995) Identification and inhibition of the ICE/CED-3 protease necessary for mammalian apoptosis, *Nature* **376,** 37–43.

39. Tewari, M., Quan, L. T., O'Rourke, K., Desnoyersm, S., Zeng, Z., Beidler, D. R., Poirier, D. R., Salvesen, G. S., and Dixit, V. M. (1995) YAMA/CPP32β, a mammalian homolog of CED-3, is a CrmA-inhibitable protease that cleaves the death substrate poly (ADP-ribose) polymerase, *Cell* **81,** 801–809.

40. Faucheu, C., Diu, A., Chan, E., Blanchet, A., Miossec, C., Herve, F., Collard-Dutilleul, V., Gu, Y., Aldape, R. A., Lippke, J. A., Rocher, C., Su, M., Livingston, D. J., Hercend, T., and Lalanne, J. (1995) A novel human protease similar to the interleukin-1β converting enzyme induces apoptosis in transfected cells, *EMBO J.* **14(9),** 1914–1922.

41. Voekel-Johnson, C., Entingh, A. J., Wold, W., Gooding, L. R., and Laster, S. M. (1995) Activation of intracellular proteases is an early event in TNF-induced apoptosis, *J. Immunol.* **154,** 1707–1716.

42. Brancolini, C., Benedetti, M., and Schneider, C. (1995) Microfilament reorganization during apoptosis: the role of Gas2, a possible substrate for ICE-like proteases, *EMBO J.* **14(21),** 5179–5190.

43. Bredesen, D. E. (1995) Neural apoptosis, *Ann. Neurol.* **38,** 839–851.
44. Martin, S. J. and Cotter, T. G. (1994) Apoptosis of human leukemia: induction, morphology, and molecular mechanisms, in *Current Communications in Cell and Molecular Biology* (Tomei, L. D. and Cope, F. O., eds.), Cold Spring Harbor Laboratory, Cold Spring Harbor, NY, pp. 185–229.
45. Boudreau, N., Sympson, C. J., Werb, Z., and Bissell, M. J. (1995) Suppression of ICE and apoptosis in mammary epithelial cells by extracellular matrix, *Science* **267,** 891–893.
46. Los, M., Van de Craen, M., Penning, L. C., Schenk, H., Westendorp, M., Baeuerie, P. A., Droge, W., Krammer, P. H., Fiers, W., and Schulze-Osthoff, K. (1995) Requirement of an ICE/CED-3 protease for FAS/APO-1-mediated apoptosis, *Nature* **375,** 81–83.
47. Enari, M., Hug, H., and Nagata, S. (1995) Involvement of an ICE-like protease in FAS-mediated apoptosis, *Nature* **375,** 78–81.
48. Kerr, J. F. R. and Harmon, B. V. (1991) Definition and incidence of apoptosis: an historical perspective, in *Current Communications in Cell and Molecular Biology* (Cope, L. D. T. a. F. O., ed.), Cold Spring Harbor Laboratory, Cold Spring Harbor, NY, pp. 5–29.
49. Lazebnik, Y., Cole, S., Cooke, C., Nelson, W., and Earnshaw, W. (1993) Nuclear events of apoptosis in vitro in cell-free mitotic extracts: a model system for analysis of the active phase of apoptosis, *J. Cell. Biol.* **123(1),** 7–22.
50. Wyllie, A. (1980) Glucocorticoid-induced thymocyte apoptosis is associated with endogenous endonuclease activation, *Nature* **284,** 555,556.
51. Walker, R. P., Kokileva, L., LeBlanc, J., and Sikorska, M. (1993) Detection of the initial stages of DNA fragmentation in apoptosis, *Biotechniques* **15(6),** 1032–1040.
52. Raff, M., Barres, B., Burne, J., Coles, H., Ishizaki, Y., and Jacobson, M. (1993) Programmed cell death and the control of cell survival: lessons from the nervous system, *Science* **262,** 695–699.
53. Rubin, L., Gatchalian, C., Rimon, G., and Brooks, S. (1994) The molecular mechanisms of neuronal apoptosis, *Curr. Opinion Neurobiol.* **4,** 696–702.
54. Silos-Santiago, I., Greenlund, L., Johnson, E., and Snider, W. (1995) Molecular genetics of neuronal survival, *Curr. Opinion Neurobiol.* **5,** 42–49.
55. Pittman, R. N., Wang, S., DiBenedetto, A. J., and Mills, J. C. (1993) A system for characterizing cellular and molecular events in programmed neuronal cell death, *J. Neurosci.* **13(9),** 3669–3680.
56. Edwards, S. N., Buckmaster, A. E., and Tolkovsky, A. M. (1991) The death program in cultured sympathetic neurones can be suppressed at the posttranslational level by nerve growth factor, cyclic AMP, and depolarization, *J. Neurochem.* **57(6),** 2140–2143.
57. Deckwerth, T. and Johnson, E. (1993) Temporal analysis of events associated with programmed cell death (apoptosis) of sympathetic neurons deprived of nerve growth factor, *J. Cell. Biol.* **123,** 1207–1222.
58. Edwards, S. and Tolkovsky, A. (1994) Characterization of apoptosis in cultured rat sympathetic neurons after nerve growth factor withdrawal, *J. Cell. Biol.* **124(4),** 537–546.
59. Martin, D., Ito, A., Horigome, K., Lampe, P. A., and Johnson, E. M. (1992) Biochemical characterization of programmed cell death in NGF-deprived sympathetic neurons, *J. Neurobiol.* **23,** 1205–1220.
60. Dypbukt, J. M., Ankarcrona, M., Burkitt, M., Sjoholm, A., Strom, K., Orrenius, S., and Nicoreta, P. (1994) Different prooxidant levels stimulate growth, trigger apoptosis, or produce necrosis of insulin-secreting R1Nm5F cells: the role of intracellular polyamines, *J. Biol. Chem.* **269,** 30,553–30,560.
61. Bonfoco, E., Krainc, D., Ankarcrona, M., Nicoreta, P., and Lipton, S. A. (1995) Apoptosis and necrosis: two distinct events induced respectively by mild and intense insults with *N*-methyl-D-aspartate or nitric oxide/superoxide in cortical cell cultures, *Proc. Natl. Acad. Sci. USA* **92,** 7162–7166.
62. Ankarcrona, M., Dypbukt, J. M., Bonfoco, E., Orrenius, S., Lipton, S. A., and Nicoreta, P. (1995) Glutamate-induced neuronal death: a succession of necrosis and apoptosis depending on mitochodrial function, *Neuron* **15,** 961–973.

63. LeBlanc, A. C. (1995) Increased production of 4 kDa amyloid β peptide in serum deprived human primary neuron cultures: possible involvement of apoptosis, *J. Neurosci.* **15(12),** 7837–7846.
64. Sheng, M. and Greenberg, M. E. (1990) The regulation and function of c-*fos* and other immediate early genes in the nervous system, *Neuron* **4,** 477–485.
65. Smeyne, R. J., Vendrell, M., Hayward, M., Baker, S. J., Miao, G. G., Schilling, K., Robertson, L. M., Curran, T., and Morgan, J. I. (1993) Continuous c-*fos* expression precedes programmed cell death in vivo, *Nature* **363,** 166–169.
66. Estus, S., Zaks, W., Freeman, R., Gruda, M., Bravo, R., and Johnson, E. (1994) Altered gene expression in neurons during programmed cell death: Identification of c-*jun* as necessary for neuronal apoptosis, *J. Cell. Biol.* **127(6),** 1717–1727.
67. Ham, J., Whitefield, J., Pfarr, C. M., Lallemand, J., Yaniv, M., and Rubin, L. L. (1995) A c-*jun* dominant negative mutant protects sympathetic neurons against programmed cell death, *Neuron* **14,** 927–939.
68. Merry, D. E., Veis, D. J., Hickey, W. F., and Korsmeyer, S. J. (1994) *bcl*-2 protein expression is widespread in the developing nervous system and retained in the adult PNS, *Development* **120,** 301–311.
69. Gonzalez-Garcia, M., Perez-Ballestro, R., Ding, L., Duan, L., Boise, L., and Thompson, C. B. (1995) *bcl*-x is expressed in embryonic and postnatal neural tissues and functions to prevent neuronal cell death, *Proc. Natl. Acad. Sci. USA* **92,** 4304–4308.
70. Motoyama, N., Wang, F., Roth, K. A., Sawa, H., Nakayama, K.-I., Nakayama, K., Negishi, I., Senju, S., Zhang, Q., Fujii, S., and Loh, D. Y. (1995) Massive cell death of immature hematopoietic cells and neurons in *bcl*-x-deficient mice, *Science* **267,** 1506–1510.
71. Krajewski, S., Krajewska, M., Shabaik, A., Wang, H.-G., Irie, S., Fong, L., and Reed, J. C. (1994) Immunohistochemical analysis of in vivo patterns of *bcl*-x expression, *Cancer Res.* **54,** 5501–5507.
72. Frankowski, H., Missoten, M., Fernandez, P.-A., Martinou, I., Michel, P., Sadoul, R., and Martinou, J.-C. (1995) Function and expression of the *bcl*-x gene in the developing and adult nervous system, *Neuroreport* **6,** 1917–1921.
73. Veis, D. J., Sorenson, C. M., Shutter, J. R., and Korsmeyer, S. J. (1993) *bcl*-2-deficient mice demonstrate fulminant lymphoid apoptosis, polycistic kidneys, and hypopigmented hair. *Cell* **75,** 229–240.
74. Shimizu, S., Eguchi, Y., Kosaka, H., Kamlike, W., Matsuda, H., and Tsujimoto, Y. (1995) Prevention of hypoxia-induced cell death by *bcl*-2 and *bcl*-xL, *Nature* **374,** 811–813.
75. Roth, K., Motoyama, N., and Loh, D. (1996) Apoptosis of *bcl*-x-deficient telencephalic cells in vitro, *J. Neurosci.,* **16,** 1753–1758.
76. Batistatou, A., Merry, D. E., Korsmeyer, S. J., and Greene, L. A. (1993) *bcl*-2 affects survival but not neuronal differentiation of PC12 cells, *J. Neurosci.* **13,** 4422–4428.
77. Mah, S. P., Zhong, L. T., Liu, Y., Roghani, A., Edwards, R. H., and Bredesen, D. E. (1993) The protooncogene *bcl*-2 inhibits apoptosis in PC12 cells, *J. Neurochem.* **60,** 1183–1186.
78. Garcia, I., Martinou, I., Tsujimoto, Y., and Martinou, J. (1992) Prevention of programmed cell death of sympathetic neurons by the *bcl*-2 proto-oncogene, *Science* **258,** 302–304.
79. Dubois-Dauphin, M., Frankowski, H., Tsujimoto, Y., and Huarte, J. (1994) Neonatal motorneuron overexpressing the *bcl*-2 protooncogene in transgenic mice are protected from axotomy-induced cell death, *Proc. Natl. Acad. Sci. USA* **91,** 3309–3313.
80. Martinou, J.-C., Dubois-Dauphin, M., Staple, J. K., Rodriguez, I., Frankowski, H., Missotten, M., Albertini, P., Talabot, D., Catsicas, S., Pietra, C., and Huarte, J. (1994) Overexpression of *bcl*-2 in transgenic mice protects neurons from naturally occurring cell death and experimental ischemia, *Neuron* **13,** 1017–1030.
81. Jacobson, M. D. and Raff, M. (1995) Programmed cell death and *bcl*-2 protection in very low oxygen, *Nature* **374,** 814–816.
82. Greenlund, L. J. S., Korsmeyer, S. J., and Johnston, E. M. (1995) Role of *bcl*-2 in the survival and function of developing and mature sympathetic neurons, *Neuron* **15,** 649–661.

83. Haldar, S., Jena, N., and Croce, C. M. (1995) Inactivation of *bcl*-2 by phosphorylation, *Proc. Natl. Acad. Sci. USA* **92**, 4507–4511.

84. Milligan, C. E., Prevette, D., Yaginuma, H., Homma, S., Cardwell, C., Fritz, L. C., Tomaselli, K. J., Oppenheim, R. W., and Schwartz, L. M. (1995) Peptide inhibitors of the ICE protease family arrest programmed cell death of motorneurons in vivo and in vitro, *Neuron* **15**, 385–393.

85. Hanger, D. P., Brion, J. P., Gallo, J. M., Cairns, N. J., Luthert, P. J., and Anderton, B. H. (1991) Tau in Alzheimer's disease and Down's syndrome is insoluble and abnormally phosphorylated, *Biochem. J.* **275(APR)**, 99–104.

86. Brion, J. P., Hanger, D. P., Bruce, M. T., Couck, A. M., Flamentdurand, J., and Anderton, B. H. (1991) Tau in Alzheimer neurofibrillary tangles—N-terminal and C-terminal regions are differentially associated with paired helical filaments and the location of a putative abnormal phosphorylation site, *Biochem. J.* **273**, 127–133.

87. Hamos, J., DeGennaro, L., and Drachman, D. (1989) Synaptic loss in Alzheimer's disease and other dementias, *Neurology* **39**, 355–361.

88. Davies, P. and Maloney, A. (1976) Selective loss of central cholinergic neurons in Alzheimer's disease, *Lancet* **2**, 1403.

89. Whitehouse, P., Price, D., Struble, R., Clark, A., Coyle, J., and DeLong, M. (1982) Alzheimer's disease and senile dementia: loss of neurons in the basal forebrain, *Science* **215**, 1237–1239.

90. Terry, R., Peck, A., DeTeresa, R., Schechter, R., and Horoupian, D. (1981) Some morphometric aspects of the brain in senile dementia of the Alzheimer type, *Ann. Neurol.* **10**, 184–192.

91. Barr, P. J. and Tomei, D. (1994) Apoptosis and its role in human disease, *Bio/Technology* **12**, 487–493.

92. Rose, C. D. and Henneberry, R. C. (1993) Mechanisms of programmed cell death and their implications for the brain, *Neurodegeneration* **2**, 287–298.

93. Xiong, W. and Montell, C. (1995) Defective glia induce neuronal apoptosis in the repo visual system of *Drosophila*, *Neuron* **14**, 581–590.

94. Sofroniew, M. V., Galletly, N. P., Isacson, O., and Svendsen, C. N. (1990) Survival of adult basal forebrain cholinergic neurons after loss of target neurons, *Science* **247**, 338–342.

95. LeBlanc, A. C. (1994) The role of β-amyloid peptide in Alzheimer's disease, *Metabolic Brain Disease* **9(1)**, 3–31.

96. Sherrington, R., Rogaev, E. J., Liang, Y., Rogaeva, E. A., Levesque, G., Ikeda, M., Chi, H., Lin, C., Li, G., Holman, K., Tauda, T., Mar, L., Foncin, J.-F., Bruni, A. C., Montreal, M. P., Sorbi, S., Rainero, I., Pinessi, L., Nee, L., Chumakov, I., Pollen, D., Brookes, A., Sanseau, P., Pollinsky, R. J., Wasco, W., Da Silva, H. A. R., Haines, J. L., Pericak-Vance, M. A., Tanzi, R. E., Roses, A. D., Fraser, P., Rommens, J. M., and St. George-Hyslop, P. H. (1995) Cloning of a gene bearing mis-sense mutations in early-onset familial Alzheimer's disease, *Nature* **375**, 754–760.

97. Querfurt, H. W., Wisjsman, E. M., St. George Hyslop, P., and Selkoe, D. (1995) βAPP mRNA transcription is increased in cultured fibroblasts from the familial Alzheimer's disease-1 family, *Mol. Brain Res.* **28**, 319–337.

98. Yankner, B. A., Duffy, L. K., and Kirschner, D. A. (1990) Neurotrophic and neurotoxic effects of amyloid β protein: reversal by tachykinin neuropeptides, *Science* **250**, 279–286.

99. Forloni, G., Chiesa, R., Smiroldo, S., Verga, L., Salmona, M., Tagliavini, F., and Angeretti, N. (1993) Apoptosis mediated neurotoxicity induced by chronic application of β-amyloid fragment 25-35, *Neuroreport* **4**, 523–526.

100. Loo, D., Copani, A., Pike, C. J., Whittemore, E., Walencewicz, A. J., and Cotman, C. W. (1993) Apoptosis is induced by β-amyloid in cultured central nervous system neurons, *Proc. Natl. Acad. Sci. USA* **90**, 7951–7955.

101. Mattson, M., Cheng, B., Culwell, A., Esch, F., Lieberburg, I., and Rydel, R. (1993) Evidence for excitoprotective and intraneuronal calcium-regulating roles for secreted forms of the β-amyloid precursor protein, *Neuron* **10**, 243–254.

102. Levy-Lahad, E., Wasco, W., Poorkej, P., Romano, D. M., Oshima, J., Pettingell, W. H., Yu, C., Jondro, P., Schmidt, S., Wang, K., Crowley, A., Fu, Y., Guenette, S., Galas, D., Nemens, E., Wijsman, E., Bird, T., Schellenberg, G., and Tanzi, R. (1995) Candidate gene for the chromosome 1 familial Alzheimer's disease locus, *Science* **269,** 973–977.

103. Rabizadeh, S., Gralla, E. B., Borcheldt, D., Gwinn, R., Valentine, J., Sisodia, S., Wong, P., Lee, M., Hahn, H., and Bredesen, D. (1995) Mutations associated with amyotropic lateral sclerosis convert superoxide dismutase from an antiapoptotic gene to a proapoptotic gene: studies in yeast and neural cells, *Proc. Natl. Acad. Sci. USA* **92,** 3024–3028.

104. Lassmann, H., Bancher, C., Breitschopf, H., Wegiel, J., Bobinski, M., Jellinger, K., and Wisniewski, H. (1995) Cell death in Alzheimer's disease evaluated by DNA fragmentation *in situ, Acta Neuropathol.* **89,** 35–41.

105. Su, J., Anderson, A., Cummings, B., and Cotman, C. (1994) Immunohistochemical evidence for apoptosis in Alzheimer's disease, *Neuroreport* **5,** 2529–2533.

106. Petito, C. K. and Roberts, B. (1995) Evidence of apoptotic cell death in HIV encephalitis, *Am. J. Pathol.* **146(5),** 1121–1130.

107. Zhang, P., Hirsch, E. C., Damier, P., Duyckaerts, C., and Javoy-Agid, F. (1992) c-*fos* protein-like immunoreactivity: distribution in the human brain and over-expression in the hippocampus of patients with Alzheimer's disease, *Neuroscience* **46(1),** 9–21.

108. Anderson, A. J., Cummings, B. J., and Cotman, C. W. (1994) Increased immunoreactivity of *jun*- and *fos*-related proteins in Alzheimer's disease: Association with pathology, *Exp. Neurol.* **125,** 286–295.

109. May, P. C., Lampert-Etchells, M., Johnson, S. A., Poirier, J., Masters, J. N., and Finch, C. E. (1990) Dynamics of gene expression for a hippocampal glycoprotein elevated in Alzheimer's disease and in response to experimental lesions in rat, *Neuron* **5,** 831–839.

110. Ahuja, H. S., Tenniswood, M., Lockshin, M., and Zakeri, Z. (1994) Expression of clusterin in cell differentiation and cell death, *Biochem. Cell. Biol.* **72,** 523–530.

111. Satou, T., Cummings, B. J., and Cotman, C. W. (1995) Immunoreactivity for *bcl*-2 protein within neuorns in the Alzheimer's disease brain increases with disease severity, *Br. Res.* **697(1-2),** 35–43.

112. Wisniewski, H., Wegiel, J., Wang, M., Kujawa, M., and Lach, B. (1989) Ultrastructural studies of the cells forming amyloid fibers in classical plaques, *Can. J. Neurol. Sci.* **16,** 535–542.

113. Pike, C. J., Burdick, D., Walencewicz, A. J., Glabe, C. G., and Cotman, C. W. (1993) Neurodegeneration induced by β-amyloid peptides in vitro: the role of peptide assembly state, *J. Neurosci.* **13(4),** 1676–1687.

114. Pike, C. J., Cummings, B. J., and Cotman, C. W. (1992) β-amyloid induces neuritic dystrophy in vitro: similarities with Alzheimer pathology, *Neuroreport* **3,** 769–772.

115. Anderson, A. J., Pike, C. J., and Cotman, C. W. (1995) Differential induction of immediate early gene proteins in cultured neurons by β-amyloid (Aβ): Association of c-*jun* with Aβ-induced apoptosis, *J. Neurochem.* **65,** 1487–1498.

116. Takashima, A., Noguchi, K., Sato, K., Hoshino, T., and Imahori, K. (1993) tau protein kinase I is essential for amyloid β–protein–induced neurotoxicity, *Proc. Natl. Acad. Sci. USA* **90,** 7789–7793.

117. Mattson, M. P., Cheng, B., Davis, D., Bryant, K., Lieberburg, I., and Rydel, R. E. (1992) β-amyloid peptides destabilize calcium homeostasis and render human cortical neurons vulnerable to excitotoxicity, *J. Neurosci.* **12(2),** 376–389.

118. Behl, C., Davis, J., Cole, G. M., and Schubert, D. (1992) Vitamin E protects nerve cells from amyloid β protein toxicity, *Biochem. Biophys. Res. Commun.* **186(2),** 944–950.

119. Behl, C., Davis, J., Lesley, R., and Schubert, D. (1994) Hydrogen peroxide mediates amyloid β protein toxicity, *Cell* **77,** 817–827.

120. Schubert, D., Behl, C., Lesley, R., Brack, A., Dargusch, R., Sagara, Y., and Kimura, H. (1995) Amyloid peptides are toxic via a common oxidative mechanism, *Proc. Natl. Acad. Sci. USA* **92,** 1989–1993.

121. Shearman, M., Ragan, C., and Iversen, L. (1994) Inhibition of PC12 cell redox activity is a specific, early indicator of the mechanism of β-amyloid-mediated cell death, *Proc. Natl. Acad. Sci. USA* **91,** 1470–1474.

122. Butterfield, A., Hensley, K., Harris, M., Mattson, M., and Carney, J. (1994) β-amyloid peptide free radical fragments initiate synaptosomal lipoperoxidation in a sequence-specific fashion: Implications to Alzheimer's disease, *Biochem. Biophys. Res. Comm.* **200,** 710–715.

123. Bredesen, D. (1994) Neuronal apoptosis: genetic and biochemical modulation, in *Apoptosis II* (D. T. a. F. Cope, ed.), Cold Spring Harbor Laboratory, Cold Spring Harbor, NY, pp. 397–421.

124. Rabizadeh, A., Bitler, C. M., Butcher, L. L., and Bredesen, D. E. (1994) Expression of the low-affinity nerve growth factor receptor enhances β-amyloid peptide toxicity, *Proc. Natl. Acad. Sci. USA* **91,** 10,703–10,706.

125. Gravina, S., Ho, L., Eckman, C., Long, K., Otvos, L., Younkin, L., Suzuki, N., and Younkin, S. (1995) Amyloid β peptide (Aβ) in Alzheimer's Disease brain, *J. Biol. Chem.* **270(13),** 7013–7016.

126. Busciglio, J., Lorenzo, A., Yeh, J., and Yankner, B. A. (1995) β-amyloid fibrils induce tau phosphorylation and loss of microtubule binding, *Neuron* **14,** 879–888.

127. Arispe, N., Pollard, H. B., and Rojas, E. (1993) Giant multilevel cation channels formed by Alzheimer disease amyloid β-protein [AβP-(1-40)] in bilayer membranes, *Proc. Natl. Acad. Sci. USA* **90,** 10,573–10,577.

128. Mirzabekov, T., Lin, M., Yuan, W., Marshall, P. J., Carman, M., Tomaselli, K., Lieberburg, I., and Kagan, B. L. (1994) Channel formation in planar bilayers by a neurotoxic fragment of the beta-amyloid peptide, *Biochem. Biophys. Res. Commun.* **202(2),** 1142–1148.

129. Etcheberrigaray, R., Ito, E., Kim, C. S., and Alkon, D. L. (1994) Soluble β-amyloid induction of Alzheimer's phenotype for human fibroblast K$^+$ channels, *Science* **264,** 276–279.

130. Araujo, D. M. and Cotman, C. W. (1992) β-amyloid stimulates glial cells in vitro to produce growth factors that accumulate in senile plaques in Alzheimer's disease, *Br. Res.* **559,** 141–145.

131. Meda, L., Cassatella, M., Szendrei, G., Otvos, L., Baron, P., Villalba, M., Ferrari, D., and Rossi, F. (1995) Activation of microglial cells by β-amyloid protein and interferon-gamma, *Nature* **374,** 647–650.

6

The β-Amyloid Model of Alzheimer's Disease

Conformation Change, Receptor Cross-Linking, and the Initiation of Apoptosis

Carl W. Cotman, David H. Cribbs, and Aileen J. Anderson

1. INTRODUCTION

In 1855, Virchow, looking for a link between plants and animals, discovered deposits of a substance in the brain that stained with iodine; he named this substance amyloid, after the Greek word for starch *(1)*. The amyloid in these deposits was later identified as a peptide, and subsequently recognized as the major component of senile plaques in Alzheimer's disease (AD). β-Amyloid (Aβ) has been used extensively to identify AD pathology. It was generally thought that Aβ itself was metabolically inert, lacking in biological activity, until recent studies with cultured neurons and other cells provided the first clear evidence that Aβ is an active peptide. Aβ has been shown to initiate neuronal degeneration and transiently enhance neuronal growth. These observations opened up the action of Aβ to extensive investigation and led to the key finding that the biological activity of Aβ is dependent on its transformation into a β-sheet conformation and related higher order molecular assemblies. This is of fundamental importance, because it suggests that the biological activity of Aβ is dependent on protein conformation and that the transition into this conformation generates a new biological activity. Indeed, the amount of Aβ that accumulates in the brain appears to correlate to the decline of brain function *(2)*. The consequences of such a relationship between biological activity and protein conformation are critical to understanding the role of Aβ and other β-pleated sheet protein assemblies, such as prion protein, in disease.

In this chapter, we will briefly review the state of knowledge on the amyloid model of neuronal dysfunction and degeneration in AD. We suggest that Aβ acts as a driving force that places neurons at risk for injury, damages their processes, and is one of a class of stimuli that initiates cell death via apoptosis. Specifically, we suggest that Aβ acts on neurons in a fashion analogous to a superantigen, and causes a form of apoptosis, termed activation-induced cell death, through the crosslinking of membrane receptors. Currently, cell-culture and in vivo assays are extensively employed to define the fundamental mechanisms driving Aβ-mediated neuronal dysfunction and death, and as screening assays for neuroprotective agents. Many of the morphological and molecular changes observed in vitro predict features of neuronal degeneration also found *in situ*

From: Molecular Mechanisms of Dementia *Edited by: W. Wasco and R. E. Tanzi Humana Press Inc., Totowa, NJ*

in postmortem brain tissues derived from AD subjects. In turn, features identified *in situ* have helped refine the understanding of the pathways of degeneration as defined in vitro. We will critically examine the evidence that apoptosis exists in AD brain and contributes to neuronal degeneration as predicted from in vitro experiments. We will also illustrate that Aβ can contribute to the degeneration of brain vascular smooth muscle cells, and can activate astrocytes, an effect that may represent a fundamental mechanism in the gliosis that surrounds plaques in AD. Overall, the data reviewed here converge on the hypotheses that Aβ, and its transition to higher-order molecular assemblies, is a significant organizing and driving force underlying the development of pathology in AD.

2. BIOLOGICAL ACTIVITY OF Aβ

Initial investigations into the action of Aβ in vitro revealed that Aβ stimulated process outgrowth and enhanced survival over short time intervals in cultured hippocampal neurons *(3,4)*. Concurrent studies paradoxically showed that these peptides could also enhance neuronal death in response to excitotoxins *(5)* and induce neurodegeneration in culture *(4,6–10)*, suggesting that Aβ peptides were capable of exerting multiple bioactivities, i.e., enhancing growth or inducing toxicity. Further studies have clarified this issue, demonstrating that the in vitro activity of Aβ peptides is dependent on the assembly state of these peptides *(7,8,11–13)*.

As Aβ is aged, it assembles into higher-order structures, similar to those in the AD brain, and transforms into a stimulus that initiates neuronal cell death (Fig. 1). After incubation of synthetic Aβ1–42 peptides for several days in vitro, sheet-like structures are visible at the light microscopic level and an altered electrophoresis profile is evident on reducing gels, indicating the formation of insoluble aggregates *(8,14)*. These aggregated Aβ peptides demonstrate positive Congo red and thioflavine S staining similar to that observed in the AD brain *(14,15)*. Critically, Aβ peptides that exhibit aggregation as assessed by electrophoresis or sedimentation assays demonstrate toxicity in cultured neurons, whereas Aβ peptides that do not exhibit an aggregated state by these measures do not exhibit toxicity *(7,16)*.

The finding that Aβ, once assembled into particular aggregrates, initiates neuronal cell death provided one of the first assays in the field that could generate insights into the mechanisms of neurodegeneration in AD and also serve as an assay to screen for therapeutic agents. Identifying the type of cell death induced by Aβ was necessary to progress in defining the signaling pathways and events central to Aβ toxicity. Therefore, we asked the following question: Do cells degenerate via necrotic or apoptotic pathways, and is the same mechanism operative in the AD brain?

To determine if Aβ-mediated neurodegeneration in vitro occurs by a necrotic or apoptotic pathway, we employed a battery of assays to examine the relevant morphological and biochemical features that differentiate these mechanisms *(17)*. An initial clue that the cell death initiated by Aβ peptides is apoptotic rather than necrotic was our observation that cultured neurons treated with Aβ for 24–48 h exhibit asynchronous somal condensation with maintained plasma membrane integrity *(17)*. In order to confirm these data, we employed electron microscopy to identify more stringent criteria of apoptosis, specifically blebbing of the membrane surface and condensation of nuclear chromatin. As demonstrated by scanning and transmission electron micrographs, Aβ-treated neurons exhibit the classic ultrastructural changes of apoptotic degeneration *(17,18)*.

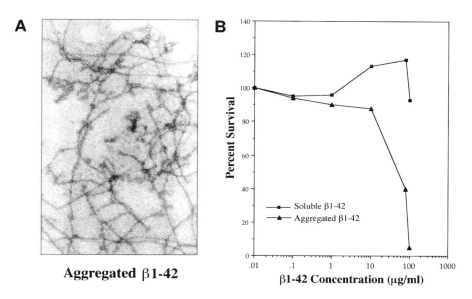

Aggregated β1-42

β1-42 Concentration (μg/ml)

Fig. 1. As Aβ is aged, it aggregates into higher-order structures and fibrils **(A)**, similar to those in the AD brain, and transforms from a stimulus that is neurotrophic-like (soluble) **(B)**, into a stimulus that initiates neuronal cell death (assembled).

A definitive biochemical feature of many cell types undergoing apoptosis is the degradation of DNA into oligonucleosome-length fragments *(19)*. Consistent with this criterion, DNA isolated from neurons treated with Aβ for 24 h exhibits a ladder of oligonucleosome-length fragments, a reproducible effect observed in both short- and long-term neuronal culture paradigms. Importantly, DNA fragmentation is not a nonspecific consequence of neuronal injury, since neurons exposed to the calcium ionophore A23187 show only random DNA degradation. Taken together, these morphological and biochemical data provide strong evidence for the hypothesis that Aβ induces degeneration in primary neuronal cultures via an apoptotic pathway, a finding also reported by Forloni et al. *(20)*.

The finding that a molecule can develop the capacity to induce degeneration over time as its conformation state changes is novel and unexpected, although consistent with the greater vulnerability of the brain to degeneration as it ages.

3. CONFORMATION-DEPENDENT ACTIVITY OF Aβ

Thus, recent studies have shown that Aβ-induced neurotoxicity in vitro is correlated with assembly into an aggregated state, and suggest that this state is reflective of that present in congo- or thioflavine-positive accumulations of Aβ in AD brain. Consistent with this suggestion, an in vivo correlate for Aβ toxicity in vitro has been observed in some studies. Injection of aggregated Aβ peptides or plaque cores isolated from AD tissue into rat brain in these studies results in the induction of some markers of AD-type pathology and neurodegeneration *(21–23)*. These observations further suggest that Aβ may serve as a stimulus leading to altered growth and/or neuronal degeneration in AD. However, it will be essential to determine the conformational state of the injected peptides to evaluate these issues of Aβ toxicity fully in future in vivo studies.

In order to understand the degenerative processes induced by Aβ, it is essential to define the characteristics of Aβ salient to its function as a neurotoxic stimulus. In a previous study, we used a series of synthetic Aβ peptides with progressively truncated carboxy-termini to demonstrate that the length of this hydrophobic region is a crucial determinant of the peptide's ability both to aggregate and induce neurotoxicity in vitro *(13)*. We have also synthesized a series of truncated Aβ peptides (Aβ4, Aβ8, Aβ12, Aβ17) to examine the effects of N-terminal heterogeneity, which occurs in vivo and in vitro, on the assembly and biological activity of Aβ. The N-terminal truncated isoforms produced enhanced aggregation into neurotoxic β-sheet fibrils, suggesting that these truncated peptides may initiate the pathological neurodegeneration in AD by acting as a nucleation site for Aβ deposition *(24)*. The proteolytic enzymes that generate these truncated Aβ peptides may be of considerable significance in the pathogenesis of AD, in particular, the α-secretase, which has been proposed to block the formation of potential amyloidogenic Aβ peptides. To define the primary structure of Aβ involved in its role as an apoptotic stimulus further, we have begun a comprehensive study in which several series of Aβ peptides will be synthesized and examined for toxicity and aggregation. Thus far, we have observed that assembled, bioactive Aβ peptides exhibit β-sheet structure, and that amino acid substitutions that disrupt Aβ assembly also prevent β-sheet structure and abolish toxicity. The use of structural modeling with such peptides will be useful in elucidating the role of specific amino acids and their side chains in both the assembly and bioactivity of Aβ.

Interestingly, other amyloidogenic peptides in addition to Aβ (e.g., prion) also appear to assemble into β-sheet fibrils and mediate toxicity in cultured neurons *(25–28)*. Not all aggregating peptides trigger toxic events, however. For example, an internal sequence of amylin, which forms aggregates (aa 20–29), does not trigger neuronal dystrophy or cell death *(13,29)*, although aggregates of full-length amylin (aa 1–37; the principal component of amyloid deposits found in the pancreases of type-2 diabetes patients) induce the degeneration of cultured neurons *(29)* and the apoptotic death of cultured pancreatic islet cells *(30)*. Thus, a shared structural feature of many nonhomologous fibrillar proteins may serve as an apoptotic stimulus mediating a common form of cell death. What is this characteristic, and does Aβ act via a common surface receptor or access a more general mechanism of programmed cell death (PCD)?

According to classic receptor pharmacology, if Aβ acts via a specific receptor similar to a classic neurotransmitter receptor, the D-stereoisomer would not be predicted to exhibit bioactivity comparable to the native all-L-peptide. For example, glutamate receptors readily discriminate L vs D antagonistic agents *(31)*. To investigate this possibility, we have examined the all-D-stereoisomer of Aβ. We have found that the all-D-stereoisomer of Aβ1–42 has a mirror image circular dichroism spectra. However, it not only forms aggregates indistinguishable from the all-L-form, but also induces neurotoxicity with a nearly identical dose–response curve, as shown in Fig. 2 *(32)*. As we *(33)* and others *(34,35)* have reported, it appears that some aspect of β-sheet structure is necessary, but there is a range of tolerance in the exact stereospecific requirements of the assembly.

Thus, we suggest that extracellular macromolecular assemblies can serve as stimuli or agonists that trigger a particular sequence of cellular reactions in neurons that initiate an apoptotic program of cell death. These agonists are characterized in part by

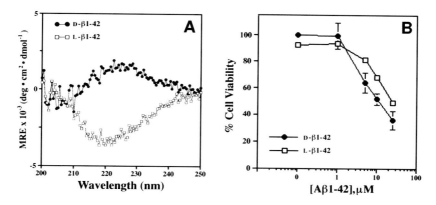

Fig. 2. The all-D-stereoisomer of β1–42 shows mirror image circular dichroism spectra to the L-isomer **(A)**, but forms aggregates indistinguishable from all-L-β1–42 and induces neurotoxicity with a nearly identical dose–response curve *(32)*.

β-sheet fibrillar structure, but in addition have the common ability to access critical signal transduction and downstream mechanisms that drive cell death. This hypothesis leads to several key questions. First, because Aβ exerts its toxicity in neurons via an apoptotic mechanism, what is known about membrane stimuli that induce apoptosis in other systems? Second, based on this information, is it possible to induce apoptosis in neurons via an agent that mimics the membrane effect that is predicted by this model of Aβ conformation–activity relationship?

4. STIMULI THAT INITIATE CELL DEATH

A large body of work on cell death has been conducted on the immune system. In this system, for example, clonal selection for T-cells ends in the induction of apoptosis by an extracellular activator in cells developmentally "programmed" to die; accordingly, apoptotic cell death in these cells is termed PCD. A common feature of extracellular activators of apoptosis is that they involve interactions with membrane proteins, and either disrupt a constitutive cellular survival signal required to suppress an intrinsic cell suicide program *(36)* or produce a novel signal that leads to PCD *(37–39)*. The loss of a constitutively required signal can occur via a reduction in the level of soluble trophic factors or a disruption of cell–cell or cell–extracellular matrix interactions *(36,40)*. The active generation of a death signal is dependent on the crosslinking of specific membrane receptors by multivalent ligands, which initiates a signal transduction event that triggers PCD, and is thus called activation-induced PCD *(41–43)*. A number of well-characterized extracellular agents that bind to the cell surface have been reported to initiate activation-induced PCD, and, in several cases, the receptor involved has been identified, e.g., bacterial superantigens *(37,38)*, the Fas ligand *(39)*, and certain viruses *(44)*. In the case of bacterial superantigens, initiation of activation-induced PCD in T-lymphocytes occurs when the superantigen binds to a major histocompatibility complex class II antigen, thus forming a complex that activates T-cells and initiates PCD when it crosslinks the T-cell antigen receptors *(38)*. A key feature of this process is that it can be mimicked with antibodies against the T-cell antigen receptor, but not with monovalent antibody fragments, which indicates that the binding event is insufficient to activate the PCD signal and that crosslinking of the receptors is required to initiate PCD *(45,46)*.

Aβ-initiated apoptosis is very similar to activation-induced PCD in two critical ways: Aβ induces PCD only when in a fibrillar β-sheet assembly state *(17,47)*, and only when in contact with neuronal surfaces. These similarities suggest that Aβ may initiate a type of activation-induced PCD in a manner analogous to superantigens and Fas receptor crosslinking.

5. CONCANAVALIN A (CON A) ACTIVATION-INDUCED CELL DEATH MODEL

Can the crosslinking of neuronal membrane receptors induce PCD in neurons? Although specific PCD-linked receptors have not yet been identified in neurons, lectins are capable of binding and crosslinking many different glycosylated membrane receptors on cells, activating the receptors and causing a wide variety of cellular responses, including the induction of cell death. We have examined the response of neurons to the lectin Con A, because neurons contain a high density of receptors for this lectin *(48)* and it is possible to examine binding with crosslinking and without crosslinking by chemically modifying the Con A.

Con A produced measurable cell death and morphological changes at concentrations >10 nM, and at 100 nM, induced massive cell death in primary neuronal cultures (Fig. 3). Con A-induced neuronal death exhibited many of the hallmarks associated with PCD, such as membrane blebbing, nuclear condensation and margination, and internucleosomal DNA cleavage *(49)*. Con A was found to induce cell death in neurons at concentrations that are mitogenic to T-lymphocytes *(43)* and thymocytes *(41)*. Interestingly, the same signals that induce proliferation and differentiation in lymphocytes can also induce PCD under different conditions, such as different activation states, developmental states, or cellular associations *(42,43,50)*. Thus, an incomplete set of signals, inappropriately timed signals, hyperactivation, or signals in an improper sequence have been proposed to result in activation-induced PCD *(42)*. This hypothesis is consistent with the results obtained with Con A and with other neuronal activators of PCD, such as Aβ, which may initiate a signaling cascade that is inappropriate for survival.

To examine the importance of receptor crosslinking in the Con A-initiated PCD, the effect of succinylated Con A was compared to that of native Con A. Succinylated Con A is a stable dimer and is much less effective at forming membrane aggregates of Con A receptors than the native Con A. Native Con A is a tetramer and binds with other tetramers to induce receptor aggregation. As shown in Fig. 4, native Con A caused a clustering of Con A receptors in agreement with previous findings. In contrast, succinylated Con A did not produce receptor clusters, nor did it produce significant cell death even at micromolar concentrations *(49)*. Thus, when the crosslinking of membrane receptors to form receptor clusters was blocked, the subsequent downstream intracellular signaling that initiates PCD was also blocked, suggesting that receptor crosslinking is a necessary part of the signal that initiates Con A-induced PCD.

The Con A model shares certain features with Aβ-induced PCD. The time-courses for both the Con A- and Aβ-induced morphological changes and the subsequent PCD are comparable *(13)*. Similar to Con A, Aβ has also been reported to increase neurite outgrowth *(3)* followed by degeneration *(16)*, under some experimental conditions.

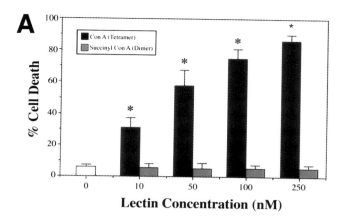

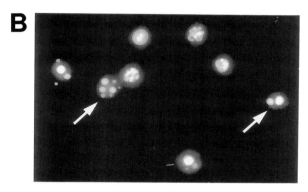

Apoptotic Nuclei

Fig. 3. Con A produces measurable cell death and morphological changes at concentrations >10 n*M*, and, at 100 n*M*, induces massive cell death in neuronal cultures **(A)**. At 24 h after Con A exposure, many of the nuclei show multiple nuclear apoptotic bodies as revealed by Syto 11 nuclear staining **(B)**.

Although most protocols for Aβ-induced cell death now employ preassembled peptide, over a much extended time-course, Aβ in the soluble form will also cause cell death. Shortly prior to cell death, the surface of the neurons exhibits clusters of the peptide (Fig. 5) *(16,51)* similar to that observed with Con A. Taken together, these findings raise the possibility that both Con A and Aβ act through a crosslinking of cell-surface molecules to initiate activation-induced PCD. Neurons may be particularly sensitive to disturbances on their surface and to the crosslinking of particular components.

It is important to note that the response of neurons to receptor crosslinking is not general to all types of neurons or brain cells. Brain vascular smooth muscle cells, for example, bind Aβ on the surface, appear to show Aβ clusters on their surface, and also show a pattern of degeneration characteristic of apoptosis *(52)*. On the other hand, some neuronal subtypes (such as GABAergic cells) are resistant to Aβ-mediated apoptosis in vitro and to degeneration in the AD brain. Similarly, astrocytes do not degenerate when exposed to Aβ, but do take on a more reactive appearance similar to their

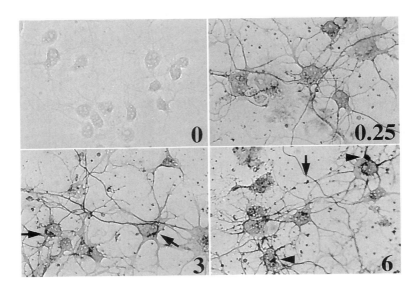

Fig. 4. Native Con A initiates time-dependent clustering of Con A receptors, which appears to precede cell death. Con A receptors on neurons were initially uniformly dispersed, but then formed receptor clusters on the plasma membrane. Biotinylated-Con A (250 nM) was used to detect the initial distribution of Con A receptors on cortical neurons and to monitor the redistribution of the receptors. At the 0-time point no detectable biotinylated Con A is present on the neurons. The Con A receptors were initially (0.25 h) evenly distributed over the entire neuronal surface. By 3 h, clusters of Con A receptors were concentrated in the region adjacent to the soma and large aggregates of receptors were also visible on the somal membranes *(arrows)*. At the 6-h-time point, clusters of Con A receptors appeared as blebs on some of the neurites *(arrows)* and very large aggregates were associated with the somal areas *(arrowheads)*.

status when associated with senile plaques *(53)*. Thus, the Aβ in vitro model exhibits many of the aspects of selectivity characteristic of the AD brain.

The temporal sequence of events that occurs in neurons following Con A-induced crosslinking of membrane receptors may provide insights into pathways that predispose neurons to PCD. The specific nature of the Con A–neuron interaction will aid in the identification of the receptors involved, and in the description of the subsequent intracellular signaling cascade and changes in gene expression relating to PCD. As additional information on the mechanism of extracellular activators of PCD becomes available, a comparison of the intracellular signaling events may provide insights into a conserved PCD activation pathway and the nature of the stimuli that place neurons at risk.

6. APOPTOSIS IN AD

To understand the stimuli and conditions that contribute to neuronal dysfunction and cell death in AD, it is essential to make comparisons between in vitro paradigms and observations in vivo. There are a number of cases where this strategy has already been beneficial in assessing the validity of in vitro models. For example, in parallel with classical AD pathology, Aβ induces the formation of dystrophic neurites in cultured neurons *(16,54)*. Similarly, reductions in glucose metabolism have been suggested to

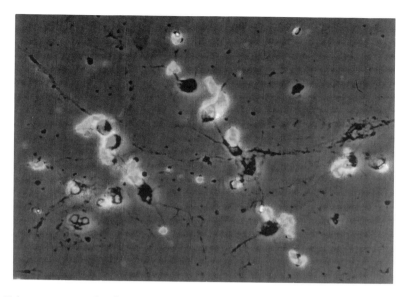

Fig. 5. Primary neuronal culture stained with antibody to Aβ. Over time, soluble Aβ appears to assemble and cluster on the neuronal surface, similar to that observed with Con A. The figure illustrates the appearance of clusters of Aβ 24 h after exposure of neurons to soluble, nonaggregated Aβ1–42.

contribute to neurodegeneration in AD *(55–59)*, and Aβ has been shown to exacerbate neurodegeneration in cultured neurons when glucose levels are reduced *(60)*. Aβ has also been shown to increase the susceptibility of neurons to excitotoxicity in both rodent *(5)* and human *(61)* neuronal cultures, and these observations have recently been confirmed in the rodent brain *(62)*. Additional evidence suggesting that Aβ may act as a stimulus to induce degeneration in vivo comes from a transgenic model overexpressing Aβ1–42, in which Aβ transgene expression was detected in a variety of peripheral tissues, but degeneration characteristic of apoptosis was restricted to regions of the brain affected in AD *(63)*. Taken together, these studies imply that Aβ can interact with other cellular insults or risk factors to exacerbate pathological mechanisms in AD or act directly to induce damage.

Does apoptosis exist as a mechanism in AD, and if so, what are the molecular pathways mediating this mechanism? Recent evidence suggests that apoptosis may be a primary mechanism in the degeneration of neurons in age-related diseases, such as AD. Although studies *in situ* are still at an early stage, data supporting a role for apoptosis in AD are accumulating. Apoptotic nuclear changes similar to those identified in vitro are also apparent in the AD brain. These observations are consistent with the hypothesis that apoptosis may be a mechanism for the removal of damaged cells in AD.

As previously mentioned, apoptosis is generally defined on the basis of strict morphological criteria and, in particular, by the cleavage of DNA into oligonucleosome-length fragments detectable by gel electrophoresis in many, but not all, models of apoptosis *(64–67)*. The process of DNA degradation produces a series of oligonucleosome-length DNA fragments that have newly generated 3'-OH ends. Conversely, normal cells have very low numbers of terminal DNA strand breaks. DNA fragmentation labeling techniques use enzymes, such as terminal deoxynucleotidyl transferase (TdT) or Klenow polymerase, to catalyze the addition of conjugated dNTPs to the 3'-OH termini of single- or double-stranded DNA, which can then be visualized immunohistochemically. Since DNA degradation occurs in both apoptosis and necrosis, both apoptotic and necrotic DNA strand breaks can be labeled by enzymes, such as TdT. Moreover, it is increasingly apparent that apoptosis and necrosis are not mutually exclusive processes, and that there may be a continuum between these pathways *(68,69)*. Thus, it is important to evaluate TdT labeling in the context of multiple morphological characteristics of apoptosis detectable at the light microscopy level and to be cautious in drawing conclusions regarding the mechanism of cell death in postmortem tissue labeled using such techniques *(47)*.

We have recently reported that cells in the AD brain exhibit labeling for DNA strand breaks using TdT, and that at the light microscopy level, the morphological distribution of this labeling in many cells is consistent with apoptosis *(70,71)*. We observed low levels of TdT labeling in control cases, but frequent TdT-positive nuclei in brain tissue from AD cases. In support of these findings, a greater than twofold increase in DNA strand breaks has been reported in AD vs control cerebral cortex using biochemical techniques *(72)*. Additionally, many TdT-labeled cells exhibited an apoptotic-like morphological distribution of DNA strand breaks, including granulated and marginated patterns of intense TdT labeling, shrunken, irregular cellular shape, and the presence of what appeared to be apoptotic bodies (Fig. 6). TdT labeling occurred in distinct cells, not in clumped groups of cells as would be expected in the case of necrosis, where cell lysis and inflammation would have resulted in the involvement of clusters of nearby cells. TdT-labeled nuclei were not found in association with histological evidence suggestive of necrosis. Importantly, although there is an increase and a change in the distribution of TdT labeling with increasing postmortem delay *(71)*, postmortem delays of under 4–6 h as employed previously *(70)* do not exhibit detectable postmortem labeling artifacts. Furthermore, comparison of conventional postmortem control and AD tissue with rapid autopsy tissue did not reveal differences in TdT labeling, again supporting the consistency and validity of TdT labeling at the postmortem delays in these studies.

We further addressed the issue of potential TdT-labeling artifacts by examining the relationship of TdT labeling to brain area *(71)*. If the large increase in TdT labeling in AD is related to disease pathology and not a nonspecific artifact, TdT labeling would be predicted to be found in brain areas typically exhibiting AD pathology and neuronal cell loss, such as entorhinal cortex, but not in areas in which such pathology is generally absent, such as cerebellum. In general, TdT labeling was absent or present at very low levels in the cerebellum as compared to the entorhinal cortex of the AD cases examined. These findings correspond with previous results regarding ultrastructural neuronal injury and the formation of AD pathology *(75,76)*, supporting the hypothesis that TdT labeling reflects AD-related pathological processes and neuronal loss. Furthermore, comparison of conventional postmortem control and AD tissue with rapid autopsy tissue did not reveal differences in TdT labeling, again supporting the consistency and validity of TdT labeling at the postmortem delays employed in these studies.

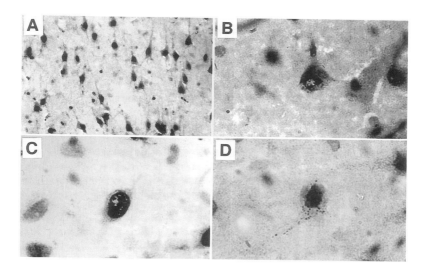

Fig. 6. Immunoreactivity for Bcl-2 appears to be elevated in AD brain, and some neurons show almost 1 to 1 colocalization between Bcl-2 and TdT labeling *(73,74)*, suggesting that Bcl-2 is in fact induced in neurons that exhibit DNA damage. **(A)** Low magnification field showing colocalization of Bcl-2 immunoreactivity in the cytoplasm (light gray) and TdT in the nucleus (black). **(B,C)** High magnification of double labeled neurons (center cells). The cells at the periphery of the field are not labeled for Bcl-2. The reproduction of the colored neurochemically stained tissue in gray scale reveals non-Bcl-2 staining cells. **(D)** Neuron associated with TdT-positive apoptotic bodies. The nucleus is Bcl-2-positive (from ref. *74; see* this paper for color reproductions of Bcl-2/TdT labeled neurons).

As we have noted, a powerful means of critically examining the validity of models and hypotheses regarding pathological mechanisms is to make comparisons across models and between in vitro and *in situ* observations. *In situ* data from autopsied AD brain tissue parallel in vitro observations from models of neuronal Aβ toxicity on both morphological and biochemical levels. The initiation of apoptosis in many systems involves the induction of a set of genes that participate in the regulation and/or control of cellular process preceding or required for the cell suicide. An additional factor to examine, therefore, is whether parallels in the initiation of such potential molecular markers for cellular apoptosis can be detected across models of Aβ toxicity and in the AD brain. The immediate early gene c-Jun has been shown to be induced during, and involved in, apoptosis, in both nonneuronal and neuronal systems *(77–79)*. In correspondence with this putative role, we have reported that neurons that initiate apoptosis in response to Aβ treatment also exhibit a selective and prolonged expression of c-Jun, whereas GABAergic neurons, which are resistant to neurodegeneration in AD *(80–84)* and have been shown to be resistant to Aβ-induced apoptosis in vitro, do not express c-Jun in this model. c-Jun is selectively induced in neurons undergoing apoptosis, but not necrosis, in this culture system *(85)*. c-Jun is also induced with a similar time-course in the Con A model of activation-induced cell death, which we propose may mimic some aspects of Aβ toxicity in cultured neurons *(49)*. In parallel with these in vitro results, we have reported increases in immunoreactivity for c-Jun in AD as compared to control brain, and the colocalization of immunoreactivity for c-Jun with neuronal pathology in AD *(86)*. Most recently, we have reported that there appears to be an association between c-Jun immunoreactivity and TdT labeling in the AD brain, suggesting that the expression of c-Jun and presence of DNA damage may be related *(71)*.

Importantly, although many of the cells labeled by TdT in the AD brain exhibit clear morphological characteristics of apoptosis, studies in AD tissue reveal a surprisingly large number of TdT-labeled nuclei in the entorhinal cortex/hippocampal formation. Gel electrophoresis of ^{32}P end-labeled genomic DNA is an extremely sensitive technique for the detection of DNA degradation, which has been successfully employed both in vitro and in vivo *(87–90)*. However, we and others have been unsuccessful in detecting DNA fragmentation with this technique in neurological disease *(71,90)*. Thus, although the morphological evidence for the presence of apoptosis in the AD brain on the basis of TdT labeling is quite strong, irrefutable evidence remains elusive. In the context of the large number of TdT-labeled cells present in the AD brain, this observation in itself may reveal information regarding the progression of DNA damage and pathology in this disease. Although DNA strand breaks detected with TdT reflect an increase in DNA damage in AD compared to control brain, this observation suggests it is unlikely that all of these cells are undergoing cell death by either apoptosis or necrosis during the disease stage captured at autopsy. Consequently, it is essential to examine critically the implications of the large difference in TdT labeling observed between control and AD brain *in situ*. One possibility is that TdT labeling in some of these cells represents an active process of DNA damage/DNA repair in cells at risk. Alternatively, reports on AD tissue have estimated cell loss in layer 2 of the entorhinal cortex as high as 87% relative to aged normal control subjects *(91)*. Thus, it remains possible that a slow or deficient clearance process is a contributing factor in the high number of TdT-labeled cells observed in AD compared to control brain.

The accumulation of DNA damage as the result of deficient DNA repair has previously been suggested to have a role in neurodegeneration in AD *(92,93)*. This accumulation could also be the result of an acceleration of DNA damage. The initiation of compensatory mechanisms in response to such events may be predicted to contribute to an active and prolonged process of DNA damage/DNA repair and cell death. Even in this case, the detection of DNA damage by TdT labeling could be used as one of the earliest markers of neuronal abnormality in AD brain and, correspondingly, reflect an increased vulnerability of neuronal cells to insult.

In this context, comparisons between in vitro and *in situ* models again contribute important information in evaluating hypotheses regarding the progression and mechanisms of AD pathology. We have previously shown that overexpression of the cell death inhibitory protein Bcl-2 blocks apoptosis induced by Aβ in cultured neurons *(94)*. To test the hypothesis that compensatory mechanisms inhibiting cell death may be initiated in the AD brain, immunoreactivity for Bcl-2 was examined in human postmortem tissue and found to be elevated in AD brain *(73)*. Furthermore, there is a strong, almost 1 to 1, colocalization between Bcl-2 and TdT labeling in AD brain *(74)*, suggesting that Bcl-2 is in fact induced in neurons that exhibit DNA damage. Interestingly, previous studies in human lymphocytes have shown that Bcl-2 exerts its protective effects at a stage downstream of the initiation of DNA strand cleavage *(95)*. This observation is consistent with the degree of TdT labeling observed in AD brain. Also, in accordance with the hypothesis that there may be an extended process of DNA damage/DNA repair and cell death in AD, the DNA repair enzyme Ref-1 is elevated in AD neurons *(95a)*. An increase in the expression of Ref-1 is particularly interesting in that this DNA repair enzyme has also been shown to regulate the DNA-binding activity of the transcriptional regulatory protein c-Jun *(96)*, which we propose to have a role in neuronal apoptosis induced by both Aβ and Con A. These proteins could be components of a dynamic and extended competition between cell death processes and compensatory responses in the AD brain.

7. CONCLUSIONS

In this chapter, we have developed the hypothesis that Aβ places neurons at risk for injury, damages processes, and can initiate cell death by apoptosis. The biological activity of amyloid depends on a change in its conformation into β-pleated sheets or related higher-order assemblies. Once in a particular conformation, Aβ initiates a series of signal transduction mechanisms that drives a cellular program to induce membrane blebbing, dispersion of polyribosomes, the induction of various genes, and apoptosis. We have further suggested that the specific mechanism of Aβ-induced apoptosis may be analogous to a form of apoptosis called activation-induced PCD, in which membrane receptor crosslinking leads to cell death. An analogous mechanism may be the induction of apoptosis by the lectin, Con A. Con A in its native form aggregates on the neuron surface, causes receptor clustering, and initiates apoptosis, whereas when Con A is modified so that it binds but does not aggregate on the surface, it does not cause cell death. Taken together, our data suggest that protein conformation and the assembly of higher-order aggregates are key factors that place neurons at risk and ultimately cause their degeneration.

An important verification of the relevance of these models for AD pathology is the parallel between observations on in vitro models of Aβ toxicity and *in situ* observations of the AD brain. In this context, data from our studies and others indicate that apoptosis may be a mechanism driving the degeneration of neurons in the brain. The AD brain shows extensive DNA damage in some neurons, nuclear morphology consistent with apoptosis, and the presence and coexpression in some cells of c-Jun as predicted from culture experiments. Thus, our studies and others indicate that apoptosis may be a mechanism driving the degeneration of neurons in the brain. It should be emphasized, however, that Aβ is only one of the stimuli that can initiate apoptosis; others may include oxidative damage *(97)* and direct DNA damage.

It is clear that research over the past several years has provided very strong evidence that the polymerization of Aβ peptides to higher-order conformations has led to the accumulation of the product and the emergence of a new biological activity. In the case of Aβ, this conformation has self-assembly characteristics that, once initiated, appear to generate more Aβ accumulation *(98)* and a cascade that places neurons at risk and, over time, contributes to their degeneration. In this respect, the Aβ model is not unique to the Aβ-peptide, but has parallels to prion disease and other forms of amyloidosis, such as pancreatic islet disease and amyloidosis in the cardiac or vascular system *(99–101)*. Taken together, Aβ appears to be a member of a family of protein conformation-dependent disorders that are both genetically and risk factor-based and which the organism must face as it ages.

REFERENCES

1. Virchow, R. (1855) Zur Cellulose-Fruge, *Virchows Arch.* **8**, 140–144.
2. Cummings, B. J. and Cotman, C. W. (1995) Image analysis of beta-amyloid load in Alzheimer's disease and relation to dementia severity, *Lancet* **346**, 1524–1528.
3. Whitson, J. S., Selkoe, D. J., and Cotman, C. W. (1989) Amyloid beta protein enhances the survival of hippocampal neurons *in vitro*, *Science* **243**, 1488–1490.
4. Yankner, B. A., Duffy, L. K., and Kirschner, D. A. (1990) Neurotrophic and neurotoxic effects of amyloid β-protein: reversal by tachykinin neuropeptides, *Science* **250**, 279–282.
5. Koh, J. Y., Yang, L. L., and Cotman, C. W. (1990) β-Amyloid protein increases the vulnerability of cultured cortical neurons to excitotoxic damage, *Brain Res.* **533**, 315–320.
6. Yankner, B. A., Dawes, L. R., Fisher, S., Villa, K. L., Oster, G. M. L., and Neve, R. L. (1989) Neurotoxicity of a fragment of the amyloid precursor associated with Alzheimer's disease, *Science* **245**, 417–420.
7. Pike, C. J., Walencewicz, A. J., Glabe, C. G., and Cotman, C. W. (1991) *In vitro* aging of β-amyloid protein causes peptide aggregation and neurotoxicity, *Brain Res.* **563**, 311–314.
8. Pike, C. J., Walencewicz, A. J., Glabe, C. G., and Cotman, C. W. (1991) Aggregation-related toxicity of synthetic β-amyloid protein in hippocampal cultures, *Eur. J. Pharmacol.* **207**, 367,368.
9. Behl, C., Davis, J., Cole, G. M., and Schubert, D. (1992) Vitamin E protects nerve cells from amyloid beta protein toxicity, *Biochem. Biophys. Res. Commun.* **186**, 944–950.
10. Takadera, T., Sakura, N., Mohri, T., and Hashimoto, T. (1993) Toxic effect of a beta-amyloid peptide (beta 22–35) on the hippocampal neuron and its prevention, *Neurosci. Lett.* **161**, 41–44.
11. Busciglio, J., Gabuzda, D. H., Matsudaira, P., and Yankner, B. A. (1993) Generation of beta-amyloid in the secretory pathway in neuronal and nonneuronal cells, *Proc. Natl. Acad. Sci. USA* **90**, 2092–2096.
12. Mattson, M. P., Tomaselli, K. J., and Rydel, R. E. (1993) Calcium-destabilizing and neuro-degenerative effects of aggregated β-amyloid peptide are attenuated by basic FGF, *Brain Res.* **621**, 35–49.
13. Pike, C. J., Burdick, D., Walencewicz, A., Glabe, C. G., and Cotman, C. W. (1993) Neuro-degeneration induced by β-amyloid peptides *in vitro*: the role of peptide assembly state, *J. Neurosci.* **13**, 1676–1687.
14. Burdick, D., Soreghan, B., Kwon, M., Kosmoski, J., Knauer, M., Henschen, A., Yates, J., Cotman, C., and Glabe, C. (1992) Assembly and aggregation properties of synthetic Alzheimer's A4/β-amyloid peptide analogs, *J. Biol. Chem.* **267**, 546–554.
15. Hilbich, C., Kisters-Woike, B., Reed, J., Masters, C. L., and Beyreuther, K. (1991) Aggregation and secondary structure of synthetic amyloid βA4 peptides of Alzheimer's disease, *J. Mol. Biol.* **218**, 149–163.
16. Pike, C. J., Cummings, B. J., and Cotman, C. W. (1992) β-amyloid induces neuritic dystrophy *in vitro*: similarities with Alzheimer pathology, *Neuroreport* **3**, 769–772.
17. Loo, D. T., Copani, A. G., Pike, C. J., Whittemore, E. R., Walencewicz, A. J., and Cotman, C. W. (1993) Apoptosis is induced by beta-amyloid in cultured central nervous system neurons, *Proc. Natl. Acad. Sci. USA* **90**, 7951–7955.
18. Watt, J., Pike, C. J., Walencewicz, A. J., and Cotman, C. W. (1994) Ultrastructural analysis of β-amyloid-induced apoptosis in cultured hippocampal neurons, *Brain Res.* **661**, 147–156.
19. Wyllie, A. H., Kerr, J. F. R., and Currie, A. R. (1980) Cell death: the significance of apoptosis, *Int. Rev. Cytol.* **68**, 251–306.
20. Forloni, G., Chiesa, R., Smiroldo, S., Verga, L., Salmona, M., Tagliavini, F., and Angeretti, N. (1993) Apoptosis mediated neurotoxicity induced by chronic application of beta amyloid fragment 25-35, *Neuroreport* **4**, 523–526.
21. Frautschy, S. A., Baird, A., and Cole, G. M. (1991) Effects of injected Alzheimer beta-amyloid cores in rat brain, *Proc. Natl. Acad. Sci. USA* **88**, 8362–8366.

22. Emre, M., Geula, C., Ransil, B. J., and Mesulam, M. M. (1992) The acute neurotoxicity and effects upon cholinergic axons of intracerebrally injected beta-amyloid in the rat brain, *Neurobiol. Aging* **13,** 553–559.
23. Kowall, N. W., McKee, A. C., Yankner, B. A., and Beal, M. F. (1992) *In vivo* neurotoxicity of beta-amyloid [beta(1–40)] and the beta(25–35) fragment, *Neurobiol. Aging* **13,** 537–542.
24. Pike, C. J., Overman, M. J., and Cotman, C. W. (1995) Amino-terminal deletions enhance aggregation of beta-amyloid peptides *in vitro, J. Biol. Chem.* **270,** 23,895–23,898.
25. Forloni, G., Angeretti, N., Chiesa, R., Monzani, E., Salmona, M., Bugiani, O., and Tagliavini, F. (1993) Neurotoxicity of a prion protein fragment, *Nature* **362,** 543–546.
26. Selvaggini, C., De, G. L., Cantu, L., Ghibaudi, E., Diomede, L., Passerini, F., Forloni, G., Bugiani, O., Tagliavini, F., and Salmona, M. (1993) Molecular characteristics of a protease-resistant, amyloidogenic and neurotoxic peptide homologous to residues 106-126 of the prion protein, *Biochem. Biophys. Res. Commun.* **194,** 1380–1386.
27. Tagliavini, F., Prelli, F., Verga, L., Giaccone, G., Sarma, R., Gorevic, P., Ghetti, B., Passerini, F., Ghibaudi, E., Forloni, G., Schmona, M., Bugiani, O., and Frangione, B. (1993) Synthetic peptides homologous to prion protein residues 106–147 form amyloid-like fibrils *in vitro, Proc. Natl. Acad. Sci. USA* **90,** 9678–9682.
28. De Gioia, L., Selvaggini, C., Ghibaudi, E., Diomede, L., Bugiani, O., Forloni, G., Tagliavini, F., and Salmona, M. (1994) Conformational polymorphism of the amyloidogenic and neurotoxic peptide homologous to residues 106–126 of the prion protein, *J. Biol. Chem.* **269,** 7859–7862.
29. May, P. C., Boggs, L. N., and Fuson, K. S. (1993) Neurotoxicity of human amylin in rat primary hippocampal cultures: similarity to Alzheimer's disease amyloid-β neurotoxicity, *J. Neurochem.* **61,** 2330–2333.
30. Lorenzo, A., Razzaboni, B., Weir, G. C., and Yankner, B. A. (1994) Pancreatic islet cell toxicity of amylin associated with type-2 diabetes mellitus, *Nature* **368,** 756–760.
31. Monaghan, D. T., Bridges, R. J., and Cotman, C. W. (1989) The excitatory amino acid receptors: their classes, pharmacology, and distinct properties in the function of the central nervous system, *Ann. Rev. Pharmacol. Toxicol.* **29,** 365–402.
32. Cribbs, D. H., Pike, C. J., Weinstein, S. L., Velazquez, P., and Cotman, C. W. (1996) All-D-enantiomers of β-amyloid exhibit similar biological properties to all-L-β-amyloids (submitted).
33. Pike, C. J., Walencewicz-Wasserman, A. J., Kosmoski, J., Cribbs, D. H., Glabe, C. G., and Cotman, C. W. (1995) Structure–activity analyses of beta-amyloid peptides: contributions of the beta 25-35 region to aggregation and neurotoxicity, *J. Neurochem.* **64,** 253–265.
34. Simmons, L. K., May, P. C., Tomaselli, K. J., Rydel, R. E., Fuson, K. S., Brigham, E. F., Wright, S., Lieberburg, I., Becker, G. W., Brems, D. N., and Li, W. Y. (1994) Secondary structure of amyloid beta peptide correlates with neurotoxic activity *in vitro, Mol. Pharmacol.* **45,** 373–379.
35. Howlett, D. R., Jennings, K. H., Lee, D. C., Clark, M. S., Brown, F., Wetzel, R., Wood, S. J., Camilleri, P., and Roberts, G. W. (1995) Aggregation state and neurotoxic properties of Alzheimer beta-amyloid peptide, *Neurodegeneration* **4,** 23–32.
36. Raff, M. C., Barres, B. A., Burne, J. F., Coles, H. S., Ishizaki, Y., and Jacobson, M. D. (1993) Programmed cell death and the control of cell survival: lessons from the nervous system, *Science* **262,** 695–700.
37. Dellabona, P., Peccoud, J., Kappler, J., Marrack, P., Benoist, C., and Mathis, D. (1990) Superantigens interact with MHC class II molecules outside of the antigen groove, *Cell* **62,** 1115–1121.
38. Marrack, P. and Kappler, J. (1990) The staphylococcal enterotoxins and their relatives (published erratum appears in *Science* 1990 Jun 1, **248**[4959]:1066) (*see* comments), *Science* **248,** 705–711.
39. Nagata, S. and Golstein, P. (1995) The Fas death factor, *Science* **267,** 1449–1456.

40. Ruoslahti, E. and Reed, J. C. (1994) Anchorage dependence, integrins, and apoptosis, *Cell* **77,** 477,478.
41. Shi, Y. F., Sahai, B. M., and Green, D. R. (1989) Cyclosporin A inhibits activation-induced cell death in T-cell hybridomas and thymocytes, *Nature* **339,** 625,626.
42. Lenardo, M. J. (1991) Interleukin-2 programs mouse alpha beta T lymphocytes for apoptosis, *Nature* **353,** 858–861.
43. Radvanyi, L. G., Mills, G. B., and Miller, R. G. (1993) Religation of the T cell receptor after primary activation of mature T cells inhibits proliferation and induces apoptotic cell death, *J. Immunol.* **150,** 5704–5715.
44. Banda, N. K., Bernier, J., Kurahara, D. K., Kurrle, R., Haigwood, N., Sekaly, R.-P., and Finkel, T. H. (1992) Crosslinking CD4 by human immunodeficiency virus gp120 primes T cells for activation-induced apoptosis, *J. Exp. Med.* **176,** 1099–1106.
45. Smith, C. A., Williams, G. T., Kingston, R., Jenkinson, E. J., and Owen, J. J. (1989) Antibodies to CD3/T-cell receptor complex induce death by apoptosis in immature T cells in thymic cultures, *Nature* **337,** 181–184.
46. Takahashi, S., Maecker, H. T., and Levy, R. (1989) DNA fragmentation and cell death mediated by T cell antigen receptor/CD3 complex on a leukemia T cell line, *Eur. J. Immunol.* **19,** 1911–1919.
47. Cotman, C. W. and Anderson, A. J. (1995) A potential role for apoptosis in neurodegeneration and Alzheimer's disease, *Mol. Neurobiol.* **10,** 19–45.
48. Cotman, C. W. and Taylor, D. (1974) Localization and characterization of concanavalin A receptors in the synaptic cleft, *J. Cell Biol.* **62,** 236–242.
49. Cribbs, D. H., Kreng, V. M., Anderson, A. J., and Cotman, C. W. (1996) Crosslinking of membrane glycoproteins by Concanavalin A induces apoptosis in cortical neurons, *Neuroscience,* in press.
50. Kang, S. M., Beverly, B., Tran, A. C., Brorson, K., Schwartz, R. H., and Lenardo, M. J. (1992) Transactivation by AP-1 is a molecular target of T cell clonal anergy, *Science* **257,** 1134–1138.
51. Busciglio, J., Lorenzo, A., and Yankner, B. A. (1992) Methodological variables in the assessment of beta amyloid neurotoxicity, *Neurobiol. Aging* **13,** 609–612.
52. Davis-Salinas, J., Saporito-Irwin, S. M., Cotman, C. W., and Van Nostrand, W. E. (1995) Amyloid beta-protein induces its own production in cultured degenerating cerebrovascular smooth muscle cells, *J. Neurochem.* **65,** 931–934.
53. Pike, C. J., Cummings, B. J., Monzavi, R., and Cotman, C. W. (1994) Beta-amyloid-induced changes in cultured astrocytes parallel reactive astrocytosis associated with senile plaques in Alzheimer's disease, *Neuroscience* **63,** 517–531.
54. Fraser, P. E., Levesque, L., and McLachlan, D. R. (1994) Alzheimer Aβ amyloid forms an inhibitory neuronal substrate, *J. Neurochem.* **62,** 1227–1230.
55. Haxby, J. V. and Rapoport, S. I. (1986) Abnormalities of regional brain metabolism in Alzheimer's disease and their relation to functional impairment, *Prog. Neuropsychopharmacol. Biol. Psychiatry* **10,** 427–438.
56. McGeer, P. L., Kamo, H., Harrop, R., Li, D. K., Tuokko, H., McGeer, E. G., Adam, M. J., Ammann, W., Beattie, B. L., Calne, D. B., Martin, W. R. W., Pate, B. D., Rogers, J. G., Ruth, T. J., Sayre, C. I., and Stoessl, A. J. (1986) Positron emission tomography in patients with clinically diagnosed Alzheimer's disease, *Can. Med. Assoc. J.* **134,** 597–607.
57. Hoyer, S., Oesterreich, K., and Wagner, O. (1988) Glucose metabolism as the site of the primary abnormality in early-onset dementia of Alzheimer type? *J. Neurol.* **235,** 143–148.
58. Beal, M. F., Hyman, B. T., and Koroshetz, W. (1993) Do deficits in mitochondrial energy metabolism underlie the pathology of neurodegenerative diseases? *TINS* **16,** 178–184.
59. Goto, I., Taniwaki, T., Hosokawa, S., Otsuka, M., Ichiya, Y., and Ichimiya, A. (1993) Positron emission tomographic (PET) studies in dementia, *J. Neurol. Sci.* **114,** 1–6.
60. Copani, A., Koh, J., and Cotman, C. W. (1991) β-amyloid increases neuronal susceptibility to injury by glucose deprivation, *Neuroreport* **2,** 763–765.

61. Mattson, M. P., Cheng, B., Davis, D., Bryant, K., Lieberberg, I., and Rydel, R. E. (1992) β-amyloid peptides destabilize calcium homeostasis and render human cortical neurons vulnerable to excitotoxicity, *J. Neurosci.* **12,** 376–389.

62. Dornan, W. A., Kang, D. E., McCampbell, A., and Kang, E. E. (1993) Bilateral injections of βA(25–35)+IBO into the hippocampus disrupts acquisition of spatial learning in the rat, *NeuroReport* **5,** 165–168.

63. LaFerla, F. M., Tinkle, B. T., Bieberich, C. J., Haudenschild, C. C., and Jay, G. (1995) The Alzheimer's A beta peptide induces neurodegeneration and apoptotic cell death in transgenic mice, *Nature Genet.* **9,** 21–30.

64. Duke, R. C., Chervenak, R., and Cohen, J. J. (1983) Endogenous endonuclease-induced DNA fragmentation: an early event in cell-mediated cytolysis, *Proc. Natl. Acad. Sci. USA* **80,** 6361–6365.

65. Wyllie, A. H., Morris, R. G., Smith, A. L., and Dunlop, D. (1984) Chromatin cleavage in apoptosis: association with condensed chromatin morphology and dependence on macromolecular synthesis, *J. Pathol.* **142,** 67–77.

66. Tepper, C. G. and Studzinski, G. P. (1992) Teniposide induces nuclear but not mitochondrial DNA degradation, *Cancer Res.* **52,** 3384–3390.

67. Zakeri, Z. F., Quaglino, D., Latham, T., and Lockshin, R. A. (1993) Delayed internucleosomal DNA fragmentation in programmed cell death, *FASEB J.* **7,** 470–478.

68. Lennon, S. V., Martin, S. J., and Cotter, T. G. (1991) Dose-dependent induction of apoptosis in human tumour cell lines by widely diverging stimuli, *Cell Proliferation* **24,** 203–214.

69. Kunimoto, M. (1994) Methylmercury induces apoptosis of rat cerebellar neurons in primary culture, *Biochem. Biophys. Res. Commun.* **204,** 310–317.

70. Su, J. H., Anderson, A. J., Cummings, B. J., and Cotman, C. W. (1994) Immunohistochemical evidence for DNA fragmentation in neurons in the AD brain, *Neuroreport* **5,** 2529–2533.

71. Anderson, A. J., Su, J. H., and Cotman, C. W. (1996) DNA damage and apoptosis in Alzheimer's disease: colocalization with c-*Jun* immunoreactivity, relationship to brain area, and effect of postmortem delay, *J. Neurosci.* **16,** 1710–1719.

72. Mullaart, E., Boerrigter, M. E. T. I., Ravid, R., Swaab, D. F., and Vijg, J. (1990) Increased levels of DNA breaks in cerebral cortex of Alzheimer's disease patients, *Neurobiol. Aging* **11,** 169–173.

73. Satou, T., Cummings, B. J., and Cotman, C. W. (1995) Immunoreactivity for BCL-2 protein within neurons in the Alzheimer's disease brain increases with disease severity, *Brain Res.* **697,** 35–43.

74. Su, J. H., Satou, T., Anderson, A. J., and Cotman, C. W. (1996) Up-regulation of Bcl-2 is associated with neuronal DNA damage in Alzheimer's disease, *Neuroreport* **7,** 437–440.

75. Yamazaki, T., Yamaguchi, H., Nakazato, Y., Ishiguro, K., Kawarabayashi, T., and Hirai, S. (1992) Ultrastructural characterization of cerebellar diffuse plaques in Alzheimer's disease, *J. Neuropathol. Exp. Neurol.* **51,** 281–286.

76. Li, Y. T., Woodruff, P. D., and Trojanowski, J. Q. (1994) Amyloid plaques in cerebellar cortex and the integrity of Purkinje cell dendrites, *Neurobiol. Aging* **15,** 1–9.

77. Colotta, F., Polentarutti, N., Sironi, M., and Mantovani, A. (1992) Expression and involvement of c-*fos* and c-Jun protooncogenes in programmed cell death induced by growth factor deprivation in lymphoid cell lines, *J. Biol. Chem.* **267,** 18,278–18,283.

78. Estus, S., Zaks, W. J., Freeman, R. S., Gruda, M., Bravo, R., and Johnson, E. M. (1994) Altered gene expression in neurons during programmed cell death: identification of c-Jun as necessary for neuronal apoptosis, *J. Cell Biol.* **126,** 1717–1727.

79. Ham, J., Babij, C., Whitfield, J., Pfarr, C. M., Lallemand, D., Yaniv, M., and Rubin, L. L. (1995) A c-*Jun* dominant negative mutant protects sympathetic neurons against programmed cell death, *Neuron* **14,** 927–939.

80. Spillane, J. A., White, P., Goodhardt, M. J., Flack, R. H. A., Bowen, D. M., and Davison, A. N. (1977) Selective vulnerability of neurones in organic dementia, *Nature* **266,** 558–559.

81. Rossor, M. N., Garrett, N. J., Johnson, A. L., Mountjoy, C. Q., Roth, M., and Iverson, L. L. (1982) A post-mortem study of the cholinergic and GABA systems in senile dementia, *Brain* **105**, 313–330.

82. Smith, C. C., Bowen, D. M., Sims, N. R., Neary, D., and Davison, A. N. (1983) Amino acid release from biopsy samples of temporal neocortex from patients with Alzheimer's disease, *Brain Res.* **264**, 138–141.

83. Mountjoy, C. Q., Rossor, M. N., Iversen, L. L., and Roth, M. (1984) Correlation of cortical cholinergic and GABA deficits with quantitative neuropathological findings in senile dementia, *Brain* **107**, 507–518.

84. Lowe, S. L., Francis, P. T., Procter, A. W., Palmer, A. M., Davison, A. N., and Bowen, D. M. (1988) Gamma-aminobutyric acid concentration in brain tissue at two stages of Alzheimer's disease, *Brain* **111**, 785–799.

85. Anderson, A. J., Pike, C. J., and Cotman, C. W. (1995) Differential induction of immediate early gene proteins in cultured neurons by beta-amyloid (Aβ): association of c-Jun with Aβ-induced apoptosis, *J. Neurochem.* **65**, 1487–1498.

86. Anderson, A. J., Cummings, B. J., and Cotman, C. W. (1994) Increased immunoreactivity for *Jun*- and *Fos*-related proteins in Alzheimer's disease: association with pathology, *Exp. Neurol.* **125**, 286–295.

87. Rosl, F. (1992) A simple and rapid method for detection of apoptosis in human cells, *Nucleic Acids Res.* **20**, 5243.

88. Tilly, J. L. and Hsueh, A. J. (1993) Microscale autoradiographic method for the qualitative and quantitative analysis of apoptotic DNA fragmentation, *J. Cell. Physiol.* **154**, 519–526.

89. Beilharz, E. J., Williams, C. E., Dragunow, M., Sirimanne, E. S., and Gluckman, P. D. (1995) Mechanisms of delayed cell death following hypoxic-ischemic injury in the immature rat: evidence for apoptosis during selective neuronal loss, *Brain. Res. Mol. Brain. Res.* **29**, 1–14.

90. Portera-Cailliau, C., Herdeen, J. C., Price, D. L., and Koliatsos, V. E. (1995) Evidence for apoptotic cell death in Huntington disease and excitotoxic animal models, *J. Neurosci.* **15**, 3775–3787.

91. Lippa, C. F., Hamos, J. E., Pulaski, S. D., DeGennaro, L. J., and Drachman, D. A. (1992) Alzheimer's disease and aging: effects on perforant pathway perikarya and synapses, *Neurobiol. Aging* **13**, 405–411.

92. Boerrigter, M. E., Wei, J. Y., and Vijg, J. (1992) DNA repair and Alzheimer's disease, *J. Gerontol.* **47**, B177–184.

93. Mazzarello, P., Poloni, M., Spadari, S., and Focher, F. (1992) DNA repair mechanisms in neurological diseases: facts and hypotheses, *J. Neurol. Sci.* **112**, 4–14.

94. Cribbs, D. H., Martinou, J. C., Knowles, J., and Cotman, C. W. (1996) Overexpression of bcl-2 protects against β-amyloid toxicity in cultured hippocampal neurons (submitted).

95. Reed, J. C. (1994) Bcl-2 and the regulation of programmed cell death, *J. Cell Biol.* **124**, 1–6.

95a. Anderson, A. J., Su, J. H., and Cotman, C. W. (1996) Increase in immunoreactivity for the DNA repair enzyme Ref-1 in Alzheimer's disease brain, submitted.

96. Xanthoudakis, S., Miao, G., Wang, F., Pan, Y., and Curran, T. (1992) Redox activation of Fos-Jun DNA binding activity is mediated by a DNA repair enzyme, *EMBO J.* **11(9)**, 3323–3335.

97. Whittemore, E. R., Loo, D. T., and Cotman, C. W. (1994) Exposure to hydrogen peroxide induces cell death via apoptosis in cultured rat cortical neurons, *Neuroreport* **5**, 1485–1488.

98. Cribbs, D. H., Davis-Salinas, J., Cotman, C. W., and vanNostrand, W. E. (1995) β-Amyloid induces increased expression and processing of the amyloid precursor protein in cortical neurons, *Alzheimer's Res.* **1**, 197–200.

99. Wetzel, R. (1994) Mutations and off-pathway aggregation of proteins, *Trends Biotechnol.* **12**, 193–198.

100. Kelly, J. W. (1996) Alternative conformations of amyloidogenic proteins govern their behavior, *Curr. Opinion Struct. Biol.* **6**, 11–17.

101. Taubes, G. (1996) Misfolding the way to disease, *Science* **271**, 1493–1495.

7

Energy/Glucose Metabolism in Neurodegenerative Diseases

John P. Blass

1. INTRODUCTION

That disorders in energy/glucose metabolism can cause neurological and psychiatric disorders has been known for over a century. After the work of Claude Bernard on the importance of glucose metabolism, the German-speaking neurologists, psychiatrists, and pathologists ("alienists") recognized on neuropathological grounds that impairing the supply of glucose and oxygen to the brain could cause a variety of neurological syndromes *(1,2)*. That impairments of energy/glucose metabolism were important causes of diseases of the brain remained conventional wisdom through the 1950s. Among the evidence in support of this view were:

1. Extensive studies in aviation medicine, documenting the sensitivity of higher brain functions to reductions in oxygen tension *(3)*;
2. The widespread use of hypoglycemic (insulin) shock therapy in the treatment of psychoses; and
3. The recognition from even early neurochemical studies that (a) mammalian brain has a second-to-second dependence on glucose/energy metabolism to maintain function, and (b) impairments of cerebral glucose/energy metabolism typically impair brain function.

For instance, Judah Quastel *(4)* wrote in 1932:

The mental symptoms accompanying anoxaemia (as, for instance, that following ascent to high altitudes) are well known. They include loss of judgement and memory, disorientation for time, irritability, and emotional instability. Abnormal mental symptoms accompany carbon monoxide poisoning, and there appears to be little question that anoxaemia of the brain leads to irrational behavior. Anoxaemia may not only be created by lack of oxygen, however, but by conditions which render the oxygen unavailable for oxidative processes. Hence disturbances in the nervous system which result in diminished rates of oxidation will be as productive of mental disorder as lack of oxygen alone.

Subsequent neurochemical studies have continued to support Quastel's prescient proposal. For instance, delirium ("metabolic encephalopathy") is characteristically associated with decrements in the rate of cerebral glucose metabolism (CMR_{glu} and CMR_{O_2}), with consequent impairment of cholinergic transmission *(5)*. Since the mid-1960s, investigators have tended to favor the view that diseases of the brain are more

From: Molecular Mechanisms of Dementia *Edited by:* W. Wasco and R. E. Tanzi Humana Press Inc., Totowa, NJ likely related to genes that are expressed only or primarily in the brain, including "rare" message (mRNA), than in genes the expression of which occurs not only in neurons, but also in other types of cells. However, more recent molecular neurobiological and molecular genetic data have supported the suggestion that impairments of brain glucose/energy metabolism can be important causes of diseases of the brain.

The data from molecular neurobiology include data from studies of transgenic "knockout" mice. Although there have been some striking successes in modeling human neurological diseases in knockout mice, surprisingly often the knockout of a gene/gene product previously considered critical for brain function has not been associated with detectable pathology in the transgenic mouse carrying that knockout. The surprising absence of signs and symptoms in mice lacking these molecules may reflect redundancy in the nervous system in the pathways/mechanisms in which these molecules participate, particularly if the molecules are missing during neural development. For instance, it is well established that a number of neurotransmitters and growth/maintenance factors can converge on a relatively limited number of intracellular signaling mechanisms. In sharp contrast, there is no redundancy in the main pathways of glucose/energy metabolism. To a limited extent and under special conditions, glycolysis (the breakdown of glucose to pyruvate and lactate) can be bypassed by a high-fat, highly ketonemic diet *(6)*. However, there are no quantitatively significant pathways that bypass the Krebs tricarboxylic acid cycle and electron transport in mammalian brain. These old pathways, which are similar in plants and animals and in most bacteria, are essential to mammalian life and specifically to brain function. These observations suggest that intrinsic impairments in these pathways could be a fertile area for genetic causes of neurological and psychiatric disorders *(7–10)*.

In fact, molecular genetics has supported that hypothesis. Studies over the last 35 yr have documented many neurological disorders associated with functionally significant mutations in the pathways of glucose/energy metabolism in association with neurological disease *(8)*. Mutations associated with disease of the nervous system have been reported in all the major pathways of glucose/energy metabolisms *(8)*. These data indicate that functionally significant mutations in the components of these nonredundant pathways are compatible with extrauterine life. The extensive data include demonstrations of specific mutations at the genomic level, in both nuclear genes *(11)* and in mtDNA *(12)*.

Of great interest is a recent report that polyglutamines, such as those found in the proteins produced from the genes for Huntington's disease (HD) and dentorubralpallidoluysian atrophy (DRPLA), can bind to a highly regulated enzyme of carbohydrate catabolism, glyceraldehyde-3-phosphate dehydrogenase (GAPDH) *(13)*. These recent data suggest an interesting mechanism linking mutations in genes other than those of glucose/energy metabolism to the development of intrinsic impairments in these critical pathways.

The neurochemical data for the presence and importance of abnormalities of glucose/energy metabolism have been extensively reviewed, particularly in relation to Alzheimer's disease (AD) *(7–10)*. The discussion below briefly:

1. Reviews these data, emphasizing newer findings;
2. Discusses the genetic data; and
3. Briefly reviews the pathophysiological relevance of these findings to AD, HD, and DPRLA, including a brief discussion of the "slow excitotoxic hypothesis."

2. NEUROCHEMICAL DATA

The neurochemical data supporting the role of glucose/energy metabolism in AD and HD come from both in vivo and in vitro studies; in spinocerebellar ataxias (of which DRPLA is one), the data are primarily in vitro.

In vivo studies since the late 1940s have consistently shown impairments in glucose and oxidative metabolism in a variety of disorders that impair mentation, including specifically AD/"senile dementia" (*see* ref. *14* for review). Originally, these reductions in CMR_{glu} and CMR_{O_2} were thought to be important contributors to the brain dysfunction and damage. Subsequent measurements, although confirming the deficits, indicated that autoregulation was maintained and that oxygen extraction fraction was normal, and were interpreted to indicate that the decrease in cerebral metabolic rate was secondary to a combination of atrophy and dysfunction. However, three types of evidence favor the earlier interpretation—namely that the reductions in glucose/energy metabolism contribute to the brain damage. First, quantitatively, the amount of atrophy and decreased electrophysiologic function cannot account for the magnitude of the metabolic decrease *(14)*. Metabolic rate is measured per unit remaining tissue, so the decreases in metabolic rate could only be explained by atrophy if there were selective atrophy of cells and structures that had a high metabolic rate compared to the remaining tissue. In fact, the metabolic rate of neurons and synapses is only moderately higher than that of glia, and the loss of neurons in AD brain is not great enough to account for the quantitative decrease in overall brain metabolism in AD *(14)*. The decrease in metabolic rate in AD can be as great as that in insulin coma, but occurs in AD patients who are walking around and often agitated, and whose only EEG abnormality is mild nonspecific slowing. Second, the observation that autoregulation and oxygen extraction are normal in AD is relevant to the role of cerebrovascular disease, but it does not bear one way or the other on the presence of intrinsic abnormalities in the cellular metabolic machinery for oxidizing glucose to CO_2 and water.

Third, and perhaps most important, studies during the last five years have indicated that impairments of cerebral glucose metabolism precede the development of behavioral, electrophysiologic, or anatomic damage in patients at high risk for AD *(15–17)*. Convincing data have been presented for patients who are ApoE 4/ApoE 4 homozygotes *(15)*, and for patients in kindreds with familial AD *(16,17)*. It is, of course, possible to hypothesize that the techniques presently available are too insensitive to detect some subtle anatomic or physiological changes in these nonsymptomatic individuals at high risk to develop AD. However, there is no compelling evidence for that hypothesis. Impairment of cerebral glucose metabolism is a well-known cause of neuronal damage and death, including neuronal death in a pattern of selective vulnerability, as in the four-vessel occlusion rat stroke model used by Sims and Pulsinelli *(18)*. The straightforward interpretation of the recent PET scan data is that the decrements in cerebral glucose/energy metabolism contribute to subsequent brain damage in the presymptomatic patients at high risk for AD.

In HD, PET studies also indicate a decrement in cerebral glucose/energy metabolism in the brains, and specifically in the caudate nuclei, in patients who are still presymptomatic and do not yet have impressive caudate or cerebral atrophy *(19)*. Again, the most straightforward interpretation of these data is that the decrement in cerebral glucose/energy metabolism contributes to the death of nerve cells, particularly in caudate, in presymptomatic patients at high risk for HD.

In spinocerebellar ataxias, metabolic studies have shown a shift in glucose metabolism that is consistent with a decrease in oxidative metabolism and an increase in glycolysis (20). However, investigations are less extensive than in AD and HD.

In vitro studies over the last 20+ yr have documented the existence of deficiencies in the activities of major enzymes of carbohydrate/energy metabolism in AD, HD, and spinocerebellar diseases.

In AD, robust reductions occur in the activities of the pyruvate dehydrogenase complex (PDHC) and of the a-ketoglutarate dehydrogenase complex (KGDHC) (10,14). Both PDHC and KGDHC are large, multienzyme complexes, which can be considered to be submitochondrial structures rather than discrete enzymes. Both complexes have been well characterized chemically, notably by Reed and his coworkers (21). PDHC catalyzes the conversion of pyruvate (primarily derived from glucose by glycolysis) to acetyl-coenzyme A and CO_2, with the concomitant generation of NADH. The PDHC catalyzed reaction is quantitatively the important step by which the products of glucose metabolism enter the Krebs tricarboxylic acid cycle. KGDHC is an enzyme of the Krebs cycle, catalyzing the conversion of α-ketoglutarate to succinyl-coenzyme and CO_2, with concomitant generation of NADH. The KGDHC-catalyzed reaction appears to be the rate-limiting step in the Krebs tricarboxylic acid cycle in mammalian brain. The substrate of KGDHC, α-ketoglutarate, is generated not only through the Krebs cycle, but also from glutamate by transamination and by the glutamate dehydrogenase (GDH) catalyzed reaction. Therefore, KGDHC can be thought of as a component of glutamate metabolism as well as of glucose metabolism (14). This consideration is particularly interesting with regard to "excitotoxic" theories of neurodegenerative diseases (see Section 4.2.).

Decreased activity of Complex IV, a component of the electron transport chain, has also been reported in AD brain (22). Electron transport is the process by which reducing equivalents generated in metabolism, and notably in the Krebs tricarboxylic acid cycle, are oxidized to water. Complex IV, also called cytochrome oxidase, catalyzes the terminal step, which utilizes molecular oxygen with the production of water. The decrease in Complex IV activity is not as robust as those in PDHC and KGDHC. For instance, unlike the deficiencies in PDHC and KGDHC, that in Complex IV is found primarily in neuropathologically damaged areas of AD brain and not in anatomically normal areas (22,23). Rapport (23) has suggested that the decrease in Complex IV activity in AD is secondary to the disease process. Complex IV contains both proteins coded on the nuclear genome and on the mitochondrial genome (mtDNA). Krystal and coworkers (24) have shown that decreased transcription of mtDNA is an early response to a variety of insults to cells. The data of Krystal and coworkers (24) are in accord with Rapport's (23) proposal regarding the mechanism of decrease of Complex IV activity in AD.

In HD, decreased activity of PDHC has been reported in autopsy brain (25). Decreased activity of Complex I of the electron transport chain has also been reported in HD brain (26). Since components of Complex I are coded on mtDNA, the same cautions are relevant in interpreting the decrease in Complex I activity in HD as for Complex IV in AD.

In spinocerebellar ataxias, deficiencies have been reported in the activity of KGDHC (27). More extensive studies have been done in nonneural cells, as discussed below.

Nonneural cells, including cultured skin fibroblasts, have also been used to demonstrate deficiencies in glucose/energy metabolism in AD and, more controversially, in HD and in spinocerebellar ataxias. The theory behind these studies has been that molecules that are identical in the brain and in nonneural tissues can be studied in the more accessible peripheral tissues as well as in samples of brain; furthermore, cellular processes in which those molecules are involved can also be studied in the nonneural cells. Since most, although not all, of the molecules of glucose/energy metabolism are the same in brain and nonneural tissues, this hypothesis has proven particularly useful in the study of glucose/energy metabolism in neurodegenerative disease *(14)*. This assumption has been called, perhaps somewhat misleadingly, the "systemic disease hypothesis" of AD and other neurodegenerative diseases *(7,8)*.

In AD, glucose metabolism is abnormal in cultured skin fibroblasts *(28,29)*, and oxygen uptake has been reported to be decreased in cultured skin fibroblasts *(28)*. In disrupted AD fibroblasts, activity of KGDHC has been found to be decreased *(30,31)*, but that of PDHC and other mitochondrial enzymes was found to be at least normal *(30)*. Immunoblotting studies suggested the possible existence of an abnormality in the E2k component of KGDHC in AD *(30)*. Deficient activity of Complex IV has been reported in AD platelets *(32)*, but this finding was not confirmed in another study *(33)*.

In HD, the literature on the properties of cultured skin fibroblasts is extensive, confusing, and controversial *(34,35)*. A possible explanation may lie in the evidence for a PDHC deficit in HD (brain) and in the recent studies of Burke et al. *(13)*. Cultured human fibroblasts can use glutamine even more efficiently than they do glucose as a substrate. Both the studies of Sorbi et al. *(25)* and those of Burke et al. *(13)* suggest that Huntington cells may use glucose as a substrate less efficiently than they do glutamine. Glutamine is chemically unstable at physiological pH, slowly hydrolyzing to glutamate and NH_3. Standard technique for culturing human fibroblasts requires the periodic addition of freshly made up glutamine to the culture medium. However, in practice, the meticulousness with which this replenishment is done varies remarkably among laboratories. It will be of interest to compare systematically the properties of HD fibroblasts cultured in the presence and absence of added glutamine, compared to non-HD controls.

In spinocerebellar ataxias, the existence of defects in the activity of glutamate dehydrogenase (GDH) in fibroblasts from a subgroup of patients is widely accepted *(36)*. Defects in the activity of PDHC and KGDHC were reported in cultured skin fibroblasts from patients with spinocerebellar ataxia in 1976 *(37)*. The hypothesis was put forward that there might be a defect in the protein common to these two dehydrogenase complexes, namely their E3 component, lipoamide dehydrogenase (LAD). Subsequent studies of LAD in ataxias were controversial, with both claims of deficiencies *(38)* and refutations of those claims *(39)*. Deficiency of PDHC itself has, however, been confirmed in spinocerebellar ataxias *(40)*. Sorbi and coworkers *(41)* have shown the existence of deficiencies in the activities of mitochondrial enzymes of glucose/energy metabolism in patients with spinocerebellar ataxia. The common theme that appears to emerge is that impairment of glucose/energy metabolism is frequently and perhaps typically a part of the cellular lesion in hereditary ataxias.

3. MOLECULAR GENETIC DATA

Molecular genetic data supporting a significant role for deficiencies in glucose/ energy metabolism in AD, HD, and spinocerebellar ataxias are of three types. First, genetic defects in the major pathways of glucose/energy metabolism can exist and cause disease *(8)*. These defects have been documented on the genomic level—for instance, a variety of mutations in the αE1 component of PDHC *(42)*. Second, incomplete data support the possibility that a genetic abnormality in a component of KGDHC is associated with increased risk of later-onset AD *(43)*. The gene is DLST, which codes for the E2k component of KGDHC. E2k also known as dihydrolipoyl succinyltransferase, is the core protein component of the complex. The gene is found on chromosome 14q24.3, about one million base pairs away from the presenilin 1 gene for early onset familial Alzheimer's disease (FAD) *(44,45)*. The gene is approx 30 Kb in size and includes 15 exons *(45)*. Five common polymorphisms have been recognized in it (Sarkar et al., unpublished data). There is also a pseudogene on chromosome 1 that contains several single base deletions and insertions, which lead to the premature termination of translation *(45,46)*. The pseudogene is, however, transcribed; indeed, in cultured human fibroblasts, the level of the mRNA from the pseudogene is approximately the same as the level of the mRNA from the true gene (Sheu, unpublished observations). Studies including Northern blotting and PCR must take into account the presence of the transcribed pseudogene in order to avoid misleading artifacts.

DLST is not a gene for early onset, chromosome 14-linked FAD. The weak associations between polymorphisms of DLST and early onset, C14-linked FAD appear to be owing to linkage of the DLST gene to the nearby gene for presenilin 1.

DLST may be the gene associated with late-onset AD. Studies of late onset AD were undertaken primarily to complete the ruling out of an abnormality in this gene as a cause for the well-documented KGDHC deficiency in AD. Surprisingly, an association between polymorphisms of DLST and the occurrence of AD appeared to be present *(43)*. At the time of this writing, the odds ratio for the best-studied polymorphism in the best-studied ethnic group is 10.8. A pathogenic mutation has not, however, been identified as yet. Further studies with much larger series of patients and age, sex, and ethnically matched controls are in progress. If these findings prove correct, they will constitute "proof of principle" that abnormalities in glucose/energy metabolism can predispose to the occurrence of AD.

Third, recent findings by Burke and colleagues *(13)* indicate that polyglutamines can bind to at least one major enzyme of glucose/energy metabolism, namely the GAPDH. Polyglutamines occur in the abnormal proteins produced from the abnormal genes in Huntington's disease ("huntingtin") and in DRPLA. The polyglutamine sequences result from the CAG repeats characteristic of these abnormal genes. Clearly, further studies are required to clarify the possible binding of the polyglutamines to other proteins, including other dehydrogenases, and the functional significance of such binding, and explanation of the different neuropathological patterns of diseases associated with CAG repeats in specific gene. The report of Burke et al. *(13)* is, however, certainly provocative and may prove seminal in the understanding of the biochemistry of neurodegenerative diseases associated with CAG repeats.

4. PATHOPHYSIOLOGICAL CONSIDERATIONS

The potential pathophysiological significance of abnormalities in glucose/energy metabolism in neurodegenerative diseases has been the subject of a number of recent reviews *(9,10,14)*. For instance, in AD, disordered energy metabolism can contribute to the accumulation of amyloid precursor protein *(47)*, cytoskeletal disorganization, including the appearance of epitopes associated with paired helical filaments, abnormalities of signal transduction, deficiencies in cholinergic transmission, and neuronal and synaptic loss in a pattern of selective vulnerability (*see* refs. *10* and *14* for reviews and original references). The following discussion deals with only three facets of cellular pathophysiology in these diseases, namely the relation of disorders in glucose/energy metabolism to: the maintenance of cellular homeostasis; to excitotoxicity; and to free radical metabolism.

4.1. Cellular Homeostasis

This requires the continuous provision of energy, since cells maintain themselves in a nonequilibrium steady state. The energy-requiring functions include repair and renewal of cellular constituents, secretion, compartmentation, and ion homeostasis between the intracellular and extracellular milieu. The latter is particularly important in excitable cells, such as neurons. The rate of glucose/energy metabolism necessary depends on the functional demands put on a cell. Anesthesia or lowering body temperature is well established to afford partial protection against the effects of impairments of glucose/energy metabolism. On the other hand, excessive metabolic demands, such as those occurring in experimental or clinical status epilepticus, can outrun the metabolic capacity of even normal cells *(48)*. Furthermore, impairments of glucose/energy metabolism that do not appear harmful to resting cells can lead to cell damage and death when the metabolic demands on the cells are increased *(49,50)*. In the current context, a striking example is the persistence of glucose-deprived fetal neurons in culture under basal conditions and their rapid degeneration and death when toxic fragments of APP or free-radical generators are added to the culture medium *(51)*.

A point that needs emphasis is that a number of deleterious changes can occur with impairment of glucose/energy metabolism before measurable changes in ATP levels or energy charge potential is detected. These include changes in signal transduction *(52)*, in cellular calcium homeostasis *(53)*, and probably in the electromotive force across the mitochondrial membrane *(54)*. Fall in ATP levels tends to occur late, when cells are dying. Experimental data disprove the older idea that alterations in glucose/energy metabolism can be important only by affecting ATP levels.

Another often unrecognized point is that impairment of glucose/energy level can cause the death of neurons in patterns of selective vulnerability. A number of experimental and clinical examples have been reviewed previously *(10,14)*. Two provide particularly clear examples directly relevant to this discussion. In the experimental, four-vessel occlusion rat stroke model of Pulsinelli and coworkers *(18)*, controlled total brain ischemia leads to selective loss of neurons in caudate and 2 d later in hippocampus. In the hippocampus, CA1 neurons are lost, but CA2 neurons are spared—exquisite selective neuronal vulnerability resulting from total brain ischemia. Another example is the vulnerability of the caudate nucleus to the systemic injection of the antimetabolite 3-nitropropionic acid *(55)*. Thus, experimental data disprove the older assumption that significant impairments of glucose/energy metabolism must lead to diffuse, nonspecific brain dysfunction.

4.2. Excitotoxicity

This can be thought of as a special case of the general principle that metabolic demands can outrun the capacity of cellular glucose/energy metabolism to support homeostatic mechanisms. Excitation of a cell by glutamate or other excitotoxin is toxic rather than physiological when the cell is driven beyond its capacity to maintain homeostasis. Direct, robustly replicable experimental evidence indicates that impairments in glucose/energy metabolism that do not appear to harm resting neurons can lead to death of the cells when they are exposed to levels of excitotoxins, which do not harm similar cells in which glucose/energy metabolism is normal *(49–51)*. These considerations are particularly interesting regarding "slow excitotoxic injury." In slow excitotoxic injury, neurons exposed to relatively low levels of glutamate or other excitatory neurotransmitters are believed to degenerate and die prematurely. Thus, in "slow excitotoxic injury," the level of excitation exceeds the capacity of the excited neurons to maintain homeostasis. This may be owing to excessive excitation, but it could also be resulting from inadequate ability of the neurons to mobilize mechanisms to maintain homeostasis. Specifically, genetic impairments of the cellular machinery for glucose/energy metabolism, which may appear to be harmless polymorphisms in short-term studies, may turn out to predispose to "slow excitotoxic death" in neurodegenerative diseases. At least this formulation is consistent with currently available data.

4.3. Free Radicals

The pioneering studies of Harmon *(56)* and, more recently, of other workers *(50,51,57)* have demonstrated that free radicals are involved in aging and in a number of diseases of the nervous system. Excessive free radical action appears to occur in AD brain *(57)*. Since free radical mechanisms are part of the mechanisms of apoptosis and of inflammation, the presence of excessive free radicals in areas of histological damage in AD *(57)* may be at least in part biomarkers for the presence of processes well recognized to occur as part of this disease.

However, impairment of glucose/energy metabolism may impair the ability of neurons to reduce the levels of ("scavenge") free radicals *(50,51)*. Chemically, removal of free radicals involves their reduction. The quantitatively major source of reducing equivalents in the brain is glucose metabolism, with the resultant formation of NADH and NADPH. These adenine nucleotides can be used to maintain sulfhydryl groups in the reduced form, including, for instance, the sulfhydryl group in the free radical scavenger glutathione. Impairment of glucose catabolism could be expected to impair the generation of reducing equivalents and therefore their chemical activity. Although this proposal needs to be tested experimentally, it does provide a plausible mechanism by which impairments of glucose/energy metabolism could potentiate the action of free radicals in aging and neurodegenerative diseases.

4.4. Interactions Among Mechanisms

This discussion has focused on the role of impairments in glucose/energy metabolism in neurodegenerative diseases and, specifically, in AD, HD, and spinocerebellar ataxias. However, this discussion should not be construed to imply that other pathophysiological mechanisms in these diseases are not important. Indeed, as discussed, the major role of the impaired glucose/energy metabolism in these diseases may be to limit the ability of nerve cells to maintain homeostasis when metabolic demands are increased resulting from other pathophysiologically important stressors. This point has been discussed in detail elsewhere *(10,14)*. The well-established impairments in glucose/energy metabolism in these diseases may contribute to the causation of the diseases by potential damage from other causes. These considerations may be particularly important in AD, which is now recognized to be a heterogeneous disorder *(58)* that can be thought of as the "Alzheimer's syndrome" *(14)*.

REFERENCES

1. Blass, J. P., Hoyer, S., and Nitsch, R. (1992) Binswanger disease: in reply, *Arch. Neurol.* **49,** 799,800.
2. Blass, J. P., Hoyer, S., and Nitsch, R. (1991) A translation of Otto Binswanger's article, The Delineation of the Generalized Progressive Paralyses, *Arch. Neurol.* **48,** 961–972.
3. Gibson, G. E., Pulsinelli, W. A., and Blass, J. P. (1981) Brain dysfunction in mild to moderate hypoxia, *Am. J. Med.* **70,** 1247–1254.
4. Quastel, J. (1932) Anoxaemia and neurological disease, *Lancet* **2,** 14–16.
5. Gibson, G. E., Blass, J. P., Huang, H.-M., and Freeman, G. B. (1991) The cellular basis of delirium and its relevance to age related disorders including Alzheimer's disease, *International Psychoger.* **3,** 373–396.
6. Falk, R. E., Cederbaum, S. D., Blass, J. P., Pruss, R. J., and Carrel, R. E. (1976) Effects of a ketogenic diet in two brothers with pyruvate dehydrogenase deficiency, *Pediatrics* **58,** 713–721.
7. Blass, J. P., Gibson, G. E., Shimada, M., Kihara, T., Watanabe, M., and Kurinioto, K. (1980) Brain carbohydrate metabolism and dementia, in *Biochemistry of Dementia* (Burman, D. and Pennock, C. A., eds.), Wiley, London, pp. 121–134.
8. Blass, J. P., Sheu, K.-F. R., and Cederbaum, J. M. (1988) Energy metabolism in disorders of the nervous system, *Rev. Neurol. (Paris)* **144,** 543–563.
9. Beal, M. F. (1992) Does impairment of energy metabolism result in excitotoxic neuronal death in neurodegenerative diseases? *Ann. Neurol.* **31,** 119–123.
10. Blass, J. P., Sheu, K.-F. R., and Tanzi, R. (1996?) α-Ketoglutarate dehydrogenase in Alzheimer's disease, in *Energy Metabolism in Neurodegenerative Diseases* (Fiskum, G., ed.), Plenum, New York, pp. 185–192.
11. Chun, K., MacKay, N., Petrova-Benedict, R., Federico, A., Fois, A., Cole, D. E., Robertson, E., and Robinson, B. H. (1995) Mutations in the X-linked E1α subunit of pyruvate dehydrogenase: exon skipping, insertion of duplicate sequence, and missense mutations leading to the deficiency of the pyruvate dehydrogenase complex, *Am. J. Hum. Genet.* **56,** 558–569.
12. Wallace, D. C. (1994) Mitochondrial DNA sequence variation in human evolution and disease, *Proc. Natl. Acad. Sci. USA* **91,** 8739–8746.
13. Burke, J. R., Enghild, J. J., Martin, M. E., Jou, Y.-S., Myers, R. M., Roses, A. D., Vance, J. M., and Strittmater, W. J. (1996) Huntingtin and DRPLA proteins selectively interact with the enzyme GAPDH, *Nature Med.* **2,** 347–350.
14. Blass, J. P. (1993) Pathophysiology of the Alzheimer syndrome, *Neurology* **43(Suppl. 4),** S25–S38.
15. Reiman, E. M., Caselli, R. J., Yun, L. S., Chen, K., Bandy, D., Minoshima, S., Thibodeau, S. N., and Osborne, D. (1996) Preclinical evidence of Alzheimer's Disease in persons homozygous for the ε4 allele for apolipoprotein E, *N. Engl. J. Med.* **334,** 752–758.
16. Small, G. W., Mazziotta, J. C., and Collins, M. T. (1995) Apolipoprotein E type 4 allele and cerebral glucose metabolism in relatives at risk for familial Alzheimer's disease, *J. Am. Med. Assoc.* **273,** 942–947.

17. Kennedy, A. M., Frackowiak, R. S. J., and Newman, S. K. (1995) Deficits in cerebral glucose metabolism demonstrated by positron emission tomography in individuals at risk of familial Alzheimer's disease, *Neurosci. Lett.* **186,** 1270.

18. Sims, N. R. and Pulsinelli, W. A. (1987) Altered mitochondrial respiration in selectively vulnerable brain subregions following transient forebrain ischemia in the rat, *J. Neurochem.* **49,** 1367–1374.

19. Grafton, S. T., Maziotta, J. C., and Pahl, J. J. (1992) Serial changes of cerebral glucose metabolism and caudate size in persons at risk for Huntington's disease, *Arch. Neurol.* **49,** 1161–1167.

20. Gilman, S., Junck, L., Markel, D. S., Koeppe, R. A., and Kluin, K. J. (1990) Cerebral glucose hypermetabolism in Friedreich's ataxia detected with positron emission tomography, *Ann. Neurol.* **28,** 750–757.

21. Reed, L., Petit, F., and Yeaman, S. (1978) Pyruvate dehydrogenase complex: structure, function, and regulation, in *Microenvironments and Metabolic Compartmentation* (Srere, P. A. and Estabrook, R. W., eds.), Academic, New York, pp. 305–321.

22. Mutisya, E. M., Bowling, A. C., and Beal, M. F. (1994) Cortical cytochrome oxidase activity is reduced in Alzheimer's disease, *J. Neurochem.* **63,** 2179–2184.

23. Chandrasakaran, K., Giordano, T., Brady, D. R., Stoll, J., Martin, J., and Rapport, S. I. (1994) Impairment in mitochondrial cytochrome oxidase gene expression in Alzheimer's disease, *Brain Res. (Mol. Brain Res.)* **24,** 336–340.

24. Krystal, B. S., Chen, J., and Yu, B. P. (1994) Sensitivity of mitochondrial transcription to different free radical species, *Free Radicals in Biology and Medicine* **16,** 323–329.

25. Sorbi, S., Bird, E. D., and Blass, J. P. (1983) Decreased pyruvate dehydrogenase complex activity in Huntington and Alzheimer brain, *Ann. Neurol.* **13,** 72–78.

26. Parker, W. D., Boyson, S. J., and Luder, A. S. (1990) Evidence for a defect in NADH: ubiquinone oxidoreductase (complex I) in Huntington's disease, *Neurology* **40,** 1231–1234.

27. Mastrogiacomo, F. and Kish, S. J. (1994) Cerebellar α-ketoglutarate dehydrogenase activity is reduced in spinocerebellar ataxia type 1, *Ann. Neurol.* **5,** 624–626.

28. Sims, N. R., Finegan, J. M., and Blass, J. P. (1987) Altered metabolic properties of cultured skin fibroblasts in Alzheimer's Disease, *Ann. Neurol.* **21,** 451–457.

29. Peterson, C. and Goldman, J. E. (1986) Alterations in calcium content and biochemical processes in cultured skin fibroblasts from aged and Alzheimer donors, *Proc. Natl. Acad. Sci. USA* **83,** 2758–2762.

30. Sheu, K.-F. R., Cooper, A. J. L., Lindsay, J. G., and Blass, J. P. (1994) Abnormality in the α-ketoglutarate dehydrogenase complex in fibroblasts from familial Alzheimer's disease, *Ann. Neurol.* **35,** 312–318.

31. Sorbi, S., personal communication.

32. Parker, W. D., Filley, C. M., and Parks, J. K. (1990) Cytochrome oxidase deficiency in Alzheimer's disease, *Neurology* **40,** 1302–1304.

33. Van Zuylen, A. J., Bosman, G. J. C. G. M., and Ruitenbeck, W. (1992) No evidence for reduced thrombocyte cytochrome oxidase activity in Alzheimer's disease, *Neurology* **42,** 1246–1250.

34. Bondy, S. C. (1995) The relation of oxidative stress and hyperexcitation to neurological disease, *Proc. Soc. Exp. Biol. Med.* **208,** 337–345.

35. Gusella, J. F. and MacDonald, M. E. (1995) Huntington's disease, *Semin. Cell Biol.* **6,** 21–28.

36. Plaitakis, A., Berl, S., and Yahr, M. (1982) Abnormal glutamate metabolism in an adult-onset degenerative disorder, *Science* **216,** 193–196.

37. Blass, J. P., Kark, R. A. P., Menon, N., and Harris, S. H. (1976) Decreased activities of the pyruvate and ketoglutarate dehydrogenase complexes in fibroblasts from five patients with Friedreich's ataxia, *N. Engl. J. Med.* **295,** 62–66.

38. Rodriguez-Budelli, M. and Kark, R. A. P. (1978) The potential of lipoamide dehydrogenase kinetics for genetic counseling and preclinical diagnosis in certain inherited ataxias, *Neurology* **27,** 359–361.

39. Stumpf, D. A. and Parks, J. A. (1979) Friedreich ataxia II: Normal kinetics of lipoamide dehydrogenase, *Neurology* **29**, 820–826.

40. Cederbaum, J. M. and Blass, J. P. (1986) Mitochondrial dysfunction and spinocerebellar degeneration, *Neurochem. Pathol.* **4**, 43–46.

41. Sorbi, S., Piacentini, S., Fani, C., Tonini, S., Marini, P., and Amaducci, L. (1989) Abnormalities of mitohondrial enzymes in hereditary ataxias, *Acta Neurol. Scand.* **80**, 103–110.

42. Chun, K., MacKay, N., Petrova-Benedict, R., Federico, A., Fois, A., Cole, D. E., Robertson, E., and Robinson, B. H. (1995) Mutations in the X-linked E1α subunit of pyruvate dehydrogenase: exon skipping, insertion of double sequence, and missense mutations leading to the deficiency of the pyruvate dehydrogenase complex, *Am. J. Hum. Genet.* **56**, 558–569.

43. Sheu, K.-F. R., Sarkar, P., Wasco, W., Tanzi, R., and Blass, J. P. (1995) A gene locus of dihydrolipoyl succinyltransferase (DLST) is associated with Alzheimer's Disease, *J. Neurochem.* **66**, S10B.

44. Ali, G., Wasco, W., Cai, X., Szabo, P., Sheu, K.-F., Cooper, A. J., et al. (1994) Isolation, cloning, and localization of the gene for the E2k component of the human α-ketoglutarate dehydrogenase complex, *Somatic Cell Mol. Genet.* **20**, 99–104.

45. Nakano, K., Takase, C., and Sakomoto, T. (1994) Isolation, characterization, and structural organization of the gene and pseudogene for the dihydrolipoylamide succinyltransferase component ofthe 2-oxoglutarate dehydrogenase complex, *Eur. J. Biochem.* **224**, 179–186.

46. Cai, X., Szabo, P., Ali, G., and Blass, J. P. (1994) A pseudogene of dihydrolipoyl succinyltransferase (E2k) found by PCR amplification and direct sequencing in rodent-human cell hybrid DNAs, *Somatic Cell Mol. Genet.* **20**, 339–343.

47. Gabuzda, D., Busciglio, J., and Chen, L. B. (1994) Inhibition of energy metabolism alters the processing of amyloid precursor protein and induces a potentially amyloidogenic derivative, *J. Biol. Chem.* **269**, 13,628–13,635.

48. Ankarcrona, M., Dypbukt, J. M., Bonfoco, E., Zhivotovsky, B., Orrenius, S., Lipton, S. A., and Nicotera, P. (1995) Glutamate-induced neuronal death: a succession of necrosis or apoptosis depending on mitochondrial function, *Neuron* **15**, 961–973.

49. Henneberry, R. A. (1989) The role of energy in the toxicity of excitatory amino acids, *Neurobiol. Aging* **10**, 611–616.

50. Beal, M. F. (1995) Aging, energy, and oxidative stress in neurodegenative diseases, *Ann. Neurol.* **38**, 357–366.

51. Mattson, M. P. (1994) Mechanism of neuronal degeneration and preventive approaches: Quickening the pace of AD research, *Neurobiol. Aging* **15(Suppl. 2)**, S121–S125.

52. Gibson, G. E., Shimada, M., and Blass, J. P. (1978) Alterations in acetylcholine synthesis and in cyclic nucleotides in mild cerebral hypoxia, *J. Neurochem.* **31**, 757–760.

53. Huang, H.-M., Toral-Barza, L., and Gibson, G. E. (1991) Cytosolic free calcium and ATP in synaptosomes after ischemia, *Life Sci.* **48**, 1439–1445.

54. Blass, J. P. and Gibson, G. E. (1979) Consequences of mild, graded hypoxia, in *Advances in Neurology* (Fahn, S., ed.), Raven, New York, pp. 229–250.

55. Brouillet, E., Hantraye, P., Ferrante, R. J., Dolan, R., Leroy-Willig, A., Kowall, N. W., and Beal, M. F. (1995) Chronic mitochondrial energy impairment produces selective striatal degeneration and abnormal choreiform movements in primates, *Proc. Natl. Acad. Sci. USA* **92**, 7105–7109.

56. Harmon, D. (1995) Role of antioxidant nutrients in aging: Overview, *Age* **18**, 51–62.

57. Hensley, K., Hall, N., Subramaniam, R., Cole, P., Harris, M., Askenova, M., Gabbita, S. P., Wu, J. F., and Carney, J. M. (1995) Brain regional correspondence between Alzheimer's disease histopathology and biomarkers of protein oxidation, *J. Neurochem.* **65**, 2146–2156.

58. Schellenberg, G. D. (1995) Genetic dissection of Alzheimer disease, a heterogenous disorder, *Proc. Natl. Acad. Sci. USA* **92**, 8552–8559.

8

Calcium Homeostasis and Free Radical Metabolism as Convergence Points in the Pathophysiology of Dementia

Mark P. Mattson, Katsutoshi Furukawa, Annadora J. Bruce, Robert J. Mark, and Emmanuelle Blanc

1. INTRODUCTION

Realization that calcium and free radicals are key mediators of neuronal injury and death initially came from studies of acute neurodegenerative insults, such as ischemia or excitotoxic injury (*see* refs. *1* and *2* for review). At that time, many were skeptical (and some remain so) regarding the relevance of ischemic and excitotoxic injury to such disorders as Alzheimer's disease (AD). Nevertheless, it is becoming increasingly appreciated that "final common pathways" of cell death are very similar in both acute and chronic neurodegenerative conditions. Central to such final common pathways are calcium and free radicals, which can be considered transducers of cell death in both acute and chronic neurodegenerative conditions. There also existed somewhat of a dichotomy among researchers focusing on mechanisms of "necrotic" and "apoptotic" cell death, wherein "apoptologists" believed that there existed fundamental mechanistic differences that distinguished apoptosis from necrosis. That is, apoptosis was considered a process of cellular suicide involving induction of the expression of "cell death genes," whereas necrosis was a passive process resulting from an uncontrollable avalanche of ion influx and cell lysis (*see* ref. *3* for review). However, the more that mechanisms of cell death were studied, the more evident it became that calcium and free radicals are key mediators of both necrosis and apoptosis, and that the distinction between the two manifestations of cell death depended more on the quantity (severity and duration of the insult) than the quality of the insult. It is therefore critical that we understand the various genetic and environmental factors that influence neural calcium homeostasis and free radical metabolism. This translates into the following tacks of investigation:

1. Determining how mutations linked to specific neurodegenerative disorders impact on calcium regulation and free radical metabolism;
2. Identifying environmental factors that may compromise calcium homeostasis and promote free radical accumulation, and determining the specific molecular cascades involved; and

From: Molecular Mechanisms of Dementia Edited by: W. Wasco and R. E. Tanzi Humana Press Inc., Totowa, NJ

3. Elucidating the mechanisms whereby the brain normally resists neuronal degeneration (e.g., neurotrophic factor signal transduction pathways and acute response pathways).

Research along these three lines of investigation is the subject of this chapter.

2. CELLULAR CALCIUM HOMEOSTASIS IN NEURONS

The ability of neurons to maintain low rest levels of intracellular free calcium ($[Ca^{2+}]_i$), and to modulate $[Ca^{2+}]_i$ rapidly (spatially, temporally, and quantitatively) is conferred by an intricate set of membrane-associated and cytosolic calcium-regulating proteins (Fig. 1; and *see* ref. *4* for review). The concentration of calcium outside of nerve cells is typically in the 1–2 mM range, whereas $[Ca^{2+}]_i$ within the cytoplasm under resting conditions it ranges from 50 to 200 nM. This large transmembrane calcium concentration gradient is maintained largely by the plasma membrane calcium ATPase (PMCA), an energy-driven calcium pump. When neurons are stimulated (e.g., by glutamate released at a synapse or during an action potential), the $[Ca^{2+}]_i$ can rapidly (in seconds) rise to concentrations of well over 10 μM. The $[Ca^{2+}]_i$ is then rapidly removed from the cytoplasm by at least three different mechanisms. One mechanism involves activity of the plasma membrane Na^+/Ca^{2+} exchanger, which has a very high capacity. A second mechanism involves activity of a smooth endoplasmic reticulum Ca^{2+}-ATPase (SERCA), which pumps Ca^{2+} into the lumen of that organelle. A third mechanism involves cytoplasmic Ca^{2+}-binding proteins that may sequester Ca^{2+} and/or promote activation of membrane Ca^{2+} removal proteins, such as the PMCA; an example of such a Ca^{2+}-binding protein is calbindin D28k. In addition, mitochondria can sequester large amounts of calcium. Finally, the plasma membrane Na^+/K^+-ATPase serves an indirect role in maintenance of low $[Ca^{2+}]_i$ by maintaining the Na^+ gradient across the membrane, thereby discouraging Ca^{2+} influx through voltage-dependent channels. The major routes of calcium entry into the cytoplasm include voltage-dependent (VDCC) and ligand-gated (LGCC) calcium channels in the plasma membrane, and channels in the membrane of the endoplasmic reticulum. The VDCC include several different subtypes classified by their biophysical and pharmacological properties: T-type channels, which inactivate rapidly; L-type channels, which are high-conductance and remain open for long time periods following depolarization (L channels are blocked by organic blockers such as nifedipine); and N-type channels, which are intermediate conductance and are blocked by Ω conotoxin. A prominent LGCC is the *N*-methyl-D-aspartate (NMDA) glutamate receptor. The NMDA receptor is widely expressed in the brain, where it is particularly concentrated in regions (e.g., hippocampus) that play central roles in learning and memory processes. The NMDA channel requires membrane depolarization in order for it to open in response to glutamate binding. In addition to influx through plasma membrane channels, calcium can enter the cytoplasm through channels in the membrane of the endoplasmic reticulum. One class of such channels is activated by inositol triphosphate (IP$_3$), a product of inositol phospholipid hydrolysis released in response to stimuli that activate phospholipase C (PLC). For example, certain muscarinic acetylcholine receptors are linked to a GTP-binding protein called G_{q11}, which, in turn, can activate PLC. PLC then cleaves phosphatidylinositol 4,5-bis-phosphate to release diacylglycerol and IP$_3$. The diacylglycerol activates protein kinase C, whereas the IP$_3$ activates a calcium channel in the endoplasmic reticulum.

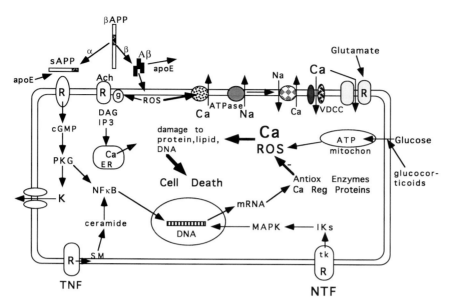

Fig. 1. Mechanisms, relevant to the pathogenesis of dementia, that destabilize or stabilize neuronal calcium homeostasis and free radical metabolism. Factors that tend to destabilize neuronal calcium homeostasis resulting in elevation of $[Ca^{2+}]_i$ include glutamate, reduced energy availability, and amyloid β-peptide (Aβ). Glutamate induces calcium influx by activating NMDA receptors, which themselves conduct calcium, and by activating AMPA and kainate receptors, which depolarize the membrane, resulting in opening of VDCC. Reduced glucose availability to neurons occurs in AD and presumably results in ATP depletion, compromise of Na^+/K^+-ATPase activity, and increased vulnerability to excitotoxicity; glucocorticoids may exacerbate energy depletion by impairing glucose transport into neurons. Aβ arises from βAPP via enzymatic processing involving β-secretase (β). Aβ forms fibrils and induces membrane oxidation, resulting in lipid peroxidation and impairment of Na^+/K^+-ATPase and Ca^{2+}-ATPase activities; this results in membrane depolarization, calcium influx, and increased sensitivity to excitotoxicity. Glutamate and energy deprivation induce several ROS, including superoxide anion radical, hydrogen peroxide, and NO; generation of these ROS appears to result from elevation of $[Ca^{2+}]_i$. On the other hand, induction of ROS by Aβ appears to be a primary event that occurs prior to elevation of $[Ca^{2+}]_i$. Elevation of $[Ca^{2+}]_i$ and ROS both contribute to damage to proteins, lipids, and DNA, and ultimately cell death. Subtoxic levels of membrane oxidation induced by Aβ can impair coupling of receptors, such as muscarinic acetylcholine receptors (ACh R), to the GTP-binding proteins (g) they activate. Neuroprotective signaling pathways that stabilize $[Ca^{2+}]_i$ and suppress accumulation of ROS include NTF, which activate receptor tyrosine kinases (tk R); a cascade of phosphorylation reactions involving intermediate kinases (IK) and mitogen-activated protein kinases (MAPK) results in activation of transcription factors. Genes whose expression is induced by NTF include proteins involved in regulation of $[Ca^{2+}]_i$ (e.g., calcium-binding proteins) and antioxidant enzymes (e.g., superoxide dismutases and catalase). TNF binds to a receptor (R), the activation of which results in hydrolysis of sphingomyelin, release of ceramide, and activation of the transcription factor NFκB. NFκB mediates induction of calcium-regulating proteins and antioxidant enzymes. Secreted forms of βAPP (sAPP) are liberated from βAPP as the result of neuronal activity. The sAPPs bind to a putative receptor linked to elevation of cGMP levels. The cGMP then activates a cGMP-dependent protein kinase, which may activate a protein phosphatase resulting in activation of a particular type of high-conductance potassium (K) channel. In this way, sAPPs hyperpolarize the membrane and counteract the depolarizing actions of glutamate, energy failure, and Aβ.

Differential expression of one or more of these proteins in nerve cells can have profound effects on their vulnerability to insults relevant to the pathogenesis of dementing disorders, including AD. For example, neurons expressing high levels of NMDA receptors are selectively vulnerable to injury induced by cerebral ischemia. Conversely, neurons expressing high levels of calbindin (e.g., dentate granule neurons of the hippocampus) are not vulnerable to excitotoxic and metabolic insults, and are preserved within neuronal populations in which surrounding neurons are killed (e.g., ischemia, epileptic seizures, and AD) *(5,6)*.

3. FREE RADICAL METABOLISM IN NEURONS

It has been known for a long time that free radicals, molecules with one or more unpaired electrons, can damage tissues and kill organisms *(7)*. However, during the last 10 yr, we have come to appreciate the many different sources of free radicals in cells, interrelationships of cellular signal transduction pathways and free radicals, and the many ways in which cells squelch reactive oxygen species (ROS). From the perspective of neurodegenerative disorders, studies of the involvement of free radicals in neuronal dysfunction and death have taken center stage with the discoveries that some inherited forms of neurodegenerative disease result from mutations in proteins involved in free radical metabolism *(8)* and that many mediators of neuronal injury act by inducing free radical production (*see* refs. *9* and *10* for review). A major site of free radical production in cells is mitochondria, where ROS, including superoxide radical ($O_2\cdot^-$), hydrogen peroxide (H_2O_2), and hydroxyl radical (OH·), are formed during the reduction of oxygen and its conversion to water (Fig. 2). Hydrogen peroxide and/or superoxide radical interacts with transition metals, such as iron, resulting in formation of the highly reactive OH·. ROS also arise from the arachidonic acid cascade of phospholipid metabolism, and self-oxidation reactions involving catecholamines, flavins, and ferridoxins. Unsaturated bonds of fatty acids are sites of free radical attack where lipid peroxides form and perpetuate an autocatalytic process of lipid peroxidation. Proteins and DNA are also damaged by free radical attack, which can compromise many homeostatic systems in cells, including those involved in Ca^{2+} regulation.

When prolonged elevation of Ca^{2+} or free radical levels occurs in neurons, a vicious feed-forward cycle ensues, such that Ca^{2+} induces free radical formation and vice versa. For example, activation of NMDA receptors induces Ca^{2+} influx, and the calcium stimulates phosphoinositol hydrolysis by activating phospholipases (PLC and PLA_2 in particular), leading to accumulation of arachidonic acid, and subsequent oxidation by cyclooxygenase (COX) and lipoxygenase (LOX) *(11,12)*. In addition, calcium influx through NMDA receptors mediates production of hydrogen peroxide *(13)* and nitric oxide (NO) via calmodulin-mediated activation of NO synthase (NOS) *(14)*. NO may further react with superoxide anion, resulting in the formation of peroxynitrite, a highly destructive radical *(15)*. In addition to inducing calcium influx, activation of glutamate receptors in a neuronal cell line impaired cystine uptake, resulting in glutathione depletion and accumulation of free radicals *(16)*. Addition of glutathione to cultures protected neurons against NMDA receptor-mediated toxicity *(17)*. It is, however, not clear that glutathione depletion is a key element of the excitotoxic mechanism, because very high (millimolar) levels of glutamate are required to impair cystine uptake markedly and deplete glutathione levels. Data from cell-culture studies of primary neurons

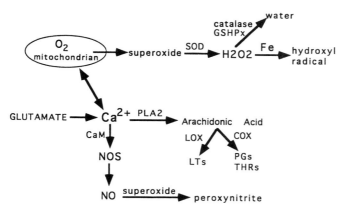

Fig. 2. Some key mechanisms involved in generation and removal of reactive oxygen species in neural cells. Superoxide anion radical is produced during the electron transport process in the mitochondria. SOD converts superoxide to hydrogen peroxide (H_2O_2). H_2O_2 can be converted to water by the enzymes catalase and glutathione peroxidase (GSH-Px). Alternatively, highly reactive hydroxyl radical can be produced via Fenton chemistry in the presence of iron (Fe). Elevation of intracellular Ca^{2+} levels induced, for example, by glutamate or amyloid β-peptide, promotes production of several different ROS. Ca^{2+} binds calmodulin and thereby activates nitric oxide synthase (NOS), resulting in the generation of NO; NO interacts with superoxide resulting in formation of peroxynitrite, which can damage proteins. In addition, Ca^{2+} promotes phospholipid hydrolysis via activity of phospholipase-A_2 (PLA_2). PLA_2 induces release of arachidonic acid, which is then attacked by LOX and COX with resultant oxyradical formation. Elevated cytoplasmic Ca^{2+} levels also alter mitochondrial transmembrane potential, which can lead to increased superoxide anion radical production. LT, leukotrienes; PG, prostaglandins; THRs, thromboxanes.

have clearly shown that neurons from several different brain regions can be killed by 10–100 μ*M* glutamate acting at NMDA and/or AMPA receptors, and by NMDA and kainate (which do not compete for cystine uptake). Since pharmacological blockade of NMDA and/or AMPA receptors attenuates or prevents neuronal injury in a variety of paradigms of glutamate toxicity (*see* Section 2.), it seems likely that glutamate inhibition of cystine uptake is of minor importance under those circumstances.

4. CALCIUM AND NEURONAL INJURY IN AD

Correlations between expression of particular Ca^{2+}-regulating proteins and selective neuronal vulnerability have been established that are consistent with roles for calcium dyshomeostasis in the pathophysiology of AD and related dementias. For example, studies of postmortem human brain have revealed interesting correlations between populations of neurons expressing particular calcium-binding proteins and their vulnerability in neurodegenerative disorders (*see* ref. 6 for review). For example, in the hippocampus, dentate granule cells express high levels of calbindin and do not degenerate in AD, whereas CA1 neurons express little or no calbindin and are vulnerable. Similarly, Parkinson's patients exhibit a marked decrease in dopaminergic neurons in the substantia nigra, but the number of calbindin-containing neurons remains constant *(18)*. The neurons that degenerate early in the course of AD (e.g., entorhinal cortex layer II cells and hippocampal CA1 neurons) express high levels of glutamate receptors, particularly those of the NMDA type *(19)*.

Clinical and epidemiological data also suggest roles for altered Ca^{2+} homeostasis and excitotoxicity in the pathogenesis of AD. A neurodegenerative syndrome concentrated on a few Western Pacific islands exhibits several features of AD, including neurofibrillary degeneration of neurons in hippocampus, entorhinal cortex, and several associated cortices *(20,21)*. Severe dementia occurs in these patients, although superimposed on the dementia are Parkinsonian- and amyotrophic lateral sclerosis-like symptoms that are directly related to degeneration of nigral dopaminergic and spinal cord motor neurons, respectively. Neurofibrillary tangles in these patients exhibit elevated levels of Ca^{2+} *(22)* consistent with the possibility that elevation of $[Ca^{2+}]_i$ plays a role in the demise of the neurons. This disorder does not have a genetic basis, and the two major hypotheses for its etiology both invoke dysregulation of Ca^{2+} homeostasis as the cause of neuronal degeneration. One hypothesis is that the natives consume an excitotoxin that is concentrated in one of their main food sources *(23)*. The other hypothesis invokes a dietary calcium/aluminum imbalance leading to secondary hyperparathyroidism *(24)*. An excitotoxic contribution to AD is also suggested by studies of excitotoxin intoxication, the best-documented example being an occurrence in Canada in which persons ingested mussels containing high levels of domoic acid. Several individuals developed dementia essentially indistinguishable from AD *(25)*. Administration of domoic acid to monkeys induced selective degeneration of many of the same neuronal populations in hippocampus and surrounding structures that degenerate in AD *(26)*.

Considerable experimental evidence supports the hypothesis that elevation of $[Ca^{2+}]_i$ is causally involved in neuronal degeneration in AD and related dementias. Much of the data have been summarized in recent reviews *(27,28)*, and some of the most compelling previous data and emerging findings will be focused on here. There is no doubt that prolonged elevation of $[Ca^{2+}]_i$ can kill neurons, and that Ca^{2+} plays a central role in the injury and death of neurons under excitotoxic and ischemic conditions (*see* ref. *29* for review). The definition of a central role for Ca^{2+} in excitotoxic and ischemic cell death was possible because of the existence of clearly defined cell-culture and animal models, the ability to monitor directly $[Ca^{2+}]_i$ in living neurons, and the development of pharmacological means to suppress elevation of $[Ca^{2+}]_i$ induced by excitotoxic and metabolic insults. In the case of AD, however, the models are less well developed.

One line of evidence supporting a role for dysregulation of Ca^{2+} homeostasis in the pathogenesis of AD is that several of the features of neuronal cell death in AD are similar to those observed in paradigms of Ca^{2+}-mediated neuronal injury. For example, exposure of rat and human primary brain cell cultures to glutamate or calcium ionophores resulted in alterations in the neuronal cytoskeleton similar to those seen in the neurofibrillary tangles of AD. The alterations included loss of microtubules, accumulation of 8–15 nm straight filaments, antigenic changes in τ and accumulation of τ in neuronal somata, proteolysis of microtubule-associated protein-2 (MAP2), and accumulation of ubiquitin immunoreactivity *(30,207)*. Sautiere et al. *(31)* also reported that glutamate induces tangle-like antigenic alterations in τ in cultured neurons. Although paired helical filaments (PHFs) were not observed in the latter studies, DeBoni et al. *(32)* reported that chronic exposure of cultured human spinal neurons to glutamate resulted in the appearance of PHF-like filamentous structures. In vivo studies showed that administration of kainic acid to adult rats induced cytoskeletal alterations in hippocampal pyramidal neurons similar to those seen in neurofibrillary tangles, including antigenic changes in τ, and proteolysis of MAP2 and spectrin *(33,34)*. Although the cause of neurofibrillary tangle formation in AD has not been definitively established, Busciglio et al. *(35)* recently provided a convincing demonstration that amyloid β-peptide (Aβ) can induce PHF-like epitopes associated with loss of microtubule binding to τ in cultured human cortical neurons, strongly implicating Aβ in the process of neurofibrillary tangle formation. In the latter study, it was also shown that the induction of the cytoskeletal alterations was tightly correlated with Aβ fibril formation, which is consistent with the pathology in AD brain (i.e., Aβ fibrils associated with neuritic pathology and diffuse Aβ not associated with pathology).

Studies that examined the mechanism of Aβ neurotoxicity also support a role for altered Ca^{2+} homeostasis and an excitotoxic mechanism of neuronal injury in AD. Exposure of cultured human cortical or rat hippocampal neurons to Aβ25–35, Aβ1–38, or Aβ1–40 caused a slow progressive elevation of rest $[Ca^{2+}]_i$ *(36,37)*. An even more striking finding was that neurons pretreated with Aβ exhibit greatly enhanced $[Ca^{2+}]_i$ responses to excitatory amino acids and membrane depolarization. Both the direct neurotoxicity of Aβ and the enhanced vulnerability to excitotoxicity were attenuated when cells were incubated in Ca^{2+}-deficient medium, indicating that Ca^{2+} influx was causally involved in the cell damage and death induced by Aβ *(36,37)*. In subsequent studies, Muller and colleagues found that Aβ increases the sensitivity of cultured mouse cortical neurons *(38)* and human lymphocytes *(39)* to signals that elevate $[Ca^{2+}]_i$. In addition, Weiss et al. *(40)* reported that the calcium channel blocker nimodipine can attenuate Aβ neurotoxicity in cultured neocortical cells.

Calbindin and calretinin are Ca^{2+}-binding proteins that may serve a neuroprotective function. Hippocampal neurons expressing calbindin are relatively resistant to excitotoxic insults in vivo and in cell culture *(5,41)*. Calcium imaging studies showed that neurons expressing calbindin in primary hippocampal cultures exhibit attenuated $[Ca^{2+}]_i$ responses to glutamate and a calcium ionophore *(41)*. In addition, it was recently reported that $[Ca^{2+}]_i$ responses are reduced in neurons injected with calbindin *(42)*. Of relevance to AD, neurons expressing calbindin in hippocampal cell cultures are relatively resistant to Aβ toxicity (Fig. 3), and trophic factors and cytokines that induce expression of calbindin in neurons protect them from Aβ toxicity *(37,43,44)*. More recently, we provided direct evidence that calbindin can protect cells against Aβ toxicity (Fig. 4). C6 glioma cells were transfected with calbindin cDNA, and clones expressing high levels of calbindin were selected. The cells expressing high levels of calbindin were resistant to the toxicities of a calcium ionophore and Aβ compared to cells expressing low levels of calbindin. Forloni et al. *(45)* and Loo et al. *(46)* reported that Aβ neurotoxicity manifests as apoptosis. On the other hand, Behl et al. *(47)* found that Aβ induced necrosis, and that the antiapoptotic gene product *bcl*-2 did not protect against Aβ toxicity *(48)*. We found that the toxicity of Aβ in the C6 glioma cells manifests as apoptosis and that calbindin-expressing B6 cells were protected against apoptosis (Fig. 4). In a rat model of selective damage to entorhinal cortex layer II cells, Peterson et al. *(19)* recently showed that calbindin-expressing neurons are spared. An increasing number of findings suggest that calretinin also plays a neuroprotective role. For example, Pike and Cotman *(49)* reported that cultured hippocampal neurons expressing calretinin are resistant to Aβ toxicity.

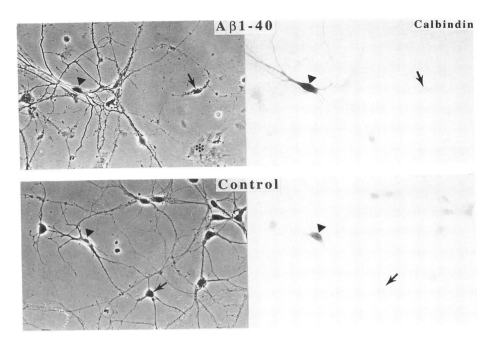

Fig. 3. Primary hippocampal neurons expressing calbindin are resistant to Aβ toxicity. Embryonic rat hippocampal cell cultures (8 d in culture) were exposed to 10 μM Aβ1–40 or vehicle (control) for 24 h. The cells were then fixed and immunostained with an antibody to calbindin D28k. Phase-contrast (left) and bright-field (right) micrographs of a field in the Aβ-treated culture and the control culture are shown. Note that in the Aβ-treated culture the calbindin-containing neuron was undamaged (arrowhead), whereas neurons not expressing calbindin degenerated (e.g., arrow). The * marks an aggregate of Aβ on the culture surface.

On a more global scale, it is important to note that the best-documented alterations in AD patients fit nicely into the Ca^{2+} hypothesis of dementia. For example, reduced glucose uptake/utilization in AD brain has been repeatedly documented and appears to occur early on in the disease, and may precede neuronal loss (*see* ref. *50* for a review). Reduced glucose availability to neurons is known to predispose neurons to excitotoxicity and Aβ toxicity *(51,52)*, both of which are Ca^{2+}-mediated processes *(27)*. Microvascular alterations have been repeatedly documented in AD brain *(53,54)* and would be expected to contribute to ischemia-like conditions, overactivation of glutamate receptors, and calcium-mediated injury to neurons. Calcium is also implicated in neuronal injury in dementias other than AD. In the case of multi-infarct dementia, the events leading to neuronal injury are almost surely similar to those that occur in ischemia, which have been extensively studied and involve energy depletion, failure of ion pumps, glutamate and K^+ release, activation of glutamate receptors, Ca^{2+} influx, proteolysis, generation of free radicals, and so on.

5. INSTIGATORS OF NEURONAL DEGENERATION IN AD

5.1. Aβ

The initial identification of β-amyloid precursor protein (βAPP) as the source of the 40–42 amino acid Aβ that constitutes the major amyloid component of Alzheimer's

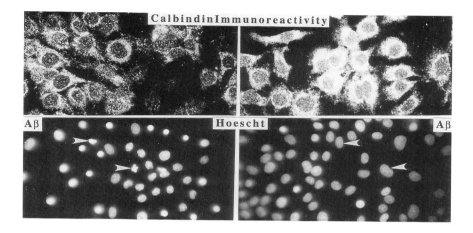

Fig. 4. Calbindin protects cells from apoptosis induced by Aβ. C6 glioma cells were transfected with calbindin cDNA. Lines expressing low (upper left panel) and high (upper right panel) levels of calbindin were selected. Cells were exposed for 20 h to 50 μ*M* Aβ25–35 and then stained with Hoescht dye to label DNA (lower panels). Many cells in the line expressing low levels of calbindin exhibited DNA condensation and signs of fragmentation (e.g., arrowheads), whereas DNA in cells in the line expressing high levels of calbindin remained diffuse, indicating resistance to apoptosis.

plaques strongly implicated βAPP in the pathogenesis of AD, and, during subsequent years, a rapidly growing body of evidence has added support for a primary role for βAPP in AD (*see* refs. *55–57* for review). For example, the βAPP gene was localized to chromosome 21, the chromosome causally involved in Down's syndrome, a disorder in which essentially all patients develop AD-like neuropathology. In a recent study, Busciglio and Yankner *(58)* showed that cortical neurons taken from Down's syndrome fetuses spontaneously undergo apoptosis following differentiation in culture in contrast to cortical neurons from normal fetuses. Moreover, they showed that the Down's syndrome neurons exhibit a marked increase in ROS production and lipid peroxidation prior to apoptosis, suggesting that altered oxyradical metabolism contributes to their demise. The latter findings demonstrate that very early in brain development, trisomy 21 makes neurons inherently vulnerable to altered environmenal conditions that tend to promote oxidative stress. The causal linkage of several different βAPP mutations to familial forms of AD provided a direct demonstration of the central role of βAPP in the pathogenesis of at least some AD cases. The mechanism whereby βAPP mutations lead to Aβ deposition and neuronal degeneration is not yet established. However, experimental studies in which human mutant βAPPs were expressed in cultured cells have indicated that the processing of βAPP is altered such that the cells produce greater levels of Aβ or more of the long form of Aβ (Aβ1–42) *(59–61)*. In vitro data indicate that Aβ1–42 aggregates more readily than Aβ1–40 and may therefore be more likely to accumulate as plaques in the brain *(62)*. The isolation of Aβ and elucidation of its amino acid sequence allowed the development of specific Aβ antibodies. Use of such antibodies in combination with stains for β-pleated sheet structure (i.e., amyloid) revealed the presence of two distinguishable forms of Aβ in AD brain, a diffuse

noncongophilic form (not associated with neuronal pathology) and a compact fibrillar form associated with silver stain-positive degenerating neurites and somata. These
basic observations provided a clue concerning the possible role of peptide aggregation in the neurotoxic activity of Aβ. Yankner and coworkers *(63)* demonstrated that
synthetic Aβ can be directly toxic to cultured rat hippocampal neurons and that the
neurotoxic activity resided in an 11-mer fragment of the peptide (amino acids 25–
35). Subsequently, several laboratories demonstrated that the neurotoxic potency of a
particular batch of synthetic Aβ was related to the "ability" of the peptide to form
aggregates *(37,58,64)*.

Much effort has been placed on developing transgenic mouse models of AD based
on overexpression of normal forms of βAPP, expression of fragments of βAPP, or
expression of human mutant forms of βAPP *(65–69)*. In the vast majority of cases, the
transgenic mice did not exhibit Aβ deposits, and if they did, no neurodegeneration
occurred. Recently, Games et al. *(70)* reported characterization of a transgenic mouse
line that exhibits age-related deposition of Aβ, synapse loss, and neuronal degeneration. A human minigene containing the V717F mutant form of βAPP was expressed
under the control of a platelet-derived growth factor-β (PDGF-β) promoter. Examination of brains of these mice revealed no abnormalities until the mice were about 4 mo
of age, at which time deposits of diffuse Aβ began to appear in hippocampus and cortical regions. By 7 mo, the V717F mice exhibited both diffuse and fibrillar (congo red
and thioflavin-positive) Aβ deposits. By 10 mo, marked synapse loss and neuronal
degeneration had occurred in brain regions where Aβ is deposited (hippocampus and
cortex), but not in brain regions lacking Aβ (e.g., cerebellum). The association of Aβ
deposits with neuronal degeneration in the V717F mice is striking and clearly makes
these mice the best animal model of AD to date. These mice will prove valuable in
establishing roles of calcium and free radicals in the pathogenesis of Aβ-induced neuronal injury in vivo.

The chemical basis and structural requirements for peptide aggregation are beginning to be elucidated. Studies of the effects of pH on peptide aggregation showed that
Aβ can aggregate at physiological pH, but that it aggregates more readily at more acidic
pHs *(71–73)*. Other conditions that promote aggregation of Aβ include an oxidizing
environment *(74,75)* and the presence of certain metals, including zinc *(76)*. Circular
dichroism analysis of different batches of Aβ and correlations with neurotoxic activity
of the same batches of peptide revealed a strong correlation between propensity of the
peptide to form β-sheet structure and neurotoxic profile *(77)*. The ability of Aβ to form
fibrils appears to be critical for neurotoxicity because congo red, which inhibited fibril
formation, also prevented the toxicity of Aβ *(78)*. Following the initial report of Yankner
and coworkers *(63)* that an 11 amino acid peptide fragment of Aβ (amino acids 25–35)
can be neurotoxic, many studies have confirmed the toxicity of Aβ25–35 and shown
that it aggregates in a manner similar to full-length Aβ *(63)*. Pike et al. *(79)* recently
reported data from studies in which individual amino acids of Aβ25–35 were systematically removed and/or replaced with other amino acids, and then the aggregation and
neurotoxic properties of the peptides examined. The data indicate that methionine 35
of Aβ plays a key role in both peptide aggregation and neurotoxicity.

A novel chemistry of Aβ that can account for many of the properties of Aβ just
described was recently revealed in electron paramagnetic resonance (EPR) spectros-

copy studies of synthetic Aβs *(80,81)*. The EPR method employs a (normally nonparamagnetic) spin-trapping compound that, on interaction with a free radical moiety, forms a spin adduct that is paramagnetic and can be detected in an EPR spectroscope. When synthetic Aβ25–35 or Aβ1–40 was incubated in physiological saline in the presence of the spin-trapping compound tert-butyl-phenylnitrone (PBN), a clear three-line radical signal was detected. The signal did not occur when the solution was purged with nitrogen, indicating a requirement for molecular oxygen *(75)*. Incubation of Aβ25–35 or Aβ1–40 with enzymes sensitive to free radical-induced damage showed that Aβ inactivates the enzymes in an oxygen-dependent manner *(75)*. More recent amino acid substitution analyses showed that removal of methionine 35 eliminates the EPR signal (*see* Chapter 7). Based on these findings and the considerable data indicating that Aβ induces free radical production in neurons in an aggregation-related manner (*see below*), it seems reasonable to consider that the formation of free radical species on certain amino acids of Aβ itself is a key event in both covalent crosslinking of the peptide to form fibrillar aggregates and neurotoxicity of the peptide. Neither the chemistry underlying formation of free radical Aβ peptides nor the environmental factors that can modulate this process are clear. However, Schubert and Chevion *(82)* and Goodman and Mattson *(89)* reported that iron facilitates Aβ toxicity, suggesting a role for this metal in Aβ aggregation and toxicity. It will be of considerable interest to determine whether amyloidogenic peptides other than Aβ (e.g., amylin, β2-microglobulin, and cystatin C) also form free radical peptides, particularly in light of recent data showing that different amyloidogenic peptides share a similar mechanism of cytotoxicity involving generation of free radicals in cells *(83–86)*.

An important question concerning the protein chemistry of Aβ toxicity is whether it is the three-dimensional conformation of Aβ fibrils that is necessary for damaging neurons, or whether it is a chemical reaction associated with the formation of fibrils that damages neurons. Although much effort has been placed on elucidating the secondary and tertiary structure of Aβ fibrils, it has not yet been established that the secondary structure of the fibrils, *per se*, is critical for peptide toxicity *(87)*. However, what has not been considered is that it is not the structure of the fibrils that confers toxic activity, but rather a chemical reaction involved in fibril formation that propagates to and damages neurons. Several observations are consistent with the latter novel hypothesis. First, the relationship between extent of aggregation of Aβ and its neurotoxic activity is that of a bell-shaped curve in which soluble Aβ is not toxic, moderately aggregated Aβ is toxic, and extensively aggregated peptide is less toxic (*75*; Mattson, unpublished data). Moreover, when Aβ is added to a "sandwich" culture in which neurons are grown on two horizontal coverslips separated by several millimeters (cells grow on the lower surface of the top coverslip and the upper surface of the bottom coverslip), neurons on each coverslip are damaged to a similar extent despite the fact that large Aβ aggregates accumulate only on the cells on the lower coverslip (Fig. 5). Based on these data and additional unpublished data, we propose that it is free radicals generated during (and causally involved in) fibril formation that propagate to neuronal membranes where they damage proteins and lipids.

When Aβ encounters cultured primary hippocampal neurons, it induces lipid peroxidation and accumulation of hydrogen peroxide *(81,88–90)*. Sagara et al. *(91)* showed that cell lines resistant to Aβ toxicity exhibited higher levels of antioxidant

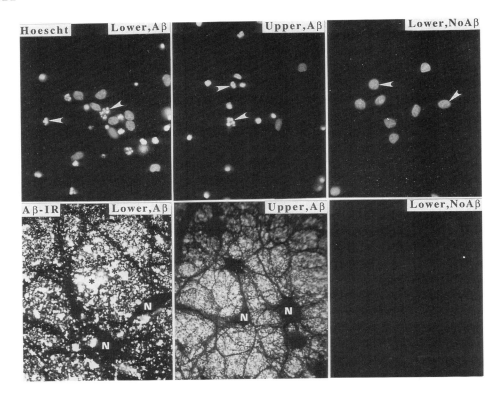

Fig. 5. Apoptosis induced by Aβ is related to the process, and not the product, of peptide aggregation. Primary "sandwich" cultures of hippocampal cells consisting of two coverslips, in horizontal orientation and separated by a space of approx 3 mm, were prepared in which cells grew on the top of the lower coverslip and the bottom of the upper coverslip. Aβ1–40 or vehicle (NoAβ) was then added to the cultures, and 24 h later, the cultures were fixed in paraformaldehyde and stained with either Hoescht dye to label DNA (top three panels) or a monoclonal antibody (MAb) to Aβ to localize the peptide (bottom three panels). Micrographs show fluorescence images of DNA staining (upper) or Aβ immunoreactivity (lower; confocal laser scanning microscope images). Note that a similar fraction of neurons grown on either the lower or upper coverslip exhibited DNA condensation and fragmentation, despite the fact that much larger aggregates of Aβ were present on the lower coverslip, indicating that the size of the aggregates is not directly related to neurotoxic activity.

enzymes, findings that suggest a role for differences in antioxidant defense systems in selective neuronal vulnerability in AD. The most likely cellular site at which Aβ induces oxidative processes is the plasma membrane, because when Aβ is added to the cultures, aggregates form and accumulate on the cell surface *(37)*. Oxidative damage to the plasma membrane appears to play a key role in disruption of ion homeostasis by Aβ described in Section 2. Mark et al. *(92)* reported that exposure of cultured rat hippocampal neurons to Aβ results in impairment of Na$^+$/K$^+$-ATPase activity, which precedes elevation of [Ca^{2+}]$_i$ and cell degeneration. Impairment of Na$^+$/K$^+$-ATPase activity and resultant membrane depolarization contributed to subsequent elevation of [Ca^{2+}]$_i$ and cell death, because manipulations that reduce Na$^+$ influx protected neurons. Moreover, selective inhibition of Na$^+$/K$^+$-ATPase with ouabain induced an elevation of [Ca^{2+}]$_i$ and apoptotic cell death *(92)*. The ability of Aβ to impair ion-motive ATPase activities was suppressed in cultures pretreated with antioxidants, indicating that free radicals mediated impairment of the pump activities. This mechanism of Aβ toxicity is likely to occur in human brain, because exposure of synaptosomes taken from neurologically normal aged humans to Aβ resulted in a highly significant impairment of both Na^+/K^+- and Ca^{2+}-ATPase activities *(92)*. The specific sequence of molecular events involved in ROS production and impairment of ion-motive ATPase activities has not yet been defined. Although these findings suggest the plasma membrane to be an important cellular site of damage induced by Aβ, the work of Shearman et al. *(93)* indicates that mitochondrial impairment is an early event in the toxicity of Aβ, and it will be of interest to determine the roles of oxyradicals in such mitochondrial alterations.

The data described immediately above suggest that the mechanism whereby Aβ disrupts calcium homeostasis is by first inducing free radicals, which then impair systems that regulate calcium homeostasis. However, Aβ may more directly promote calcium influx. For example, Arispe et al. *(94)* reported that Aβ1–40 itself forms large conductance cation channels in bilayer membranes, suggesting that the peptide may act as an ionophore. Consistent with the latter study, Furukawa et al. *(95)* reported that Aβ induces irreversible inward currents in cultured rat cortical neurons. It is not known whether these actions of Aβ involve free radical production.

Recent data suggest that Aβ may impair signal transduction mechanisms prior to neuronal degeneration. Cholinergic systems are disrupted in AD brain, but it is unclear whether deficits in cholinergic signaling occur prior to neuronal degeneration *(96)*. Experiments on postmortem brain tissue obtained from AD patients have shown evidence of impaired coupling of muscarinic receptors to G-proteins. For example, Flynn et al. *(97)* reported a reduction in the proportion of M_1 muscarinic receptors existing in the high-affinity (G-protein-coupled) state in AD frontal cortex, compared to age-matched controls. These and other data *(98,99)* suggest that this defect may, in part, explain the lack of efficacy of cholinergic agents in ameliorating cognitive symptoms of AD. In a recent study, Kelly et al. *(100)* reported that relatively brief (20 min to 4 h) exposures of cultured rat neocortical neurons to Aβ25–35 or Aβ1–40 resulted in a loss of responsiveness of the neurons to the muscarinic agonist carbachol. Thus, whereas carbachol normally induced membrane-associated GTPase activity, inositol phosphate release, and elevation of $[Ca^{2+}]_i$, none of these responses were observed in cultures pretreated with 1–50 μ*M* Aβ. Ligand-binding studies indicated that Aβ did not interfere with the binding of carbachol to receptors, suggesting that Aβ's action involved "uncoupling" of the receptor from the G-protein. Disruption of this signaling pathway may involve generation of free radicals because vitamin E attenuated the effect of Aβ. These data suggest that Aβ could disrupt muscarinic signaling pathways in early stages of AD prior to cell loss.

Although much attention has focused on the actions of Aβ on neurons, it is important to understand effects of Aβ on nonneuronal cells and how they might contribute to the pathogenesis of AD. Astrocytes and microglia are two cell types that are associated with plaques in AD brain. Cell-culture studies have revealed responses of each of these cell types to Aβ. For example, although astrocytes are quite resistant to cytotoxic actions of Aβ, they exhibit morphological responses to Aβ consistent with induction of a "reactive" state *(101)*. Glutamate transport in astrocytes may also be disrupted by Aβ as indicated by studies showing that ROS impair astrocyte glutamate transport *(102)*. Aβ was reported also to induce activation of microglia with resultant release of cytokines from these cells including tumor necrosis factor (TNF) *(103)*. Data from the latter study also indicated that Aβ induced release of an unidentified neurotoxic substance from the microglia. Previous studies indicate that the toxic substance may kill neurons by an excitotoxic mechanism involving elevation of intracellular calcium levels *(104)*. Cultured microglia can also be killed by Aβ *(105)*. Cells of the cerebral vasculature may also be adversely affected by Aβ. As evidence, Davis-Salinas et al. *(106)* reported that vascular smooth muscle cells can be damaged by Aβ. In an elegant set of recent experiments, Thomas et al. *(107)* showed that Aβ can damage and kill endothelial cells in blood vessel rings, and that the damage is prevented by superoxide dismutase. In studies of endothelial cell monolayer cultures, we have found that Aβ can disrupt glucose transport and barrier functions of these cells (Blanc, et al., manuscript submitted). Aβ toxicity toward the cultured endothelial cells manifests as apoptosis (Fig. 6). These kinds of data clearly indicate that Aβ can adversely affect multiple cell types in the brain and suggest that such actions could contribute to multiple aspects of the pathophysiology of dementia in AD, including disruption of the blood–brain barrier.

5.2. Secreted Forms of βAPP

Although direct evidence that alterations in the function of βAPP play a causal role in AD is lacking, recent findings concerning the normal functions of secreted forms of βAPP (sAPPs) and the effects of mutations on βAPP processing suggest possible roles for altered function of βAPP in the pathogenesis of AD. Important information concerning the ways in which βAPP is metabolized in cells and the normal functions of βAPP is rapidly accumulating. βAPP is produced, via alternative splicing, in several forms, including those lacking (e.g., APP695) or containing (e.g., APP751 and APP770) a kunitz protease inhibitor domain (*see* ref. *56* for review). In the brain, neurons produce predominately the 695 form, and glial cells produce 751 and 770 forms. βAPP is believed to be situated in cells in a transmembrane configuration with a short C-terminal intracellular region and a much larger extracellular N-terminus. The Aβ sequence is situated partially in the extracellular milieu and partially within the plasma membrane. Alternative enzymatic processing pathways have been identified that result in cleavage either within the Aβ sequence (α-secretase cleavage between amino acids 16 and 17 of Aβ) or at the N-terminus of Aβ (β-secretase cleavage). Both processing pathways occur normally in neural cells, because both α-secretase βAPP products (sAPPs) and intact soluble Aβ circulate in CSF in picomolar to nanomolar concentrations *(108,109)*. Of considerable importance for understanding the normal function of βAPP are data showing that full-length βAPP is axonally transported *(110)*, that βAPP accumulates in presynaptic terminals *(111)* and axonal growth cones *(112)*, and that βAPPs are released from neuronal cells in an activity-driven manner (i.e., excitatory transmitters and action potentials induce sAPP release; *113,114*) (Fig. 7). Several biologically active domains of sAPPs have been identified, including a five amino acid segment (amino acids 328–332 of APP695) that has been shown by Saitoh and coworkers to promote proliferation of mitotic cells, neurite outgrowth of cultured neurons, and synaptogenesis in vivo *(115,116)*. A region of sAPP just N-terminal to the Aβ sequence has been shown to exhibit neuroprotective activities *(117)*.

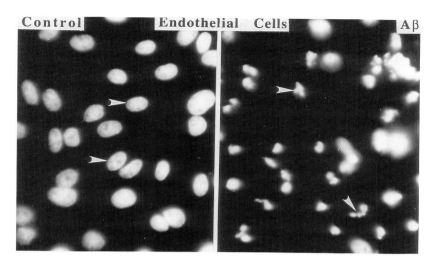

Fig. 6. Vascular endothelial cells exposed to Aβ undergo apoptosis. Cultured endothelial cells from porcine pulmonary artery were exposed to vehicle (control) or 20 μg/mL Aβ25–35 for 18 h. The cells were then fixed and stained with Hoescht dye to label DNA. Nuclei of cells in the control culture exhibited diffuse DNA staining characteristic of healthy cells (e.g., arrowheads), whereas DNA in the cells exposed to Aβ was condensed and showed signs of fragmentation (e.g., arrowheads).

Secreted APPs (sAPP695 and sAPP751) protected cultured human cortical and rat hippocampal neurons against glutamate toxicity and glucose deprivation-induced damage; the elevation of $[Ca^{2+}]_i$ normally induced by glutamate was attenuated in neurons pretreated with sAPPs *(112,117)*. These actions of sAPPs were blocked by antibodies directed against the C-terminal region of sAPP. The signal transduction pathway mediating the neuroprotective actions of sAPPs may involve generation of the second messenger cyclic GMP (cGMP), because studies of cultured hippocampal neurons showed that: sAPPs induce cGMP production; 8-bromo-cGMP mimics the $[Ca^{2+}]_i$-lowering and neuroprotective actions of sAPPs; and a cGMP-dependent protein kinase inhibitor blocked the $[Ca^{2+}]_i$-lowering and neuroprotective actions of sAPPs *(118)*. The sAPPs apparently activate a particulate (membrane-associated guanylate cyclase), because sAPPs induced cGMP production in isolated membranes from hippocampal cells, and inhibitors of NO synthesis did not block sAPP actions *(118,119)*.

Because sAPPs rapidly reduced rest $[Ca^{2+}]_i$ and attenuated $[Ca^{2+}]_i$ responses to glutamate, we tested the hypothesis that sAPPs affect ion currents via a cGMP-mediated mechanism *(120)*. Whole-cell patch-clamp recordings were performed using the nystatin-perforated patch technique. As described previously, cultured embryonic hippocampal neurons were synaptically connected and fired action potentials in response to above-threshold stimulation from synaptic inputs. Under current-clamp conditions, the frequency of action potentials was significantly reduced during application of 1 n*M* sAPP, and after a time lag of 2–3 min following washout of sAPP action potential, frequency recovered to basal levels (Fig. 8). Because activation of K+ channels reduces excitability, we tested the hypothesis that sAPPs activate K+ channels. In voltage-clamp mode, outward currents were recorded at potentials more positive than –80 mV. Neu-

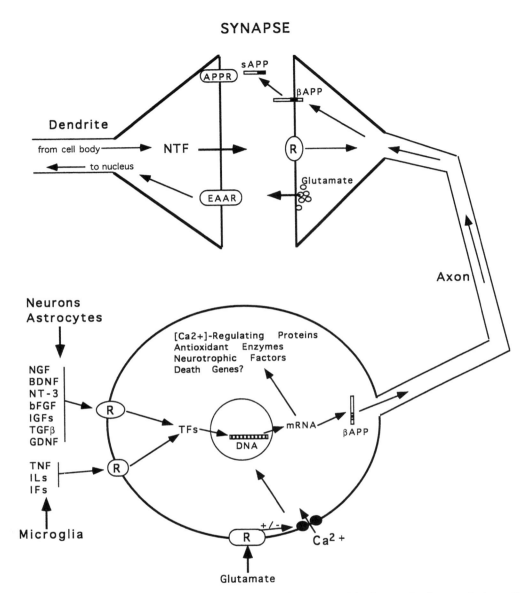

Fig. 7. Interactive roles of glutamate, βAPP, and neurotrophic factors in the regulation of neuronal plasticity. Activity induces release of glutamate from axon terminals at excitatory synapses. Glutamate binds to postsynaptic receptors, resulting in membrane depolarization and calcium influx; when activation of glutamate receptors reaches a certain threshold intensity, an action potential occurs in the postsynaptic neuron. βAPP is axonally transported, accumulates in axonal terminals, and sAPPs are also released in response to activity (i.e., action potentials). Activation of postsynaptic sAPP receptors results in membrane hyperpolarization and a reduction in calcium influx; sAPPs suppress responses to glutamate and increase the threshold for action potential generation. A variety of neurotrophic factors (e.g., NGF, BDNF, NT-3, bFGF, IGFs, TGFβ, and GDNF) and cytokines (e.g., TNF, interleukins, and interferons) are produced by neural cells (neurons, astrocytes, and/or microglia). Glutamate can induce expression and release of NTF (e.g., activation of AMPA receptors induces BDNF expression and release). *See text* for additional description.

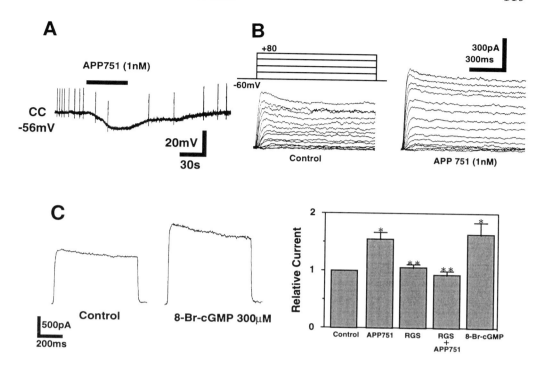

Fig. 8. Secreted forms of APP suppress neuronal excitability by activating potassium channels. **(A)** Spontaneous action potentials recorded in current-clamp (CC) mode in a neuron prior to, during, and following exposure to sAPP751. Note that the sAPP reversibly reduced firing rate and elicited a transient hyperpolarization. **(B)** Representative current recordings in a neuron prior to (control) and 5 min following exposure to sAPP751. The pulses were applied in voltage steps from −60 to +80 mV. **(C)** (Left) Current recordings in a neuron prior to and 2 min following application of 300 μM 8-bromo-cGMP. (Right) Currents were recorded 2 min following exposure to the following treatments: sAPP751, 1 nM; RGS (cGMP-dependent protein kinase inhibitor), 30 μM; 30 μM RGS + 1 nM sAPP751; 8-bromo-cGMP, 300 μM. Values are expressed relative to the control value (1.0) and represent the mean and SEM of determinations made in 5–8 neurons. $*p < 0.01$ compared to Control value. $**p < 0.01$ compared to APP751 value.

rons had a resting membrane potential of −67.4 ± 4.5 mV ($n = 14$) under current-clamp, and exposure to sAPP induced a reversible hyperpolarization. The sAPP evoked an outward current under voltage-clamp conditions at V_{HS} from −80 to −20 mV, with a reversal potential of −85, which is essentially identical to the K^+ equilibrium potential of −86 mV. A tenfold change in $(K^+)_o$ caused the reversal potential to change by 57 mV and the sAPP-induced outward current was blocked by 4-aminopyridine and charybdotoxin, demonstrating that K^+ channels were responsible. The maximum increase in outward current occurred within 60–90 s of exposure to sAPP, was maintained during continued exposure to sAPP, and recovered to baseline levels within 3–5 min of sAPP removal. The sAPPs were effective in activating the potassium channels at concentrations from 10 pM to 10 nM. Pharmacological studies and single-channel recordings demonstrated that the channels activated by sAPPs were high-conductance, Ca^{2+}-activated K^+ channels *(120)*. A selective inhibitor of cGMP-dependent protein kinase blocked the activation of I_K by sAPPs, and 8-bromo-cGMP mimicked the activation of I_K by sAPPs. Together with additional patch-clamp and calcium imaging data, we concluded that sAPPs activate K^+ channels via a cGMP-mediated mechanism. Because K^+ channels play key roles in learning and memory processes (121), the ability of sAPPs to activate K^+ channels provides an explanation for reported effects of βAPP on synaptogenesis and synaptic plasticity (112,116). The data also suggest that abnormalities in βAPP processing or sAPP activity could explain aberrant K^+ channel properties observed in AD (122), and could contribute to the neurodegenerative process by increasing neuronal vulnerability to excitotoxicity and Aβ toxicity (89).

In addition to modulating neuronal excitability and calcium homeostasis, sAPPs may also induce antioxidant mechanisms in neural cells. This is suggested by the observations that pretreatment of hippocampal cultures with sAPPs confers on neuron resistance to oxidative insults, including exposure to $FeSO_4$ and Aβ (89). Direct measurements of hydrogen peroxide levels in the cultured neurons showed that sAPPs can attenuate Aβ-induced accumulation of hydrogen peroxide. The signal transduction mechanism by which sAPPs suppress accumulation of ROS is not known. However, we have recently shown that sAPPs can activate the transcription factor NFκB and induce expression of antioxidant enzymes in cultured hippocampal cells (123). As will be described, there is evidence that this NFκB signaling pathway may mediate neuroprotective responses to several environmental stimuli, including TNFs and ROS themselves. The various data just described concerning trophic activities of sAPPs suggest that a shift in βAPP processing in AD to increased β-secretase products might (in addition to increasing the level of Aβ) reduce levels of trophic sAPPs.

5.3. Alterations in Genes Other than βAPP

Some familial AD (FAD) cases have been linked to mutations on genes that reside in chromosomes 14 and 1. A novel gene bearing several different missense mutations was cloned from chromosome 14q24.3 in seven pedigrees; the deduced amino acid sequence of the encoded protein predicts an integral membrane protein with seven-membrane spanning domains (93). Subsequent cloning of the gene residing in chromosome 1(q31–42) revealed high homology with S182; a single mutation in this gene was shown to occur in the Volga German family with this inherited form of AD (124). The Volga German gene, designated STM2, is also predicted to encode a protein with seven-trans-membrane-spanning (STM) regions. Although the function of these proteins is not yet known, their apparent structure suggests several possible ways in which they could be involved in regulation of neuronal calcium homeostasis. Families of proteins with similar STM domains were previously cloned and the functions of some of those proteins are fairly well understood. Such proteins are known to function as receptors that transduce signals to GTP-binding proteins (125,126). If S182 and STM2 serve as G-protein-coupled receptors, then there are many ways in which altered function of these proteins could result in perturbed calcium homeostasis. Indeed, many G-protein-linked receptors affect calcium homeostasis by mediating inositol phospholipid hydrolysis and calcium release. For example, metabotropic acetylcholine and glutamate receptors are linked to such pathways (127). S182 and STM proteins might also more directly regulate calcium channel function (125). Another putative function of STM proteins is in protein trafficking and processing. It was therefore suggested that mutations in

S182 and STM2 could affect metabolism of βAPP *(128)*. If mutations in S182 and STM2 promote increased production and/or deposition of Aβ, then this would lead to disruption of neuronal calcium homeostasis by the Aβ-mediated mechanisms described in Section 2.

Recent data show that presenilins are localized to endoplasmic reticulum *(129)*. We have found that the expression of a PS-1 mutation (L286V) in culutred neurons exaggerates Ca^{2+} responses to agonists (carbachol and bradykinin) that induce Ca^{2+} release from IP_3-sensitive endoplasmic reticulum stores (Guo et al., manuscript submitted). Neurons expressing L286V showed increased susceptibility to Aβ toxicity and apoptosis induced by trophic factor withdrawal. The heightened vulnerability of neurons expressing the PS-1 mutation involved oxidative stress and disruption of calcium homeostasis and, accordingly, antioxidants and calcium blockers counteracted the adverse consequences of this PS-1 mutation. By disrupting Ca^{2+} homeostasis, PS-1 mutations may sensitize neurons to age-related accumulation of Aβ and reduced trophic support.

5.4. Vascular Alterations

Although Aβ appears to play a primary causal role in some inherited forms of AD, it is less clear that it plays an initiating role in the more common sporadic forms of AD. Data from a variety of sources suggest that alterations in the vasculature are involved in initiation of neurodegenerative processes in AD. First is the strong correlation between aging and vascular alterations (atherosclerosis and microvascular damage) on the one hand *(130)*, and aging and AD on the other hand. Second, alterations in the microvasculature including damage to endothelial cells and vascular smooth muscle cells have been consistently documented in studies of AD brain *(131–133)*. Third, there is reduced energy availability to neurons in AD brain, which may occur very early in the disease process *(134)*. Fourth, increased apolipoprotein E 4 (ApoE 4) allele dosage increases the probabilities of developing atherosclerosis *(135,136)* and AD *(137)*. Fifth, brain regions that are most severely affected in AD have a relatively reduced vascular supply compared to nonvulnerable regions (*see* any basic neuroanatomy textbook). These different lines of evidence suggest that vascular alterations and AD pathogenesis may be mechanistically linked. Damage to brain microvessels would be expected to result in impaired blood flow and reduced availability of energy substrates to brain cells. Reduced energy availability would, in turn, increase neuronal vulnerability to excitotoxicity and Aβ toxicity.

Whether vascular alterations precede or follow Aβ deposition is an open question, and evidence supporting either possibility can be gleaned from the literature. For example, Aβ is produced by smooth muscle cells and endothelial cells in the vasculature *(138–140)*. Aβ is deposited in blood vessels in AD brain *(54,141)*, and, as described in Section 5.1., can damage vascular smooth muscle cells *(106)* and endothelial cells *(107)* (Fig. 6). On the other hand, diminished energy availability to cells, which could occur as the result of vascular alterations, may promote deposition of Aβ, as suggested by Gabuzda et al. *(142)*, who reported that inhibition of energy metabolism with mitochondrial poisons results in a shift in proteolytic processing of APP in a way that greatly increases production of potentially amyloidogenic C-terminal fragments. Perhaps the most likely scenario is one in which a feed-forward cascade occurs such that vascular alterations increase deposition of Aβ, which further damages vessels leading to accelerated Aβ deposition, further damage to vessels, and a further decrement in energy availability. Consideration of this scenario in AD suggests a possible mechanistic link between vascular dementia and AD.

6. ACCOMPLICES IN THE NEURODEGENERATIVE PROCESS IN AD

6.1. Steroids—Glucocorticoids and Estrogens

Clinical, epidemiolgical, and experimental data suggest that both glucocorticoids and estrogens play roles in the development and/or progression of the neurodegenerative process in AD. In the case of glucocorticoids, it has been shown that AD patients have alterations in regulation of the hypothalamic–pituitary–adrenal system *(143)* and that glucocorticoid endangerment of hippocampal neurons increases with increasing age *(144)*. Moreover, it has been shown that glucocorticoids exacerbate cytoskeletal alterations and cell death in hippocampal neurons of adult rats exposed to the excitatory amino acid kainate *(33)* or physiological stress *(34)*. In the latter studies, the cytoskeletal alterations included proteolysis of spectrin and MAP2, and accumulation of τ in neuronal somata. Glucocorticoids also increased neuronal vulnerability to Aβ toxicity *(145)*, providing further relevance of glucocorticoid actions to the pathophysiology of AD. One mechanism whereby glucocorticoids endanger neurons is by reducing cellular glucose uptake mechanisms *(146)*. This mechanism is consistent with the fact that other manipulations that impair energy availability also increase neuronal vulnerability to excitotoxicity and Aβ toxicity. Evidence that physiological levels of glucocorticoids can endanger neurons includes the findings that administration of metyrapone, an inhibitor of glucocorticoid production, to adult rats protects hippocampal neurons against damage induced by focal and global cerebral ischemia, and kainic acid *(147)*.

Postmenopausal women receiving estrogen replacement therapy have a reduced incidence of AD *(80)*. Several possible mechanisms whereby estrogens protect against AD can be proposed based on published findings. One possibility is that estrogens suppress the development of atherosclerosis *(148)* and so retard development of age-related vascular alterations that may contribute to reduced energy availability to the brain. Another possibility is that estrogens directly affect brain cells in a neuroprotective manner. Cell-culture studies have shown that 17β-estradiol can promote long-term neuronal survival *(149)*, and in vivo data suggest that estrogens stimulate production of neurotrophic factors in the brain *(150)*. Moreover, it was recently reported *(145,151)* that 17β-estradiol can protect cultured neurons against Aβ toxicity and oxidative insults. We showed that 17β-estradiol and estriol protect cultured hippocampal neurons against excitotoxicity and oxidative insults by suppressing lipid peroxidation and stabilizing calcium homeostasis *(145)* (Fig. 9). Interestingly, these actions of estrogens in neural cells are similar to the antioxidant activities of estrogens previously reported in studies of nonneuronal cells. For example, estrogens suppressed lipid peroxidation in liver microsomes *(152)* and protected endothelial cells from damage induced by oxidized low-density lipoprotein *(153)*.

6.2. ApoE

A link between ApoE alleles and predisposition for developing AD at an early age was recently established *(137,154)*. As described, the same ApoE allele that increases risk for AD (ApoE 4) also increases the risk of developing atherosclerosis. However,

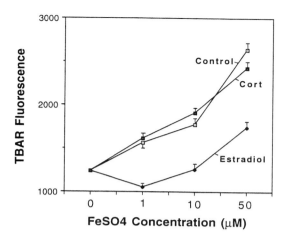

Fig. 9. Estradiol suppresses lipid peroxidation in neural membranes. Levels of thiobarbituric acid reactive substances (TBAR) were quantified in crude rat cortical membrane preparations pretreated for 30 min with vehicle (control) or 50 μM 17β-estradiol or corticosterone, and then exposed to the indicated concentrations of $FeSO_4$ for 20 min. Values represent the mean and SEM ($n = 4$–6). Values for membranes pretreated with estradiol were significantly less than values for control and corticosterone-treated membranes exposed to 1, 10, or 50 μM $FeSO_4$ ($p < 0.001$).

many investigators believe that the influence of ApoE on development of AD is owing to direct actions on neural cells rather than being simply a vascular effect. There is evidence that apolipoproteins serve important functions in neural cells. Astrocytes produce ApoE *(155)*, and it was recognized many years ago that apolipoproteins are expressed in brain and that they can influence neuronal development (*see* ref. *156* for review). When the link between ApoE and AD was established, many different laboratories began to test their pet hypotheses of how the expression of different ApoE isoforms might influence neuronal survival. As we write, articles describing various effects of ApoEs on βAPP processing, Aβ aggregation, τ biology, cell adhesion, trophic factor signaling pathways, and so on are being reported. It is likely to take some time to sort out which of these different actions of ApoEs are real, which occur in vivo, and which are important for the pathogenesis of AD. Nevertheless, several intriguing observations merit consideration in the context of the calcium/free radical hypothesis of AD.

Because of the central role of βAPP in AD, possible interactions of ApoE isoforms with βAPP and Aβ have been looked for and found. ApoE promoted fibril formation of synthetic Aβ preparations with ApoE 4 being more effective than ApoE 3 *(157)*. On the other hand, essentially opposite results were reported by Evans et al. *(158)*, who found that ApoE 3 inhibited Aβ fibril formation. In support of an inhibitory action of ApoE on fibrillogenesis, Whitson et al. *(159)* found that ApoE protected cultured neurons against Aβ toxicity. Obviously, if ApoE does affect Aβ fibril formation and neurotoxicity, then it will impact on neuronal calcium homeostasis and free radical metabolism indirectly, because Aβ toxicity involves generation of free radicals and disruption of calcium homeostasis. ApoE may also interact with and affect the function of sAPPs. As evidence, Barger et al. *(160)* recently reported that ApoEs potentiate the $[Ca^{2+}]_i$-lowering and neuroprotective activities of sAPPs in hippocampal cell cultures. In the latter studies, the order of potency of the different ApoE isoforms in potentiating the actions of sAPPs was E 2 > E 3 > E 4, suggesting the possibility that ApoE 2 and E 3 isoforms protect against neurodegeneration in AD by promoting trophic activities of sAPPs. An additional protein relevant to AD with which ApoE may interact is τ *(137)*. Finally, a quite different possible role for ApoE in neurodegenerative process was suggested by Crutcher et al. *(161)*, who reported that synthetic peptides containing the ApoE amino acid 141–155 sequence caused degeneration of neurites in cultured sympathetic neurons.

6.3. Inflammatory Processes

Evidence for an inflammatory component to the neurodegenerative process in AD is accumulating. Studies of postmortem AD brain have revealed the presence of a variety of inflammation-related molecules in association with plaques and degenerating neurons *(162)*. For example, opsonizing components of complement and complement activators, including Aβ, thrombin, ApoE, and amyloid P component, are all present in diffuse and senile plaques *(163)*. Activated microglial cells are also associated with plaques, and some of their roles in inflammatory processes are well known, including their ability to produce large amounts of superoxide anion and hydrogen peroxide. Both complement proteins *(164)* and ROS *(89)* were demonstrated to potentiate Aβ toxicity in cultured neurons. Thus, some of the inflammatory alterations in AD could contribute to accumulation of free radicals and calcium in neurons. In support of the latter hypothesis, recent clinical data suggest that use of nonsteroidal anti-inflammatory agents may reduce the risk of developing AD *(165)*. In addition, inhibitors of the arachidonic acid cascade (a pathway activated in many inflammatory conditions) protected cultured neurons against Aβ toxicity *(90)*. Nevertheless, it is far from clear that all of the events that occur as the result of activation of various cells involved in inflammation are "bad" for neurons. Indeed, many of the molecules associated with plaques are known to exhibit neurotrophic activities, and their presence at sites of injury implies they are there for a purpose, which will now be considered.

7. CRIME STOPPERS: NEUROPROTECTIVE SIGNALING MECHANISMS

7.1. Neurotrophic Factors

A complex array of neuroprotective signal transduction pathways is emerging from studies of cellular responses of the brain to injury. The expression of a remarkable variety of neurotrophic factors and cytokines increases in response to brain injury (*see* ref. *166* for a review). In experimental studies of traumatic, ischemic, and excitotoxic brain injury in rats, a short list includes: basic fibroblast growth factor (bFGF), nerve growth factor (NGF), brain-derived neurotrophic factor (BDNF), insulin-like growth factor-1 (IGF-1), transforming growth factor-β (TGFβ), sAPPs, TNF, interleukin-1β, and protease nexin-1 (PN-1). In support of roles for expression of the different trophic factors and cytokines in preventing neuronal death and promoting recovery, many different cell-culture and in vivo studies have shown that administration of the trophic factors or cytokines can promote neuronal survival and/or neurite outgrowth. For example, bFGF promoted neurite outgrowth and long-term survival of cultured hippocampal neurons, and protected the neurons against the toxicities of excitatory amino acids, glucose deprivation, and Aβ *(37,167–169)*. bFGF and NGF attenuated neurofibrillary tangle-like cytoskeletal alterations induced by glucose deprivation *(169)*. BDNF protected cultured hippocampal and cortical neurons against glucose deprivation-induced injury and glutamate toxicity *(170)*, and TGFβ protected cortical neurons in culture against excitotoxic injury *(171)*. bFGF, NGF, IGF-1, and TGFβ were all reported to reduce ischemic and/or excitotoxic injury to hippocampal and cortical neurons in adult rats *(171–174)*, findings that highlight the pathophysiological relevance of the prior in vitro studies.

Pretreatment of rat hippocampal cell cultures with bFGF resulted in a suppression of the elevation of rest $[Ca^{2+}]_i$ induced by Aβ, and blocked the enhancement of $[Ca^{2+}]_i$ responses to glutamate that otherwise occurred in neurons pretreated with Aβ *(37)*. The $[Ca^{2+}]_i$ responses to depolarization were also reduced in neurons pretreated with bFGF. NGF did not protect cultured hippocampal neurons against Aβ toxicity *(37)*, whereas BDNF did significantly reduce neuronal vulnerability to Aβ (Mattson, unpublished data). Chao et al. *(175)* recently reported that TGFβ can also protect cultured human neurons against Aβ toxicity. Collectively, these data suggest that several different neurotrophic factors can protect neurons against Aβ toxicity.

Studies aimed at identifying the cellular and molecular mechanisms responsible for neuroprotective actions of the various neurotrophic factors and cytokines just described have all yielded data pointing to two general mechanisms, namely, enhancement of calcium homeostasis and antioxidant pathways. Neurotrophins, bFGF, IGFs, and many other neurotrophic factors activate receptors with intrinsic tyrosine kinase activity. Once activated, a sequence of phosphorylation events ensues, which results in activation of transcription factors and/or phosphorylation of regulatory proteins. For example, activation of bFGF receptors results in receptor tyrosine phosphorylation, activation of mitogen-activated protein (MAP) kinases, and transcription factors that induce the expression of calbindin *(176)* and antioxidant enzymes *(13)*. bFGF was also shown to regulate the expression of specific glutamate receptor subtypes, suppressing expression of an NMDA receptor protein *(177)* and inducing the expression of the AMPA receptor subunit GluR1 *(178)*. In a recent study, we found that bFGF induced increases in levels of Cu/Zn-superoxide dismutase (SOD) and glutathione reductase in rat hippocampal cell cultures *(13)*, suggesting that induction of such antioxidant enzymes by bFGF may underlie its ability to protect neurons against oxidative insults *(179)*. Indeed, we found that accumulation of hydrogen peroxide in response to Aβ was significantly attenuated in neurons in hippocampal cultures pretreated with bFGF (Mattson, unpublished data). Futher evidence that neurotrophic factors (NTF) can induce expression of antioxidant enzymes comes from the work of Sampath et al. *(180)*, who showed that NGF increases catalase levels in cultured PC12 cells, and Spina et al. *(181)*, who showed that BDNF increases glutathione reductase levels in striatum.

7.2. Cytokines

TNFs can kill tumor cells and other mitogenic cells *(182)*. However, recent findings in several laboratories suggest that TNFs can protect postmitotic neurons against metabolic, excitotoxic, and oxidative insults, including Aβ toxicity. We first reported that the vulnerabilty of cultured hippocampal neurons to glutamate toxicity and glucose deprivation is reduced in cultures pretreated with TNFα or TNFβ *(43)*. We subsequently showed that TNFs can protect hippocampal neurons against Aβ toxicity and other oxidative insults *(44)*. In the latter study, it was shown that the increased intracellular levels of hydrogen peroxide and calcium induced by Aβ were suppressed in neurons pretreated with TNFs. There are two different receptors for TNF, p55 and p75, both of which are widely expressed in neural cells, including astrocytes, microglia, and neurons. The p55 TNF receptor is linked to a signal transduction pathway in which a sphingomyelinase is activated, resulting in the release of ceramide from sphingomyelin. Ceramide then activates NFκB, a transcription factor complex consisting of dimeric transcription factor and an associated inhibitory protein IκB (Fig. 1). Signals that activate NFκB do so by inducing dissociation of IκB from the p50-p65 transcription factor dimer. We found that TNFs induced κB DNA-binding activity in cultured hippocampal neurons and that IκB antisense oligonucleotides (which activated NFκB) protected the neurons against Aβ toxicity *(44)*. Moreover, exposure of hippocampal cell cultures to a membrane-permeant ceramide analog protected neurons against Aβ toxicity, and oxidative and excitotoxic insults *(183)*. TNFs *(43)* and ceramide (Fig. 10) induced expression of calbindin in cultured hippocampal neurons, suggesting that NFκB-mediated induction of calbindin transcription may be one mechanism whereby TNFs stabilize calcium homeostasis and protect neurons against excitotoxicity and Aβ toxicity. Collectively, these data indicate that the NFκB cytokine signaling pathway may serve as a neuroprotective pathway in neurons. Indeed, recent data indicate that the p75 NGF receptor may signal via the sphingomyelin–ceramide–NFκB pathway *(184)*. Interestingly, in addition to being activated in a receptor-mediated manner, there is evidence that free radicals can induce activation of NFκB more directly *(185)*. This suggests that NFκB may mediate cytoprotective responses to oxidative stress itself.

7.3. Secreted Forms of βAPP

As with many neurotrophic factors and cytokines, levels of βAPP mRNA and protein are increased at sites of injury in the brain *(186,187)*. During the last five years, many in vitro studies, as well as in vivo studies, have shown that sAPPs exhibit neurotrophic activities and can protect neurons against a variety of insults. For example, sAPPs promoted long-term survival of cultured rat cortical neurons *(188)*, and protected cultured rat hippocampal and cortical neurons against glucose deprivation, glutamate toxicity, and Aβ toxicity *(89,117)*. Expression of βAPP in cultured neuroblastoma cells increased their resistance to the neurotoxicities of glutamate and Aβ *(189)*. In vivo studies have also documented neuroprotective activities of sAPPs or overexpression of βAPP. For example, Smith-Swintosky et al. *(190)* reported that infusion of sAPPs into the lateral ventricle of adult rats protected CA1 hippocampal neurons against damage induced by transient global forebrain ischemia. Bowes et al. *(191)* reported that intrathecal infusion of an sAPP peptide into the spinal cord of rabbits enhanced functional recovery following spinal cord ischemia. Overexpression of βAPP in transgenic mice resulted in a reduction in neuronal and synaptic loss induced by the HIV coat protein gp120 *(192)*.

As detailed, data suggest that a neuroprotective pathway activated by sAPPs involves generation of cGMP and activation of potassium channels *(193)*. Recent findings suggest that sAPPs may also activate delayed neuroprotective pathways involving gene expression. For example, sAPPs may increase resistance of neurons to oxidative insults by inducing the expression of antioxidant enzymes. In hippocampal cell cultures, sAPPs

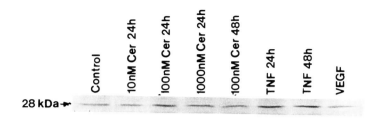

Fig. 10. TNFs and ceramide induce calbindin expression in cultured cortical neurons. Western blot analysis of calbindin levels in dissociated cell cultures that had been exposed to: vehicle (0.2% dimethylsulfoxide), Con; Cer, C2-ceramide; TNF, 100 ng/mL; VEGF, 100 ng/mL vascular endothelial cell growth factor. Note that TNF and C2 increased levels of calbindin; the mol wt of calbindin is 28 kDa.

activated NFκB *(123)* and induced expression of Cu/Zn-SOD and catalase (Mattson, unpublished data). Studies with agents that elevate cGMP levels and cGMP-dependent protein kinase inhibitors provided evidence that cGMP may mediate activation of NFκB by sAPPs *(123)*. The sAPPs may also activate MAP kinases *(194)*, which are well known as components of neurotrophic factor signaling pathways.

7.4. PN-1 and Thrombin

An intriguing set of cellular signaling cascades that may play roles in the pathogenesis of neurodegenerative disorders in general, and AD in particular, includes components of blood coagulation pathways. Over the past 10 yr, biological functions of the protease thrombin, and the thrombin inhibitor PN-1, in neural cells have begun to emerge. Thrombin receptor mRNA is quite widely expressed in the nervous system with both neurons and glia expressing the receptors *(195)*. The presence of thrombin receptors in the brain is intriguing, since thrombin is not normally found in the brain parenchyma. Nevertheless, prothrombin mRNA is expressed in the CNS, where it appears to colocalize with thrombin receptor mRNA *(195)*. This suggests that cells that are a source of thrombin in the brain may also respond to thrombin, perhaps in an autocrine manner. Thrombin influences both glial cells and neurons (*see* ref. *196* for a review). Thrombin can induce neurite retraction in cultured neuroblastoma cells and can kill cultured embryonic rat hippocampal neurons *(197,198)*. The thrombin receptor has been cloned, and is known to be a G-protein-linked receptor that induces inositol phospholipid hydrolysis and calcium release from intracellular stores *(199)*; this pathway is also operative in neurons *(200)*. Thrombin elevated rest $[Ca^{2+}]_i$ in cultured hippocampal neurons and enhanced $[Ca^{2+}]_i$ responses to glucose deprivation and Aβ *(198,201)*. Thrombin increased the vulnerability of cultured rat hippocampal neurons to glucose deprivation and Aβ toxicity.

PN-1 is a very potent thrombin inhibitor that is produced by astrocytes in the brain; PN-1 levels are increased in response to brain injury, and PN-1 is localized in plaques in AD brain (*see* ref. *196* for a review). PN-1 promotes neurite outgrowth and cell survival when added to nerve cell cultures in the absence of exogenous thrombin, suggesting that endogenous thrombin influences neuronal survival and neurite outgrowth in cultured cells. Hippocampal cultures pretreated with PN-1 were protected from both glutamate- and glucose deprivation-induced damage, apparently owing to PN-1's ability to maintain $[Ca^{2+}]_i$ homeostasis *(198)*. Pretreatment of rat hippocampal cell cultures with PN-1 resulted in significant reduction in neuronal damage induced by Aβ, and PN-1 attenuated Aβ-induced elevation of $[Ca^{2+}]_i$ and accumulation of hydrogen peroxide *(201)*. Taken together, these findings suggest that a basal level of thrombin activity may increase neuronal vulnerability to several insults, including metabolic impairment, excitotoxicity, and Aβ toxicity. PN-1 secreted locally by glial cells or neurons may bind thrombin and prevent activation of thrombin receptors in neurons, thereby reducing the vulnerability of the neurons to injury.

8. THE ROLES OF GLIAL CELLS IN THE CALCIUM/FREE RADICAL HYPOTHESIS OF DEMENTIA

Both astrocytes and microglia are present at sites of pathology in AD brain; astrocytes surround senile plaques, and microglia can often be seen infiltrating the core of the plaque *(see* ref. *163* for a review). There is no evidence that alterations in one or both of these glial cell types plays a primary role in the pathophysiology of AD, and it seems most likely that they play a modulatory role in either suppressing or enhancing neurodegenerative processes. Essentially any brain injury (e.g., traumatic, ischemic, excitotoxic) will induce "reactivity" of glial cells *(see* ref. *202* for a review). The glial cells appear to be involved in removing cellular debris at the injury site, and may also play roles in modifying both the initial damage to neurons and subsequent repair processes. At present, such roles can only be inferred from studies of neuron–glia interactions in cell culture and in vivo paradigms of neuronal injury.

Cell-culture studies have shown that astrocytes can protect neurons against several insults relevant to the pathophysiology of AD, including excitotoxicity *(168)* and Aβ toxicity *(203)*. Two mechanisms by which astrocytes may protect neurons against such insults are by producing neurotrophic factors and by enhancing removal of glutamate from the extracellular space. For example, it has been shown that astrocytes produce both bFGF and NGF in response to injuries *(204,205)*, and that each of these neurotrophic factors can protect neurons against excitotoxicity, glucose deprivation, oxidative insults, and/or Aβ toxicity *(37,167–169)*. Interestingly, Aβ induced a reactive phenotype in cultured astrocytes with several features (stellation, increased expression of glial fibrillary acidic protein (GFAP) and bFGF, and alterations in proteoglycan metabolism) similar to those seen in reactive astrocytes associated with senile plaques *(102,206)*, suggesting that Aβ deposition may be an important stimulus for the astrocyte reaction in AD.

Microglial cells respond to, and produce, several cytokines that are likely to play roles in the pathophysiology of AD. For example, TNF induces microglial activation, and activated microglia produce high levels of TNF. It was recently reported that Aβ induces TNF release from microglia in culture *(103)*, and that a substance released from such activated microglia can damage and kill neurons. The identity of the neurotoxic substance released by activated microglia has not been established, but pharmacological data indicate that glutamate receptor antagonists can protect neurons, suggesting that the substance could be an excitotoxin *(104)*. These findings indicate that, in addition to damaging neurons directly, Aβ may indirectly promote neuronal degeneration by inducing activation of microglia.

9. PHARMACOLOGICAL STRATEGIES FOR SUPPRESSING THE NEURODEGENERATIVE PROCESS IN DEMENTIAS

An important goal of research into the molecular mechanisms of neuronal degeneration that underlie AD and related dementing disorders is to identify and develop treatments that suppress the degenerative process. Table 1 is a partial list of compounds shown to protect neurons against insults relevant to the pathogenesis of AD, including Aβ toxicity, excitotoxicity, and oxidative insults. This list is based on published data, and many other compounds have undoubtedly been identified, but the data are not yet published. The list includes several different classes of compounds. Antioxidants have proven very effective in protecting neurons against many different insults in cell-culture studies, but their effectiveness in vivo remains to be established. Compounds that block Na^+ influx (e.g., phenytoin and carbamazepine) or activate K^+ channels (e.g., diazoxide and chromakalim) were effective in protecting cultured hippocampal neurons against Aβ toxicity and glutamate toxicity *(207,208)*. The latter findings are consistent with the mechanism of Aβ toxicity involving impairment of Na^+/K^+-ATPase activity and resultant membrane depolarization *(92,207)*. An intriguing class of neuroprotective compounds is the bacterial alkaloids K-252a, K-252b, and staurosporine. Picomolar concentrations of these compounds were effective in protecting cultured rat hippocampal neurons against glucose deprivation-induced injury, glutamate toxicity, and Aβ toxicity *(209,210)*. K-252a, when administered peripherally (subcutaneously or intraperitoneally) to adult rats at doses of 1–5 μg/kg body wt, protected hippocampal neurons against kainic acid-induced damage *(211)*. This alkaloid also completely ameliorated kainic acid-induced deficits in Morris watermaze tasks of visuospatial learning and memory *(211)*. The mechanism of action of the alkaloids is not completely clear, but they have been reported to induce tyrosine phosphorylation of multiple proteins, including neurotrophin receptors, focal adhesion kinase, and MAP kinases *(209,212,213)*. Another example of an agent that can protect neurons by a mechanism that appears to involve activation of an intrinsic signal transduction pathway is ceramide, which activates NFκB. Ceramide protected cultured rat hippocampal neurons against Aβ toxicity and $FeSO_4$ toxicity, indicating that it can increase resistance of neurons to oxidative insults *(183)*. As described, estrogens can also protect neurons against oxidative insults, including Aβ toxicity *(145)*.

A novel category of neuroprotective agents includes compounds that affect polymerization of actin microfilaments and microtubules. The actin-depolymerizing agent cytochalasin D protected cultured hippocampal neurons against excitotoxicity and Aβ toxicity, and also protected hippocampal neurons against seizure-induced injury in vivo *(120,214)*. The data in the latter studies suggested that the mechanism whereby cytochalasins protect neurons is by suppression of calcium influx through the NMDA receptor and voltage-dependent channels; apparently, actin filaments interact with the membrane calcium channels to promote maintenance in an open state. Microtubules may also influence calcium homeostasis and neuronal vulnerability to excitotoxicity, because taxol, which stabilizes microtubules, attenuated glutamate-induced elevation of $[Ca^{2+}]_i$ and neurotoxicity *(215)*.

Clearly, there are a wealth of compounds that have been shown to have efficacy in protecting neurons in culture and, in some cases, in vivo against insults relevant to AD. Although it remains to be determined whether these compounds or their predecessors

Table 1
Compounds that Protect Neurons Against Insults Relevant to the Pathogenesis of AD and Related Dementias

Agent	Type of insult	Mechanism of action
Vitamin E	$A\beta$, glutamate, $FeSO_4$	Chain-breaking antioxidant
Propyl gallate	$A\beta$, glutamate, $FeSO_4$	Antioxidant
Phenyl-butyl-nitrone (PBN)	$A\beta$, glutamate, $FeSO_4$	Spin-trap (antioxidant)
Nordihydroguaiaretic acid	$A\beta$, glutamate, $FeSO_4$	Antioxidant, lipoxygenase inhibitor
Nifedipine	$A\beta$, glutamate	L-type calcium channel blocker
MK-801, APV	Glutamate, $A\beta^a$	NMDA receptor antagonists
Phenytoin, carbamazepine	$A\beta$, glutamate	Sodium channel blockers (anticonvulsants)
Valproic acid	$A\beta$, glutamate	GABA agonist, sodium channel blocker
Diazoxide, pinacidil, chromakalim	$A\beta$, glutamate, $FeSO_4$	Potassium channel openers
K-252a, K-252b, staurosporine	$A\beta$, glutamate, $FeSO_4$	Activate NTF signaling pathways (tyrosine kinase cascades)
bFGF, BDNF, NGF, NT-3 NT-4/5, IGF-1, TGFβ	$A\beta$, glutamate, and/or $FeSO_4$	Tyrosine phosphorylation, MAP kinase, and gene expression
TNFα and TNFβ	$A\beta$, glutamate, $FeSO_4$	NFκB activation and gene expression
sAPPs	$A\beta$, glutamate, $FeSO_4$	Activate potassium channels and NFκB
Ceramide	$A\beta$, glutamate, $FeSO_4$	Activate NFκB
Estrogens	$A\beta$, glutamate, $FeSO_4$	Antioxidant activity
Cytochalasin D	$A\beta$, glutamate	Actin depolymerization/ decr. calcium influx
Taxol	$A\beta$, glutamate	Microtubule stAβilization/ decr. calcium influx

$^a\beta$locks excitotoxic component of $A\beta$ toxicity. *See text* for references and discussion.

will be effective in human dementias, it seems likely that, because they are effective in an array of in vitro and in vivo systems, some of these compounds and their offspring will be of benefit in humans.

10. SUMMARY

As can be appreciated from the other chapters in this volume, a great deal of valuable information has accrued concerning molecular alterations that may play roles in the pathogenesis of AD and other dementias. However, the specific ways in which such molecular alterations result in dysfunction, damage, and death of neurons have not been established. In this chapter, we considered the increasing evidence indicating that dysregulation of neuronal calcium homeostasis and free radical metabolism represent final common pathways of neuronal dysfunction and death in AD. The data described suggest that a valuable (and perhaps necessary) approach toward understanding the molecular and cellular underpinnings of AD and related dementias is to establish the mechanisms whereby different genetic mutations and age-related factors lead to free radical generation, disruption of ion homeostasis, and neuronal death in AD. Such data are accruing and range from cell-culture studies showing that Aβ induces free radical production and loss of ion homeostasis, to studies of postmortem brains of AD victims, which reveal increased protein and lipid oxidation, to studies of living AD patients demonstrating impaired glucose availability to vulnerable brain regions. Several age-related changes in the brain likely create an environment conducive to generation of free radicals and loss of Ca^{2+} homeostasis; these may include vascular alterations, reduced glucose uptake, and deposition of Aβ. On the other hand, many different neurotrophic factors and cytokines that are associated with AD pathology have recently been shown to stabilize calcium homeostasis and suppress free radical production in cultured neurons, suggesting that neuroprotective signaling pathways are activated in AD. An understanding of such signaling pathways may lead to novel preventative and therapeutic strategies for the dementias. Finally, it is predicted that mutations in different genes that are causally linked to inherited forms of AD will be found to encode proteins involved in regulation of ion homeostasis and/or free radical metabolism. Indeed, βAPP mutations appear to affect the enzymatic processing of this protein such that levels of calcium-destabilizing Aβ are increased, whereas levels of neuroprotective secreted forms of APP are reduced.

11. FUTURE DIRECTIONS OF THE CALCIUM-FREE RADICAL HYPOTHESIS

As can be appreciated from this brief review, there is certainly ample precedence for calcium and free radicals playing important roles in neurodegenerative processes in general. In fact, there are no neurodegenerative conditons, either acute or chronic, in which calcium and free radicals have been shown not to play important roles. If one accepts that calcium and free radicals are convergence points for the neurodegenerative process in AD and other dementias, then a major task is to identify the specific upstream events that disrupt calcium homeostasis and/or promote accumulation of free radicals. Some of these upstream events were enumerated above (e.g., Aβ accumulation, fibril formation, and reduced glucose availability), and it is very likely that many others will be identified. A second major area of concern is the specific molecular events involved in the neurotoxicity of Aβ and in protection by sAPPs and neurotrophic factors. For example, it is very unclear exactly how Aβ induces free radical production in neurons. Similarly, we have a very cursory knowledge of neuroprotective signal transduction pathways and how to manipulate them.

An area of investigation that we look forward to with great anticipation is the elucidation of the normal function of the proteins encoded by the chromosome 14 and chromosome 1 genes (S182 and STM2, respectively) mutated in pedigrees with early onset forms of AD *(124,128)*. The predicted structures of S182 and STM2 suggest that they are integral membrane proteins with seven-membrane-spanning domains. Such proteins often function as receptors that regulate ion channels or as ion channels themselves, or they may function in protein trafficking. It is therefore a good bet that mutations in these proteins result either directly, or indirectly, in altered calcium homeostasis and/or free radical metabolism. The elucidation of the mechanism whereby various risk factors alter calcium homeostasis and/or free radical metabolism will be another major area of interest. For example, is the influence of ApoE owing to an action directly on neurons, or is it owing to a vascular effect? How does estrogen affect the development of AD? Finally, a question often entertained, but seldom addressed with experiments at the cellular and molecular levels, is: what is aging and how does it increase the risk of so many different human diseases? Because neuroscientists study postmitotic cells, we may be in a strong position to address this ultimate question.

ACKNOWLEDGMENTS

We thank S. W. Barger, B. Cheng, and V. L. Smith-Swintosky for contributions to original research from M. P. M.'s laboratory, and D. A. Butterfield, J. Carney, S. Christakos, W. R. Markesbery, R. E. Rydel, and R. M. Sapolsky for valuable collaborations. Research was supported by grants to M. P. M. from the NIH (NINDS and NIA), the Alzheimer's Association (Evelyn T. Stone Fund and Zenith Award), and the Metropolitan Life Foundation.

REFERENCES

1. Watson, B. D. and Ginsberg, M. D. (1989) Ischemic injury in the brain. Role of oxygen radical-mediated processes, *Ann. NY Acad. Sci.* **559**, 269–281.
2. Mattson, M. (1992) Calcium as sculptor and destroyer of neural circuitry, *Exp. Gerontol.* **27**, 29–49.
3. Orrenius, S. (1995) Apoptosis: molecular mechanisms and implications for human disease, *J. Intern. Med.* **237**, 529–536.
4. Clapham, D. E. (1995) Calcium signaling, *Cell* **80**, 259–268.
5. Sloviter, R. S. (1989) Calcium-binding protein (calbindin-D28k) and parvalbumin immunocytochemistry: localization in the rat hippocampus with specific reference to the selective vulnerability of hippocampal neurons to seizure activity, *J. Comp. Neurol.* **280**, 183–196.
6. Iacopino, A. M., Quintero, E. M., and Miller, E. K. (1994) Calbindin-D_{28K}: A potential neuroprotective protein, *Neurodegeneration* **3**, 1–20.
7. Stadtman, E. R. (1992) Protein oxidation and aging, *Science* **257**, 1220–1224.
8. Rosen, D. R., Siddique, T., Patterson, D., Figlewicz, D. A., Sapp, P., Hentati, A., Donaldson, D., Goto, J., O'Regan, J. P., Deng, H.-X., Rahmani, Z., Krizus, A., McKenna-Yasek, D., Cayabyab, A., Gaston, S. M., Berger, R., Tanzi, R. E., Halperin, J. J., Herzfeldt, B., Van den Bergh, R., Hung, W.-Y., Bird, T., Deng, G., Mulder, D. W., Smyth, C., Laing, N. G., Soriano, E., Pericak-Vance, M. A., Haines, J., Rouleau, G. A., Gusella, J. S., Horvitz, H. R., and Brown, R. H., Jr. (1993) Mutations in Cu/Zn superoxide dismutase gene are associated with familial amyotrophic lateral sclerosis, *Nature* **362**, 59–62.
9. Benzi, G. and Moretti, A. (1995) Age- and peroxidative stress-related modifications of the cerebral enzymatic activities linked to mitochondria and the glutathione system, *Free Radical. Biol. Med.* **19**, 77–101.
10. Mattson, M. P. (1995) Free radicals and disruption of neuronal ion homeostasis in AD: a role for amyloid β-peptide? *Neurobiol. Aging* **16**, 679–682.
11. Sanfeliu, C., Hunt, A., and Patell, A. J. (1990) Exposure to *N*-methyl-D-aspartate increases release of arachidonic acid in primary cultures of rat hippocampal neurons and not in astrocytes, *Brain Res.* **526**, 241–248.
12. Verity, M. A. (1993) Mechanisms of phospholipase A2 activation and neuronal injury, *Ann. NY Acad. Sci.* **679**, 110–120.

13. Mattson, M. P., Lovell, M. A., Furukawa, K., and Markesbery, W. R. (1995) Neurotrophic factors attenuate glutamate-induced accumulation of peroxides, elevation of $[Ca^{2+}]_i$ and neurotoxicity, and increase antioxidant enzyme activities in hippocampal neurons, *J. Neurochem.* **65**, 1740–1751.

14. Zhang, J. and Snyder, S. H. (1995) Nitric oxide in the nervous system, *Ann. Rev. Pharmacol. Toxicol.* **35**, 213–233.

15. Lipton, S. A., Choi, Y. B., Pan, Z. H., Lei, S. Z., Chen, H. S. V., Sucher, N. J., Losaizo, J., Singd, D. J., and Stemler, J. S. (1993) A redox-based mechanism for the neuroprotective and neurodestructive effects of nitric oxide and related nitroso-compounds, *Nature* **364**, 626–632.

16. Murphy, T. H., Miyamoto, M., Sastre, A., Schnaar, R. L., and Coyle, J. T. (1989) Glutamate toxicity in a neuronal cell line involves inhibition of cystine transport and oxidative stress, *Neuron* **2**, 1547–1558.

17. Levy, D. I., Sucher, N. J., and Lipton, S. A. (1991) Glutathione prevents *N*-methyl-D-aspartate receptor-mediated neurotoxicity, *Neuropharmacol. Neurotoxicol.* **2**, 345–348.

18. Yamada, T., McGeer, P. L., Baimbridge, K. G., and McGeer, E. G. (1990) Relative sparing in Parkinson's disease of substantia nigra dopamine neurons containing calbindin-D28K, *Brain Res.* **526**, 303–307.

19. Peterson, D. A., Lucidi-Phillipi, C. A., Murphy, D. P., Ray, J., and Gage, F. H. (1996) FGF-2 protects layer II entorhinal glutamatergic neurons from axotomy-induced death, *J. Neurosci.* **16**, 886–898.

20. Garruto, R. (1991) Pacific paradigms of environmentally-induced neurological disorders: Clinical, epidemiological and molecular perspectives, *Neurotoxicol.* **12**, 347–378.

21. Hof, P. R., Nimchinsky, E. A., Buee-Scherrer, V., Buee, L., Nasrallah, J., Hottinger, A. F., Purohit, D. P., Loerzel, A. J., Steele, J. C., and Delacourte, A. (1994) Amyotrophic lateral sclerosis/Parkinsonism-dementia complex of Guam: quantitative neuropathology, immunohistochemical analysis of neuronal vulnerability, and comparison with related neurodegenerative disorders, *Acta Neuropathol.* **88**, 397–404.

22. Garruto, R. M., Fukatsu, R., Yanagihara, R., Gajdusek, D. C., Hook, G., and Fiori, C. E. (1984) Imaging of calcium and aluminum in neurofibrillary tangle-bearing neurons in Parkinsonism-dementia of Guam, *Proc. Natl. Acad. Sci. USA* **81**, 1875–1879.

23. Spencer, P. S., Nunn, P. B., Hugon, J., Ludolph, A. C., Ross, S. M., Roy, D. N., and Robertson, R. C. (1987) Guam amyotrophic lateral sclerosis—Parkinsonism—dementia linked to a plant excitant neurotoxin, *Science* **237**, 517–522.

24. Garruto, R. M., Shankar, S. K., Yanagihara, R., Salazar, A. M., Amyx, H. L., and Gajdusek, D. C. (1989) Low-calcium, high-aluminum diet-induced motor neuron pathology in cynomolgus monkeys, *Acta Neuropathol.* **78**, 210–219.

25. Zattore, R. J. (1990) Memory loss following domoic acid intoxication from ingestion of toxic mussels, *Can. Dis. Wkly. Rep.* **16(Suppl. 1E)**, 101–103.

26. Scallet, A. C., Binienda, Z., Caputo, F. A., Hall, S., Paule, M. G., Rountree, R. L., Schmued, L., Sobotka, T., and Slikker, W. (1993) Domoic acid-treated cynomolgus monkeys (M. fascicularis): effects of dose on hippocampal neuronal and terminal degeneration, *Brain Res.* **627**, 307–313.

27. Mattson, M. P., Barger, S. W., Cheng, B., Lieberburg, I., Smith-Swintosky, V. L., and Rydel, R. E. (1993) β-amyloid precursor protein metabolites and loss of neuronal calcium homeostasis in Alzheimer's disease, *Trends Neurosci.* **16**, 409–415.

28. Mattson, M. P. (1994) β-amyloid precursor protein metabolites, metabolic compromise, and loss of neuronal calcium homeostasis in Alzheimer's disease, *Ann. NY Acad. Sci.* **747**, 50–76.

29. Mattson, M. P. and Barger, S. W. (1995) Programmed cell life: neuroprotective signal transduction and ischemic brain injury, in *Cerebrovascular Diseases: The 19th Princeton Stroke Conference* (Moskowitz, M. A. and Caplan, L. R., eds.), Butterworth, Stoneham, MA, pp. 271–290.

30. Mattson, M. P. (1990) Antigenic changes similar to those seen in neurofibrillary tangles are elicited by glutamate and calcium influx in cultured hippocampal neurons, *Neuron* **4**, 105–117.

31. Sautiere, P. E., Sindou, P., Couratier, P., Hugon, J., Wattez, A., and Delacourte, A. (1992) Tau antigenic changes induced by glutamate in rat primary culture model: a biochemical approach, *Neurosci. Lett.* **140**, 206–210.

32. De Boni, U. and Crapper-McLachlan, D. R. (1985) Controlled induction of paired helical filaments of the Alzheimer type in cultured human neurons by glutamate and aspartate, *J. Neurol. Sci.* **65**, 105–118.

33. Elliott, E., Mattson, M. P., Vanderklish, P., Lynch, G., Chang, I., and Sapolsky, R. M. (1993) Corticosterone exacerbates kainate-induced alterations in hippocampal tau immunoreactivity and spectrin proteolysis in vivo, *J. Neurochem.* **61**, 57–67.

34. Stein-Behrens, B., Mattson, M. P., Chang, I., Yeh, M., and Sapolsky, R. M. (1994) Stress exacerbates neuron loss and cytoskeletal pathology in the hippocampus, *J. Neurosci.* **14**, 5373–5380.

35. Busciglio, J., Lorenzo, A., Yeh, J., and Yankner, B. A. (1995) β-amyloid fibrils induce tau phosphorylation and loss of microtubule binding, *Neuron* **14**, 879–888.

36. Mattson, M. P., Cheng, B., Davis, D., Bryant, K., Lieberburg, I., and Rydel, R. E. (1992) β-amyloid peptides destabilize calcium homeostasis and render human cortical neurons vulnerable to excitotoxicity, *J. Neurosci.* **12**, 376–389.

37. Mattson, M. P., Tomaselli, K., and Rydel, R. E. (1993) Calcium-destabilizing and neurodegenerative effects of aggregated β-amyloid peptide are attenuated by basic FGF, *Brain Res.* **621**, 35–49.

38. Hartmann, H., Eckert, A., and Muller, W. E. (1993) Beta-amyloid protein amplifies calcium signalling in central neurons from the adult mouse, *Biochem. Biophys. Res. Commun.* **194**, 1216–1220.

39. Eckert, A., Hartmann, H., and Muller, W. E. (1993) Beta-amyloid protein enhances the mitogen-induced calcium response in circulating human lymphocytes, *FEBS Lett.* **330**, 49–52.

40. Weiss, J. H., Pike, C. J., and Cotman, C. W. (1994) Ca^{2+} channel blockers attenuate β-amyloid peptide toxicity to cortical neurons in culture, *J. Neurochem.* **62**, 372–375.

41. Mattson, M. P., Rychlik, B., Chu, C., and Christakos, S. (1991) Evidence for calcium-reducing and excitoprotective roles for the calcium binding protein (calbindin-D28k) in cultured hippocampal neurons, *Neuron* **6**, 41–51.

42. Chard, P. S., Bleakman, D., Christakos, S., Fullmer, C. S., and Miller, R. J. (1993) Calcium buffering properties of calbindin D28k and parvalbumin in rat sensory neurones, *J. Physiol.* **472**, 341–357.

43. Cheng, B., Christakos, S., and Mattson, M. P. (1994) Tumor necrosis factors protect neurons against excitotoxic/metabolic insults and promote maintenance of calcium homeostasis, *Neuron* **12**, 139–153.

44. Barger, S. W., Horster, D., Furukawa, K., Goodman, Y., Krieglstein, J., and Mattson, M. P. (1995) TNFα and TNFβ protect hippocampal neurons against amyloid β-peptide toxicity: evidence for involvement of a κB-binding factor and attenuation of peroxide and Ca^{2+} accumulation, *Proc. Natl. Acad. Sci. USA* **92**, 9328–9332.

45. Forloni, G., Chiesa, R., Smiroldo, S., and Verga, L. (1993) Apoptosis mediated neurotoxicity induced by chronic application of beta amyloid fragment 25-35, *Neuroreport* **4**, 523–526.

46. Loo, D. T., Copani, A., Pike, C. J., Whittemore, E. R., Walencewicz, A. J., and Cotman, C. W. (1993) Apoptosis is induced by beta-amyloid in cultured central nervous system neurons, *Proc. Natl. Acad. Sci. USA* **90**, 7951–7955.

47. Behl, C., Davis, J. B., Klier, F. G., and Schubert, D. (1994) Amyloid beta peptide induces necrosis rather than apoptosis, *Brain Res.* **645**, 253–264.

48. Behl, C., Hovey, L., Krajewski, S., Schubert, D., and Reed, J. C. (1993) BCL-2 prevents killing of neuronal cells by glutamate but not by amyloid beta protein, *Biochem. Biophys. Res. Commun.* **197**, 949–956.

49. Pike, C. J. and Cotman, C. W. (1995) Calretinin-immunoreactive neurons are resistant to β-amyloid toxicity in vitro, *Brain Res.* **671,** 293–298.
50. Meier-Ruge, W., Bertoni-Freddari, C., and Iwangoff, P. (1994) Changes in brain glucose metabolism as a key to the pathogenesis of Alzheimer's disease, *Gerontology* **40,** 246–252.
51. Novelli, A., Reilly, J. A., Lyska, P. C., and Henneberry, R. C. (1988) Glutamate becomes neurotoxic via the *N*-methyl-D-aspartate receptor when intracellular energy levels are reduced, *Brain Res.* **451,** 205–212.
52. Copani, A., Koh, J.-Y., and Cotman, C. W. (1991) β-amyloid increases neuronal susceptibility to injury by glucose deprivation, *NeuroReport* **2,** 763–765.
53. de la Torre, J. C. (1994) Impaired brain microcirculation may trigger Alzheimer's disease, *Neurosci. Biobehav. Rev.* **18,** 397–401.
54. Perlmutter, L. S. (1994) Microvascular pathology and vascular basement membrane components in Alzheimer's disease, *Mol. Neurobiol.* **9,** 33–40.
55. Yankner, B. A. and Mesulam, M. M. (1991) β-amyloid and the pathogenesis of Alzheimer's disease, *N. Engl. J. Med.* **325,** 1849–1857.
56. Mullan, M. and Crawford, F. (1993) Genetic and molecular advances in Alzheimer's disease, *Trends Neurosci.* **16,** 398–403.
57. Selkoe, D. J. (1993) Physiological production of the β-amyloid protein and the mechanism of Alzheimer's disease, *Trends Neurosci.* **16,** 403–409.
58. Busciglio, J., Yeh, J., and Yankner, B. A. (1993) β-amyloid neurotoxicity in human cortical culture is not mediated by excitotoxins, *J. Neurochem.* **61,** 1565–1568.
59. Cai, X., Golde, T., and Youkin, S. (1993) Release of excess amyloid β protein from a mutant amyloid β protein precursor, *Science* **259,** 514–516.
60. Citron, M., Vigo-Pelfrey, C., Teplow, D. B., Miller, C., Schenk, D., Johnston, J., Winblad, B., Venizelos, N., Lannfelt, L., and Selkoe, D. J. (1994) Excessive production of amyloid β-protein by peripheral cells of symptomatic and presymptomatic patients carrying the Swedish familial Alzheimer disease mutation, *Proc. Natl. Acad. Sci. USA* **91,** 11,993–11,997.
61. Suzuki, N., Cheung, T. T., Cai, X. D., Odaka, A., Otvos, L. J., Eckman, C., Golde, T. E., and Younkin, S. G. (1994) An increased percentage of long amyloid β protein secreted by familial amyloid β protein precursor (βAPP$_{717}$) mutants, *Science* **264,** 1336–1340.
62. Lansbury, P. T., Costa, P. R., Griffiths, J. M., Simon, E. J., Auger, M., Halverson, K. J., Kocisko, D. A., Hendsch, Z. S., Ashburn, T. T., Spencer, R. G. S., Tidor, B., and Griffin, R. G. (1995) Structural model for the β-amyloid fibril: interstrand alignment of an antiparallel β sheet comprising a C-terminal peptide, *Nature Struct. Biol.* in press.
63. Yankner, B. A., Duffy, L. K., and Kirschner, D. A. (1990) Neurotrophic and neurotoxic effects of amyloid beta protein: reversal by tachykinin neuropeptides, *Science* **250,** 279–282.
64. Pike, C., Burdick, D., Walencewicz, A., Glabe, C., and Cotman, C. (1993) Neurodegeneration induced by β-amyloid peptides in vitro: the role of peptide assembly state, *J. Neurosci.* **13,** 1676–1686.
65. Quon, D., et al. (1991) Formation of β-amyloid protein deposits in brains of transgenic mice, *Nature* **352,** 239–241.
66. Mucke, L., Masliah, E., Johnson, W. B., Ruppe, M. D., Alford, M., Rockenstein, E. M., Forss-Petter, S., Pietropaolo, M., Mallory, M., and Abraham, C. R. (1994) Synaptotrophic effects of human amyloid β protein precursors in the cortex of transgenic mice, *Brain Res.* **666,** 151–167.
67. Wirak, D. O., Bayney, R., Ramabhadran, T. V., Fracasso, R. P., Hart, J. T., Hauer, P. E., Hsiau, P., Pekar, S. K., Scangos, G. A., Trapp, B. D., and Unterbeck, A. J. (1991) Deposits of amyloid beta protein in the central nervous system of transgenic mice, *Science* **253,** 323–325.
68. Sandhu, F. A., Salim, M., and Zain, S. B. (1991) Expression of the human beta-amyloid protein of Alzheimer's disease specifically in the brains of transgenic mice, *J. Biol. Chem.* **266,** 21,331–21,334.

69. De Koning, E. J. P., Morris, E. R., Hofhuis, F. M. A., Posthuma, G., Hoppener, J. W. M., Morris, J. F., Capel, P. J. A., Clark, A., and Verbeek, J. S. (1994) Intra- and extracellular amyloid fibrils are formed in cultured pancreatic islets of transgenic mice expressing human islet amyloid polypeptide, *Proc. Natl. Acad. Sci. USA* **91**, 8467–8471.

70. Games, D., Adams, D., Alessandrinl, R., Barbour, R., Berthelette, P., Blackwell, C., Carr, T., Clemens, J., Donaldson, T., Gillespie, F., Guido, T., Hagoplan, S., Johnson-Wood, K., Khan, K., Lee, M., Lelbowitz, E., McConlogue, S., Montoya-Zavala, M., Mucke, L., Paganini, L., Penniman, E., Power, M., Schenk, D., Seubert, P., Snyder, B., Soriano, F., Tan, H., Vitale, J., Wadsworth, S., Wolozin, B., and Zhao, J. (1995) Alzheimer-type neuropathology in transgenic mice overexpressing V717F β-amyloid precursor protein, *Nature* **373**, 523–527.

71. Fraser, P. E., Nguyen, J. T., Surewicz, W. K., and Kirschner, D. A. (1991) pH-dependent structural transitions of Alzheimer amyloid peptides, *Biophys. J.* **60**, 1190–1201.

72. Hilbich, C., Kisters-Woike, B., Reed, J., Masters, C. L., and Beyreuther, K. (1991) Aggregation and secondary structure of synthetic amyloid beta A4 peptides of Alzheimer's disease, *J. Mol. Biol.* **218**, 149–163.

73. Burdick, D., Soreghan, B., Kwon, M., Kosmoski, J., Knauer, M., Henschen, A., Yates, J., Cotman, C., and Glabe, C. (1992) Assembly and aggregation properties of synthetic Alzheimer's A4/Beta amyloid peptide analogs, *J. Biol. Chem.* **267**, 546–554.

74. Dyrks, T., Dyrks, E., Hartmann, T., Masters, C., and Beyreuther, K. E. (1992) Amyloidogenicity of beta A4 and beta A4-bearing amyloid protein precursor fragments by metal-catalyzed oxidation, *J. Biol. Chem.* **267**, 18,210–18,217.

75. Hensley, K., Carney, J. M., Mattson, M. P., Aksenova, M., Harris, M., Wu, J. F., Floyd, R., and Butterfield, D. A. (1994) A model for β-amyloid aggregation and neurotoxicity based on free radical generation by the peptide: relevance to Alzheimer's disease, *Proc. Natl. Acad. Sci. USA* **91**, 3270–3274.

76. Bush, A. I., Pettingell, W. H., Multhaup, G., d Paradis, M., Vonsattel, J. P., Gusella, J. F., Beyreuther, K., Masters, C. L., and Tanzi, R. E. (1994) Rapid induction of Alzheimer β-amyloid formation by zinc, *Science* **265**, 1464–1467.

77. Simmons, L. K., May, P. C., Tomaselli, K. J., Rydel, R. E., Fuson, K. S., Brigham, E. F., Wright, S., Lieberburg, I., Becker, G. W., and Brems, D. N. (1994) Secondary structure of amyloid beta peptide correlates with neurotoxic activity in vitro, *Mol. Pharmacol.* **45**, 373–379.

78. Lorenzo, A. and Yankner, B. A. (1994) β-amyloid neurotoxicity requires fibril formation and is inhibited by Congo red, *Proc. Natl. Acad. Sci. USA* **91**, 12,243–12,247.

79. Pike, C. J., Walencewicz-Wasserman, A. J., Kosmoski, J., Cribbs, D. H., Glabe, C. G., and Cotman, C. W. (1995) Structure-activity analyses of β-amyloid peptides: Contributions of the β25-35 region to aggregation and neurotoxicity, *J. Neurochem.* **64**, 253–265.

80. Henderson, V. W., Paganini-Hill, A., Emanuel, C. K., Dunn, M. E., and Buckwalter, J. G. (1994) Estrogen replacement therapy in older women. Comparisons between Alzheimer's disease cases and nondemented control subjects, *Arch. Neurol.* **51**, 896–900.

81. Butterfield, D. A., Hensley, K., Harris, M., Mattson, M. P., and Carney, J. (1994) β-amyloid peptide free radical fragments initiate synaptosomal lipoperoxidation in a sequence-specific fashion: implications to Alzheimer's disease, *Biochem. Biophys. Res. Commun.* **200**, 710–715.

82. Schubert, D. and Chevion, M. (1995) The role of iron in beta amyloid toxicity, *Biochem. Biophys. Res. Commun.* **216**, 702–707.

83. May, P. C., Boggs, L. N., and Fuson, K. S. (1993) Neurotoxicity of human amylin in rat primary hippocampal cultures: similarity to Alzheimer's disease amyloid-beta neurotoxicity, *J. Neurochem.* **61**, 2330–2333.

84. Lorenzo, A., Razzaboni, B., Weir, G. C., and Yankner, B. A. (1994) Pancreatic islet cell toxicity of amylin associated with type-2 diabetes mellitus, *Nature* **368**, 756–760.

85. Schubert, D., Behl, C., Lesley, R., Brack, A., Dargusch, R., Sagara, Y., and Kimura, H. (1995) Amyloid peptides are toxic via a common oxidative mechanism, *Proc. Natl. Acad. Sci. USA* **92**, 1989–1993.

86. Mattson, M. P. and Goodman, Y. (1995) Different amyloidogenic peptides share a similar mechanism of neurotoxicity involving reactive oxygen species and calcium, *Brain Res.* **676,** 219–224.

87. Jarrett, J. T. and Lansury, P. T. (1993) Seeding "One-dimensional crystallization" of amyloid: a pathogenic mechanism in Alzheimer's disease and scrapie? *Cell* **73,** 1055–1058.

88. Behl, C., Davis, J., Lesley, R., and Schubert, D. (1994) Hydrogen peroxide mediates amyloid β protein toxicity, *Cell* **77,** 817–827.

89. Goodman, Y. and Mattson, M. P. (1994) Secreted forms of β-amyloid precursor protein protect hippocampal neurons against amyloid β-peptide-induced oxidative injury, *Exp. Neurol.* **128,** 1–12.

90. Goodman, Y., Steiner, M. R., Steiner, S. M., and Mattson, M. P. (1994) Nordihydroguaiaretic acid protects hippocampal neurons against amyloid β-peptide toxicity, and attenuates free radical and calcium accumulation, *Brain Res.* **654,** 171–176.

91. Sagara, Y., Dargusch, R., Klier, F. G., Schubert, D., and Behl, C. (1996) Increased antioxidant enzyme activity in amyloid beta protein-resistant cells, *J. Neurosci.* **16,** 497–505.

92. Mark, R. J., Hensley, K., Butterfield, D. A., and Mattson, M. P. (1995) Amyloid β-peptide impairs ion-motive ATPase activities: evidence for a role in loss of neuronal Ca^{2+} homeostasis and cell death, *J. Neurosci.* **15,** 6239–6249.

93. Shearman, M. S., Hawtin, S. R., and Tailor, V. J. (1995) The intracellular component of cellular 3-(4, 5-Dimethylthiazol-2-yl)-2, 5-Diphenyltetrazolium bromide (MTT) reduction is specifically inhibited by β-amyloid peptides, *J. Neurochem.* **65,** 218–227.

94. Arispe, N., Pollard, H. B., and Rojas, E. (1993) Giant multilevel cation chanels formed by Alzheimer disease amyloid β-protein [AβP-(1-40)] in bilayer membranes, *Proc. Natl. Acad. Sci. USA* **90,** 10,573–10,577.

95. Furukawa, K., Abe, Y., and Akaike, N. (1994) Amyloid β protein-induced irreversible current in rat cortical neurones, *NeuroReport* **5,** 2016–2018.

96. Collerton, D. (1986) Cholinergic function and intellectual decline in Alzheimer's disease, *Neuroscience* **19,** 1–28.

97. Flynn, D. D., Weinstein, D. A., and Mash, D. C. (1991) Loss of high-affinity agonist binding to M1 muscarinic receptor in Alzheimer's Disease. Implications for failure of cholinergic replacement therapies, *Ann. Neurol.* **29,** 256–262.

98. Pearce, B. D. and Potter, L. T. (1991) Coupling of m1 muscarinic receptors to G protein in Alzheimer disease, *Alzheimer Dis. Assoc. Disord.* **5,** 163–172.

99. Warpman, U., Alafuzoff, I., and Nordberg, A. (1993) Coupling of muscarinic receptors to GTP proteins in postmortem human brain—alterations in Alzheimer's disease, *Neurosci. Lett.* **150,** 39–43.

100. Kelly, J., Furukawa, K., Barger, S. W., Rengen, M. R., Mark, R. J., Blanc, E. M., Roth, G., and Mattson, M. P. (1996) Amyloid β-peptide disrupts carbachol-induced muscarinic cholinergic signal transduction in cortical neurons, *Proc. Natl. Acad. Sci. USA* **93,** 6753–6758.

101. Pike, C. J., Cummings, B. J., Monzavi, R., and Cotman, C. W. (1994) β-amyloid-induced changes in cultured astrocytes parallel reactive astrocytosis associated with senile plaques in Alzheimer's disease, *Neuroscience* **63,** 517–531.

102. Volterra, A., Trotti, D., Floridi, S., and Racagni, G. (1994) Reactive oxygen species inhibit high-affinity glutamate uptake: molecular mechanism and neuropathological implications, *Ann. NY Acad. Sci.* **738,** 153–162.

103. Meda, L., Cassatella, M. A., Szendrei, G. I., Otvos, L., Jr., Baron, P., Villalba, M., Ferrari, D., and Rossi, F. (1995) Activation of microglial cells by beta-amyloid protein and interferon-gamma, *Nature* **374,** 647–650.

104. Lipton, S. A. (1994) AIDS-related dementia and calcium homeostasis, *Ann. NY Acad. Sci.* **747,** 205–224.

105. Korotzer, A. R., Pike, C. J., and Cotman, C. W. (1993) β-amyloid peptides induce degeneration of cultured rat microglia, *Brain Res.* **624,** 121–125.

106. Davis-Salinas, J., Saporito-Irwin, S. M., Cotman, C. W., and Van Nostrand, W. E. (1995) Amyloid beta-protein induces its own production in cultured degenerating cerebrovascular smooth muscle cells, *J. Neurochem.* **65,** 931–934.

107. Thomas, T., Thomas, G., McLendon, C., Sutton, T., and Mullan, M. (1996) β-amyloid-mediated vasoactivity and vascular endothelial damage, *Nature* **380,** 168–171.

108. Haass, C., Schlossmacher, M. G., Hung, A. Y., Vigo-Pelfrey, C., Mellon, A., Ostaszewski, B., Lieberburg, I., Koo, E. H., Schenk, D., Teplow, D. B., and Selkoe, D. J. (1992) Amyloid β-peptide is produced by cultured cells during normal metabolism, *Nature* **359,** 322–325.

109. Seubert, P., Vigo-Pelfrey, C., Esch, F., Lee, M., Dovey, H., Davis, D., Sinha, S., Schlossmacher, M., Whaley, J., Swindlehurst, C., McCormack, R., Wolfert, R., Selkoe, D. J., Lieberburg, I., and Schenk, D. (1992) Isolation and quantitation of soluble Alzheimer's β-peptide from biological fluids, *Nature* **359,** 325–327.

110. Koo, E. H., Sisodia, S. S., Archer, D. R., Martin, L. J., Weidemann, A., Beyreuther, K., Fischer, P., Masters, C. L., and Price, D. L. (1990) Precursor of amyloid protein in Alzheimer disease undergoes fast anterograde axonal transport, *Proc. Natl. Acad. Sci. USA* **87,** 1561–1565.

111. Schubert, W., Prior, R., Weidemann, A., Dircksen, H., Multhaup, G., Masters, C. L., and Beyreuther, K. (1991) Localization of Alzheimer βA4 amyloid at presynaptic terminals, *Brain Res.* **563,** 184–194.

112. Mattson, M. P. (1994) Secreted forms of β-amyloid precursor protein modulate dendrite outgrowth and calcium responses to glutamate in cultured embryonic hippocampal neurons, *J. Neurobiol.* **25,** 439–450.

113. Nitsch, R. M., Slack, B. E., Wurtman, R. J., and Growdon, J. H. (1992) Release of Alzheimer amyloid precursor derivatives stimulated by activation of muscarinic acetylcholine receptors, *Science* **258,** 304–307.

114. Nitsch, R. M., Farber, S. A., Growdon, J. H., and Wurtman, R. J. (1993) Release of amyloid beta-protein precursor derivatives by electrical depolarization of rat hippocampal slices, *Proc. Natl. Acad. Sci. USA* **90,** 5191–5193.

115. Ninomiya, H., Roch, J.-M., Sundsmo, M. P., Otero, D. A., and Saitoh, T. (1993) Amino acid sequence RERMS represents the active domain of amyloid β/A4 protein precursor that promotes fibroblast growth, *J. Cell Biol.* **121,** 879–886.

116. Roch, J. M., Masliah, E., Roch-Levecq, A. C., Sundsmo, M. P., Otero, D. A., Veinbergs, I., and Saitoh, T. (1994) Increase of synaptic density and memory retention by a peptide representing the trophic domain of the amyloid β/A4 protein precursor, *Proc. Natl. Acad. Sci. USA* **91,** 7450–7454.

117. Mattson, M. P., Cheng, B., Culwell, A., Esch, F., Lieberburg, I., and Rydel, R. E. (1993) Evidence for excitoprotective and intraneuronal calcium-regulating roles for secreted forms of β-amyloid precursor protein, *Neuron* **10,** 243–254.

118. Barger, S. W., Fiscus, R. R., Ruth, P., Hofmann, F., and Mattson, M. P. (1995) Role of cyclic GMP in the regulation of neuronal calcium and survival by secreted forms of β-amyloid precursor, *J. Neurochem.* **64,** 2087–2096.

119. Barger, S. W. and Mattson, M. P. (1995) Secreted form of the Alzheimer's amyloid precursor protein stimulates a membrane-associated guanylate cyclase, *Biochem. J.* **311,** 45–47.

120. Furukawa, K. and Mattson, M. P. (1995) Cytochalasins protect hippocampal neurons against amyloid β-peptide toxicity: evidence that actin depolymerization suppresses Ca^{2+} influx, *J. Neurochem.* **65,** 1061–1068.

121. Alkon, D. L. (1995) Molecular mechanisms of associative memory and their clinical implications, *Behav. Brain Res.* **66,** 151–160.

122. Etcheberrigaray, R., Ito, E., Kim, C. S., and Alkon, D. L. (1994) Soluble β-amyloid induction of Alzheimer's phenotype for human fibroblast K^+ channels, *Science* **264,** 276–279.

123. Barger, S. W. and Mattson, M. P. (1996) Induction of neuroprotective κB-dependent transcription by secreted forms of the Alzheimer's β-amyloid precursor, *Mol. Brain Res.* **40,** 116–126.

124. Levy-Lahad, E., Wasco, W., Poorkaj, P., Romano, D. M., Oshima, J., Pettingell, W. H., Yu, C-E., Jondro, P. D., Schmidt, S. D., Wang, K., Crowley, A. C., Fu, Y-H., Guenette, S. Y., Galas, D., Nemens, E., Wijsman, E. M., Bird, T. D., Schellenberg, G. D., and Tanzi, R. E. (1995) Candidate gene for the chromosome 1 familial Alzheimer's disease locus, *Science* **269**, 973–977.

125. Hescheler, J. and Schultz, G. (1993) G-proteins involved in the calcium channel signalling system, *Curr. Opinion Neurobiol.* **3**, 360–367.

126. Nurnberg, B., Gudermann, T., and Schultz, G. (1995) Receptors and G proteins as primary components of transmembrane signal transduction. Part 2. G proteins: structure and function, *J. Mol. Med.* **73**, 123–132.

127. Recasens, M. and Vignes, M. (1995) Excitatory amino acid metabotropic receptor subtypes and calcium regulation, *Ann. NY Acad. Sci.* **757**, 418–429.

128. Sherrington, R., Rogaev, E. I., Liang, Y., Rogaeva, E. A., Levesque, G., Ikeda, M., Chi, H., Lin, C., Li, G., Holman, K., Tsuda, T., Mar, L., Foncin, J.-F., Bruni, A. C., Montesi, M. P., Sorbi, S., Rainero, I., Pinessi, L., Nee, L., Chumakov, I., Pollen, D., Brookes, A., Sanseau, P., Polinsky, R. J., Wasco, W., DaSilva, H. A. R., Haines, J. L., Pericak-Vance, M. A., Tanzi, R. E., Roses, A. D., Fraser, P. E., Rommens, J. M., and St. George-Hyslop, P. H. (1995) Cloning of a gene bearing missense mutations in early-onset familial Alzheimer's disease, *Nature* **375**, 754–760.

129. Kovacs, D. M., Fausett, H. J., Page, K. J., Kim, T-W., Moir, R. D., Merriam, D. E., Hollister, R. D., Hallmar, O. G., Mancini, R., Felsenstein, K. M., Hyman, B. T., Tanzi, R. E., and Wasco, W. (1996) Alzheimer-associated presenilins 1 and 2: neuronal expression in brain and localization to intracellular membranes in mammalian cells, *Nature Med.* **2**, 224–229.

130. Cooper, L. T., Cooke, J. P., and Dzau, V. J. (1994) The vasculopathy of aging, *J. Gerontol.* **49**, B191–196.

131. Kawai, M., Kalaria, R. N., Cras, P., Siedlak, S. L., Velasco, M. E., Shelton, E. R., Chan, H. W., Greenberg, B. D., and Perry, G. (1993) Degeneration of vascular muscle cells in cerebral amyloid angiopathy of Alzheimer disease, *Brain Res.* **623**, 142–146.

132. Buee, L., Hof, P. R., Bouras, C., Delacourte, A., Perl, D. P., Morrison, J. H., and Fillit, H. M. (1994) Pathological alterations of the cerebral microvasculature in Alzheimer's disease and related dementing disorders, *Acta. Neuropathol.* **87**, 469–480.

133. Kalaria, R. N. and Hedera, P. (1995) Differential degeneration of the cerebral microvasculature in Alzheimer's disease, *Neuroreport* **6**, 477–480.

134. Azari, N. P., Pettigrew, K. D., Schapiro, M. B., Haxby, J. V., Grady, C. L., Pietrini, P., Salerno, J. A., Heston, L. L., Rapoport, S. I., and Horwitz, B. (1993) Early detection of Alzheimer's disease: a statistical approach using positron emission tomographic data, *J. Cereb. Blood Flow Metab.* **13**, 438–447.

135. Hixson, J. E. (1991) Apolipoprotein E polymorphisms affect atherosclerosis in young males, *Arterioscler. Thromb.* **11**, 1237–1244.

136. Frisoni, G. G., Bianchetti, A., Govoni, S., and Trabucchi, M. (1994) Association of apolipoprotein E E4 with vascular dimentia, *JAMA* **271**, 1317.

137. Strittmatter, W. J. and Roses, A. D. (1995) Apolipoprotein E and Alzheimer disease, *Proc. Natl. Acad. Sci. USA* **92**, 4725–4727.

138. Ciallella, J. R., Rangnekar, V. V., and McGillis, J. P. (1994) Heat shock alters Alzheimer's beta amyloid precursor protein expression in human endothelial cells, *J. Neurosci. Res.* **37**, 769–776.

139. Wisniewski, H. M., Frackowiak, J., Zoltowska, A., and Kim, K. S. (1994) Vascular β-amyloid in Alzheimer's disease angiopathy is produced by proliferating and degenerating smooth muscle cells, *Int. J. Exp. Clin. Invest.* **1**, 8–16.

140. Wisniewski, H. M., Frackowiak, J., and Mazur-Kolecka, B. (1995) In vitro production of beta-amyloid in smooth muscle cells isolated from amyloid angiopathy-affected vessels, *Neurosci. Lett.* **183**, 120–123.

141. Frackowiak, J., Zoltowska, A., and Wisniewski, H. M. (1994) Non-fibrillar beta-amyloid protein is associated with smooth muscle cells of vessel walls in Alzheimer disease, *J. Neuropathol. Exp. Neurol.* **53,** 637–645.

142. Gabuzda, D., Busciglio, J., Chen, L. B., Matsudaira, P., and Yankner, B. A. (1994) Inhibition of energy metabolism alters the processing of amyloid precursor protein and induces a potentially amyloidogenic derivative, *J. Biol. Chem.* **269,** 13,623–13,628.

143. Hatzinger, M., Z'Brun, A., Hemmeter, U., Seifritz, E., Baumann, F., Holsboer-Trachsler, E., and Heuser, I. J. (1995) Hypothalamic-pituitary-adrenal system function in patients with Alzheimer's disease, *Neurobiol. Aging* **16,** 205–209.

144. Landfield, P. W., Thibault, O., Mazzanti, M. L., Porter, N. M., and Kerr, D. S. (1992) Mechanisms of neuronal death in brain aging and Alzheimer's disease: role of endocrine-mediated calcium dyshomeostasis, *J. Neurobiol.* **23,** 1247–1260.

145. Goodman, Y., Bruce, A. J., Cheng, B., and Mattson, M. P. (1996) Estrogens attenuate and corticosterone exacerbates excitotoxicity, oxidative injury and amyloid β-peptide toxicity in hippocampal neurons, *J. Neurochem.* **66,** 1836–1844.

146. Sapolsky, R. M. (1994) The physiological relevance of glucocorticoid endangerment of the hippocampus, *Ann. NY Acad. Sci.* **746,** 294–304.

147. Smith-Swintosky, V. L., Pettigrew, L. C., Sapolsky, R. M., Phares, C., Craddock, S. D., Brooke, S. M., and Mattson, M. P. (1996) Metyrapone, an inhibitor of glucocorticoid production, reduces brain injury induced by focal and global ischemia and seizures, *J. Cereb. Blood Flow Metab.* **16,** 575–598.

148. Manson, J. E. (1994) Postmenopausal hormone therapy and atherosclerotic disease, *Am. Heart J.* **128,** 1337–1343.

149. Chowen, J. A., Torres-Aleman, I., and Garcia-Segura, L. M. (1992) Trophic effects of estradiol on fetal rat hypothalamic neurons, *Neuroendocrinology* **56,** 895–901.

150. Singh, M., Meyer, E. M., and Simpkins, J. W. (1995) The effect of ovariectomy and estradiol replacement on brain-derived neurotrophic factor messenger ribonucleic acid expression in cortical and hippocampal brain regions of female Sprague-Dawley rats, *Endocrinology* **136,** 2320–2324.

151. Behl, C., Widmann, M., Trapp, T., and Holsboer, F. (1995) 17-β estradiol protects neurons from oxidative stress- induced cell death in vitro, *Biochem. Biophys. Res. Commun.* **216,** 473–482.

152. Ruiz-Larrea, M. B., Leal, A. M., Liza, M., Lacort, M., and de Groot, H. (1994) Antioxidant effects of estradiol and 2-hydroxyestradiol on iron-induced lipid peroxidation of rat liver microsomes, *Steroids* **59,** 383–388.

153. Keaney, J. F., Jr., Shwaery, G. T., Xu, A., Nicolosi, R. J., Loscalzo, J., Foxall, T. L., and Vita, J. A. (1994) 17 beta-estradiol preserves endothelial vasodilator function and limits low-density lipoprotein oxidation in hypercholesterolemic swine, *Circulation* **89,** 2251–2259.

154. Saunders, A. M., Strittmatter, W. J., Schmechel, D., St. George-Hyslop, P. H., Pericak, V. M. A., Joo, S. H., Rosi, B. L., Gusella, J. F., Crapper-MacLachlan, D. R., Alberts, M. J., Hulette, C., Crain, B., Goldgaber, D., and Roses, A. D. (1993) Association of apolipoprotein E allele E4 with late-onset familial and sporadic Alzheimer's disease, *Neurology* **43,** 1467–1472.

155. Krul, E. S. and Tang, J. (1992) Secretion of apolipoprotein E by an astrocytoma cell line, *J. Neurosci. Res.* **32,** 227–238.

156. Poirier, J. (1994) Apolipoprotein E in animal models of CNS injury and in Alzheimer's disease, *Trends Neurosci.* **17,** 525–530.

157. Castano, E. M., Prelli, F., Wisniewski, T., Golabek, A., Kumar, R. A., Soto, C., and Frangione, B. (1995) Fibrillogenesis in Alzheimer's disease of amyloid beta peptides and apolipoprotein E, *Biochem. J.* **306,** 599–604.

158. Evans, K. C., Berger, E. P., Cho, C. G., Weisgraber, K. H., and Lansbury, P. T., Jr. (1995) Apolipoprotein E is a kinetic but not a thermodynamic inhibitor of amyloid formation: implications for the pathogenesis and treatment of Alzheimer disease, *Proc. Natl. Acad. Sci. USA* **2,** 763–767.

159. Whitson, J. S., Mims, M. P., Strittmatter, W. J., Yamaki, T., Morrisett, J. D., and Appel, S. H. (1994) Attenuation of the neurotoxic efect of Aβ amyloid peptide by apolipoprotein E, *Biochem. Biophys. Res. Commun.* **199,** 163–170.

160. Barger, S. W., Seubert, P., Lieberburg, I., and Mattson, M. P. (1996) Apolipoprotein E acts as a molecular switch between the activities of secreted β-amyloid precursor protein, *J. Biol. Chem.*, submitted.

161. Crutcher, K. A., Clay, M. A., Scott, S. A., Tian, X., Tolar, M., and Harmony, J. A. (1994) Neurite degeneration elicited by apolipoprotein E peptides, *Exp. Neurol.* **130,** 120–126.

162. Eikelenboom, P., Zhan, S. S., van Gool, W. A., and Allsop, D. (1994) Inflammatory mechanisms in Alzheimer's disease, *Trends Pharmacol. Sci.* **15,** 447–450.

163. McGeer, P. L., Klegeris, A., Walker, D. G., Yasuhara, O., and McGeer, E. G. (1994) Pathological proteins in senile plaques, *Tohoku J. Exp. Med.* **174,** 269–277.

164. Rogers, J., Cooper, N. R., Webster, S., Schultz, J., McGeer, P. L., Styren, S. D., Civin, W. H., Brachova, L., Bradt, B., and Ward, P. (1992) Complement activation by beta-amyloid in Alzheimer disease, *Proc. Natl. Acad. Sci. USA* **89,** 10,016–10,020.

165. Breitner, J. C. S., Gau, B. A., Welsh, K. A., Plassman, B. L., McDonald, W. M., Helms, M. J., and Anthony, J. C. (1994) Inverse association of anti-inflammatory treatments and Alzheimer's disease, *Neurology* **44,** 227–232.

166. Mattson, M. P. and Scheff, S. W. (1994) Endogenous neuroprotection factors and traumatic brain injury: mechanisms of action and implications for therapies, *J. Neurotrauma* **11,** 3–33.

167. Mattson, M. P., Murrain, M., Guthrie, P. B., and Kater, S. B. (1989) Fibroblast growth factor and glutamate: Opposing roles in the generation and degeneration of hippocampal neuroarchitecture, *J. Neurosci.* **9,** 3728–3740.

168. Mattson, M. P. and Rychlik, B. (1990) Glia protect hippocampal neurons against excitatory amino acid-induced degeneration: Involvement of fibroblast growth factor, *Int. J. Dev. Neurosci.* **8,** 399–415.

169. Cheng, B. and Mattson, M. P. (1992) Glucose deprivation elicits neurofibrillary tangle-like antigenic changes in hippocampal neurons: prevention by NGF and bFGF, *Exp. Neurol.* **117,** 114–123.

170. Cheng, B. and Mattson, M. P. (1994) NT-3 and βDNF protect CNS neurons against metabolic/excitotoxic insults, *Brain Res.* **640,** 56–67.

171. Prehn, J. H., Backhauss, C., and Krieglstein, J. (1993) Transforming growth factor-β1 prevents glutamate neurotoxicity in rat neocortical cultures and protects mouse neocortex from ischemic injury in vivo, *J. Cereb. Blood Flow Metab.* **13,** 521–525.

172. Shigeno, T., Mima, T., Takakura, K., Graham, D. I., Kato, G., Hashimoto, Y., and Furukawa, S. (1991) Amelioration of delayed neuronal death in the hippocampus by nerve growth factor, *J. Neurosci.* **11,** 2914–2919.

173. Gluckman, P., Kempt, N., Guan, J., Mallard, C., Sirimanne, E., Dragunow, M., Klempt, M., Singh, K., Williams, C., and Nikolics, K. (1992) A role for IGF-I in the rescue of CNS neurons following hypoxic-ischemic injury, *Biochem. Biophys. Res. Commun.* **182,** 593–599.

174. Koketsu, N., Berlove, D. J., Moskowitz, M. A., Kowall, N. W., Caday, C. G., and Finlestein, S. P. (1994) Pretreatment with intraventricular basic fibroblast growth factor decreases infarct size following focal cerebral ischemia in rats, *Ann. Neurol.* **35,** 451–457.

175. Chao, C. C., Hu, S., Kravitz, F. H., Tsang, M., Anderson, W. R., and Peterson, P. K. (1994) Transforming growth factor-beta protects human neurons against beta-amyloid-induced injury, *Mol. Chem. Neuropathol.* **23,** 159–178.

176. Collazo, D., Takahashi, H., and McKay, R. D. (1992) Cellular targets and trophic functions of neurotrophin-3 in the developing rat hippocampus, *Neuron* **9,** 643–656.

177. Mattson, M. P., Kumar, K., Cheng, B., Wang, H., and Michaelis, E. K. (1993) Basic FGF regulates the expression of a functional 71 kDa NMDA receptor protein that mediates calcium influx and neurotoxicity in cultured hippocampal neurons, *J. Neurosci.* **13,** 4575–4588.

178. Cheng, B., Furukawa, K., O'Keefe, J. A., Goodman, Y., Kihiko, M., Fabian, T., and Mattson, M. P. (1995) Basic fibroblast growth factor selectively increases AMPA-receptor subunit GluR1 protein level and differentially modulates Ca^{2+} responses to AMPA and NMDA in hippocampal neurons, *J. Neurochem.* **65,** 2525–2536.

179. Zhang, Y., Tatsuno, T., Carney, J., and Mattson, M. P. (1993) Basic FGF, NGF, and IGFs protect hippocampal neurons against iron-induced degeneration, *J. Cereb. Blood Flow Metab.* **13,** 378–388.

180. Sampath, D., Jackson, G. R., Werrbach-Perez, K., and Perez-Polo, J. R. (1994) Effects of nerve growth factor on glutathione peroxidase and catalase in PC12 cells, *J. Neurochem.* **62,** 2476–2479.

181. Spina, M. B., Squinto, S. P., Miller, J., Lindsay, R. M., and Hyman, C. (1992) Brain-derived neurotropic factor protects dopamine neurons against 6-hydroxydopamine and N-methyl-4-phenylpyridinium ion toxicity: involvement of the glutathione system, *J. Neurochem.* **59,** 99–106.

182. Kolesnick, R. and Golde, D. W. (1994) The sphingomyelin pathway in tumor necrosis factor and interleukin-1 signaling, *Cell* **77,** 325–328.

183. Goodman, Y. and Mattson, M. P. (1996) Ceramide protects hippocampal neurons against excitotoxic and oxidative insults, and amyloid β-peptide toxicity, *J. Neurochem.* **66,** 869–872.

184. Dobrowsky, R. T., Werner, M. H., Castellino, A. M., Chao, M. V., and Hannun, Y. A. (1994) Activation of the sphingomyelin cycle through the low-affinity neurotrophin receptor, *Science* **265,** 1596–1599.

185. Schreck, R., Albermann, K., and Baeuerle, P. A. (1992) Nuclear factor kappa B: an oxidative stress-responsive transcription factor of eukaryotic cells, *Free Radical Res. Commun.* **17,** 221–237.

186. Banati, R. B., Gehrmann, J., Wiessner, C., Hossmann, K. A., and Kreutzberg, G. W. (1995) Glial expression of the beta-amyloid precursor protein (APP) in global ischemia, *J. Cereb. Blood Flow Meta.* **15,** 647–654.

187. McKenzie, J. E., Gentleman, S. M., Roberts, G. W., Graham, D. I., and Royston, M. C. (1994) Increased numbers of beta APP-immunoreactive neurones in the entorhinal cortex after head injury, *Neuroreport* **6,** 161–164.

188. Araki, W., Kitaguchi, N., Tokushima, Y., Ishii, K., Aratake, H., Shimohama, S., Nakamura, S., and Kimura, J. (1991) Trophic effect of β-amyloid precursor protein on cerebral cortical neurons in culture, *Biochem. Biophys. Res. Commun.* **181,** 265–271.

189. Schubert, D. and Behl, C. (1993) The expression of amyloid beta protein precursor protects nerve cells from beta-amyloid and glutamate toxicity and alters their interaction with the extracellular matrix, *Brain Res.* **629,** 275–282.

190. Smith-Swintosky, V. L., Pettigrew, L. C., Craddock, S. D., Culwell, A. R., Rydel, R. E., and Mattson, M. P. (1994) Secreted forms of β-amyloid precursor protein protect against ischemic brain injury, *J. Neurochem.* **63,** 781–784.

191. Bowes, M. P., Masliah, E., Otero, D. A. C., Zivin, J. A., and Saitoh, T. (1994) Reduction of neurological damage by a peptide segment of the amyloid β-A4 protein precursor in a rabbit spinal cord ischemia model, *Exp. Neurol.* **129,** 112–119.

192. Mucke, L., Abraham, C. R., Ruppe, M. D., Rockenstein, E. M., Toggas, S. M., Mallory, M., Alford, M., and Masliah, E. (1995) Protection against HIV-1 gp120-induced brain damage by neuronal expression of human amyloid precursor protein, *J. Exp. Med.* **181,** 1551–1556.

193. Furukawa, K., Barger, S. W., Blalock, E., and Mattson, M. P. (1996) Activation of K^+ channels and suppression of neuronal activity by secreted β-amyloid precursor protein, *Nature* **379,** 74–78.

194. Greenberg, S. M., Koo, E. J., Selkoe, D. J., Qiu, W. Q., and Kosik, K. S. (1994) Secreted β-amyloid precursor protein stimulates mitogen-activated protein kinase and enhances τ phosphorylation, *Proc. Natl. Acad. Sci. USA* **91,** 7104–7108.

195. Weinstein, J. R., Gold, S. J., Cunningham, D. D., and Gall, C. M. (1995) Cellular localization of thrombin receptor mRNA in rat brain: expression by mesencephalic dopaminergic neurons and codistribution with prothrombin mRNA, *J. Neurosci.* **15**, 2906–2919.

196. Cunningham, D. D., Pulliam, L., and Vaughan, P. J. (1993) Protease nexin-1 and thrombin: injury related processes in the brain, *Thromb. Haemostasis.* **70**, 168–171.

197. Gurwitz, D. and Cunningham, D. D. (1988) Thrombin modulates and reverses neuroblastoma neurite outgrowth, *Proc. Natl. Acad. Sci. USA* **85**, 3440–3444.

198. Smith-Swintosky, V. L., Zimmer, S., Fenton, J. W., and Mattson, M. P. (1995) Protease nexin-I and thrombin modulate neuronal Ca^{2+} homeostasis and sensitivity to glucose deprivation-induced injury, *J. Neurosci.* **15**, 5840–5850.

199. Vu, T.-K. H., Hung, D. T., Wheaton, V. I., and Coughlin, S. R. (1991) Molecular cloning of a functional thrombin receptor reveals a novel proteolytic mechanism of receptor activation, *Cell* **64**, 1057–1068.

200. Mattson, M. P. and Begley, J. G. (1996) Amyloid β-peptide alters thrombin-induced calcium responses in cultured human neural cells, *Amyloid* **3**, 28–40.

201. Smith-Swintosky, V. L., Zimmer, S., Fenton, J. W., II, and Mattson, M. P. (1995) Opposing actions of thrombin and protease nexin-1 on amyloid β-peptide toxicity and on accumulation of peroxides and calcium in hippocampal neurons, *J. Neurochem.* **65**, 1415–1418.

202. Montgomery, D. L. (1994) Astrocytes: form, functions, and roles in disease, *Vet. Pathol.* **31**, 145–167.

203. Pike, C. J., Cummings, B. J., and Cotman, C. W. (1992) beta-Amyloid induces neuritic dystrophy in vitro: similarities with Alzheimer pathology, *Neuroreport* **3**, 769–772.

204. Pechan, P. A., Chowdhury, K., Gerdes, W., and Seifert, W. (1993) Glutamate induces the growth factors NGF, bFGF, the receptor FGF-R1 and c-fos mRNA expression in rat astrocyte culture, *Neurosci. Lett.* **153**, 111–114.

205. Schwartz, J. P. and Nishiyama, N. (1994) Neurotrophic factor gene expression in astrocytes during development and following injury, *Brain Res. Bull.* **35**, 403–407.

206. Hoke, A., Canning, D. R., Malemud, C. J., and Silver, J. (1994) Regional differences in reactive gliosis induced by substrate bound β-amyloid, *Exp. Neurol.* **130**, 56–66.

207. Mark, R. J., Ashford, J. W., and Mattson, M. P. (1995) Anticonvulsants attenuate amyloid β-peptide neurotoxicity and promote maintenance of calcium homeostasis, *Neurobiol. Aging* **16**, 187–198.

208. Goodman, Y. and Mattson, M. P. (1996) K^+ channel openers protect hippocampal neurons against oxidative injury and amyloid β-peptide toxicity, *Brain Res.* **706**, 328–332.

209. Cheng, B., Barger, S. W., and Mattson, M. P. (1994) Staurosporine, K-252a and K-252b stabilize calcium homeostasis and promote survival of CNS neurons in the absence of glucose, *J. Neurochem.* **62**, 1319–1329.

210. Goodman, Y. and Mattson, M. P. (1994) Staurosporine and K-252 compounds protect hippocampal neurons against amyloid β-peptide toxicity and oxidative injury, *Brain Res.* **650**, 170–174.

211. Smith-Swintosky, V. L., Kraemer, P. J., McCants, N., Maki, A., Brown, R. W., Keller, J., Goodman, Y., and Mattson, M. P. (1996) K252a, K252b and staurosporine mitigate seizure-induced hippocampal damage and memory deficits, *Exp. Neurol.* in press.

212. Knusel, B. and Hefti, F. (1992) K252 compounds: modulators of neurotrophin signal transduction, *J. Neurochem.* **59**, 1987–1996.

213. Maroney, A. C., Lipfert, L., Forbes, M. E., Glicksman, M. A., Neff, N. T., Siman, R., and Dionne, C. A. (1995) K252a induces tyrosine phosphorylation of the focal adhesion kinase and neurite outgrowth in human neuroblastoma SH-SY5Y cells, *J. Neurochem.* **64**, 540–549.

214. Furukawa, K., Smith-Swintosky, V. L., and Mattson, M. P. (1995) Evidence that actin depolymerization protects hippocampal neurons against excitotoxicity by stabilizing $[Ca^{2+}]_i$, *Exp. Neurol.* **133**, 153–163.

215. Furukawa, K. and Mattson, M. P. (1995) Taxol stabilizes $[Ca^{2+}]_i$ and protects hippocampal neurons against excitotoxicity, *Brain Res.* **689**, 141–146.

9

β-amyloid-Derived Free Radical Oxidation:
A Fundamental Process in Alzheimer's Disease

D. Allan Butterfield, Kenneth Hensley, Nathan Hall,
Ramachandran Subramaniam, Beverly J. Howard, Pamela Cole,
Servet Yatin, Michael LaFontaine, Marni E. Harris,
Marina Aksenova, Michael Aksenov, and John M. Carney

1. INTRODUCTION

Alzheimer's disease (AD) research has progressed greatly since the first description of AD by Alzheimer *(1)* very early in this century. Three pathological hallmarks of AD are:

1. The presence in certain brain regions of senile plaques (SP), entities composed of aggregated β-amyloid surrounded by dystrophic neurites and other moieties;
2. Neurofibrillary tangles (NFT), primarily composed of phosphorylated τ, a cytoskeletal protein, and other moieties; and
3. Loss of synapses *(2–4)*.

Several theories of the etiology of this dementing disorder, currently thought to affect nearly five million people in the US, have been offered (reviewed in ref. *2*). These include slow virus, trace metal imbalance, cholinergic anomalies, loss of trophic factors, and membrane disorder *(2,3)*. In addition to the pathological hallmarks of AD noted above, three observations must be accounted for in any theory of AD:

1. This is a disorder affecting the aged population;
2. There are numerous reports of multiple membrane alterations ranging from various lipid abnormalities to altered membrane enzyme, transmembrane transporter proteins, and other membrane proteins; and
3. Amyloid in SP is largely insoluble in most traditional biochemical buffers/solvent systems.

Recently, studies from our laboratory have provided strong evidence of β-amyloid (Aβ)-derived free radical damage to neurons and glial cells as a fundamental process in AD *(5)*. These β-amyloid-derived free radicals provide a unifying framework to account for the observations cited above, and it is this work that is the subject of this chapter.

In the past few years, research has demonstrated the importance of reactive free radicals, such as reactive oxygen species (ROS), in damage to membrane lipids, proteins, and nucleic acids *(6)*. An emerging theory of AD etiology is that SP are loci of elevated oxidative stress *(7)*. Suggested sources of oxidative stress in AD SPs have

From: Molecular Mechanisms of Dementia Edited by: W. Wasco and R. E. Tanzi Humana Press Inc., Totowa, NJ

included: redox metals *(8)*, defective mitochondrial electron transport systems with attendant free radical leakiness *(9,10)*, glycation end products from Maillard chemistry *(11)*, reactive microglia *(12)*, and Aβ *(5,7,13–26)*. This chapter specifically presents the evidence for the role of Aβ as a pro-oxidant, the consequences to brain cell membrane lipid and protein oxidation and alteration of function, and the involvement of Aβ-derived free radicals as a fundamental process in AD. Reviews of the molecular biology of Aβ or of other risk factors in AD are treated elsewhere *(2,27)*.

Amyloid peptides, 39–43 amino acids in length, are the central constituent of SP, which correlate regionally with neuronal damage in AD brain *(27)*. Amyloid (Table 1) is derived from the transmembrane glycoprotein, amyloid precursor protein (APP). Mutations in APP correlate with some familial forms of AD, and APP-overexpressing, transgenic mice exhibit brain pathology reminiscent of AD *(28)*. β-amyloid spontaneously aggregates in solution, over a period of hours to days, to form large (>15 kDa) structures that fail to dissociate even in the presence of urea-SDS-PAGE gel analysis *(29,30)*. Concomitant with this aggregation is the appearance of neurotoxicity. Freshly solubilized synthetic Aβ1–40 monomer is not toxic to cultured neurons; however, after an aging period, the peptide suspension develops marked neurotoxicity *(29,30)*. In contrast, certain peptide sequences within Aβ1–40, especially an 11-amino acid subset of Aβ1–40, Aβ25–35, exhibit rapid aggregation and high levels of neurotoxicity soon after dissolution of the peptide *(30,31)*.

Little has been known about the molecular mechanism(s) of Aβ aggregation and neurotoxicity. The kinetics of aggregation indicate a nucleation event dependent on the hydrophobic carboxyl-terminal residues *(32–34)*. In hippocampal neuronal cultures, Aβ aggregates tend to accumulate at or near the membrane surface, producing local microenvironments of high Aβ concentration *(29,35)*. Once aggregated, Aβ can disrupt Ca^{2+} homeostasis and lead to high intracellular accumulation of this ion *(35)*.

Synthetic Aβ peptides are potent inducers of neurotoxicity in vitro. Many of the cell-damaging effects of Aβ can be modulated by antioxidants *(18,25)*. For all these reasons, research has tended to focus on the role of Aβ peptides as mediators of cell damage and, based largely on research in our laboratory *(5,7,13–24)*, as initiators of oxyradical stress.

2. TOXIC AMYLOID PEPTIDES PROMOTE FREE RADICAL REACTIONS IN OXYGENATED BUFFER

Our group decided to examine systematically the hypothesis that Aβ could be a source of free radical damage in cultured neuronal systems, and by extension, in AD brain *(5,7,13–24)*. Since it would be unlikely to detect directly reactive unstable free radicals, we chose to employ the electron paramagnetic resonance (EPR) technique of spin trapping *(3,36,37)* to determine if Aβ-derived free radicals could be detected *(13)*.

2.1. EPR Spin-Trapping Results

In spin-trapping experiments, a nonparamagnetic species (usually a nitrone [the trap]) reacts with a transient free radical R (the spin) to produce a stable paramagnetic nitroxide (the spin adduct) (Fig. 1).

In the case of phenyl-α-*tert*-butyl-nitrone (PBN) as the trap, the reaction of a free radical to yield a spin adduct normally produces a six-line spectrum resulting from the hyperfine coupling of the magnetic moment of the free electron with the nuclear mag-

Table 1
Amino Acid Sequence of Aβ1–40

NH$_2$-Asp-Ala-Glu-Phe-Arg-His-Asp-Ser-Gly-Tyr-Glu-Val-His-His-Gln-Lys-Leu-Val-Phe-Phe-Ala-Glu-Asp-Val-<u>Gly-Ser-Asn-Lys-Gly-Ala-Ile-*Ile-Gly-Leu-Met*</u>-Val-Gly-Gly-Val-Val-OH

Aβ25–35 is underlined; Aβ32–35 is in italics.

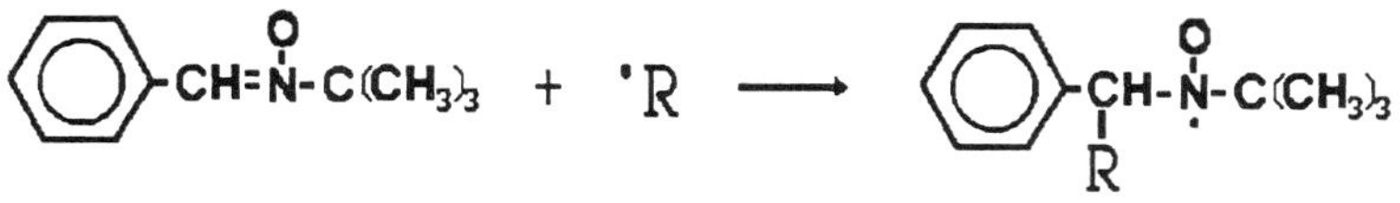

Fig. 1. Reaction between PBN and a transient free radical R*.

netic moments of the nitrogen nucleus (I = 1) and the α-hydrogen atom (I = ½). The magnitude of the doublet splitting (A$_H$) depends on several factors, including the size of the adduct *(3,36,37)*. If a radical on binding to PBN is able to cause decomposition of the trap, then a three-line (a nitroxide) or four-line (a hydronitroxide) can result *(37)*. After ascertaining that the PBN itself is unable to generate a free radical under the conditions of the experiment, an EPR spectrum is *prima fascia* evidence for the presence of a free radical. Researchers, including ourselves, have used EPR spin trapping to investigate free radical involvement in metabolism, toxicology, and pharmacology *(3,36–38)*. EPR is an extremely sensitive technique, rivaling the detection limits of fluorescence, and the EPR spectra can be easily quantified by double-integration techniques *(36)*. The power of EPR over optical methods like fluorescence involves its extreme sensitivity, the fact that opaque samples can be used (i.e., no light scattering effects), the insight into the polarity and motion of the local microenvironment near the paramagnetic center of the free radical that can be gained, and, generally, the biological system is EPR silent, i.e., only the free radical trapped by PBN gives rise to an EPR spectrum.

In addition to spin trapping, other probes, used by our group to assess Aβ-derived free radicals include: aromatic compounds, such as salicylate, that undergo electrophilic addition reaction with oxyradicals *(13)*; nitroxide spin labels, whose paramagnetism, and, hence, EPR signal intensity is lost on reaction with a free radical *(14,23)*; sensitive fluorescence or colorimetric probes that indicate protein oxidation or the presence of ROS *(18,23)*, ROS-specific enzymes viz superoxide dismutase (SOD) or catalase, to help identify the radical type *(24)*; and resident oxidatively sensitive biomolecules, such as glutamate synthetase (GS) or creating kinase (CK), as markers of ROS presence *(7,13)*.

Incubation of synthetic Aβ1–40 or its highly reactive and rapidly toxic 11-mer, Aβ25–35, with the spin-trap PBN generates EPR-detectable levels of nitroxide spin adduct that are not observed in the absence of peptide *(13,15,16)*, indicating that the peptide is the source of the radicals generated. The appearance of a three-line EPR spectrum in each case *(13)* parallels the reported time frame for neurotoxicity of these two species, i.e., hours to days for Aβ1–40 and minutes for Aβ25–35. Oxygen is required in the buffer, and the EPR signal is not inhibited by three different metal chelators *(13)*, suggesting that the Aβ-peptide-derived free radical is generated in an oxygen-dependent, but metal-independent mechanism.

Others have reported lot-to-lot variability in neurotoxicity of synthetic Aβ *(39,40)*. Consistent with these reports, we found that the EPR spectra of PBN-trapped Aβ-derived free radical species were either three- or four-line spectra, corresponding to highly toxic or moderately toxic species, respectively *(15)*. Similar three-line EPR spectra were found with a different spin-trap, 5,5-dimethylpyrroline-*N*-oxyl (DMPO), though the reaction is less vigorous and less product is observed *(15,16)*.

That PBN spin adducts of Aβ-peptide-derived free radicals did not yield traditional six-line EPR spectra is unusual. Normally, one observes hyperfine splitting by both the nitrogen atom (to give three lines), and each of these three lines split into two lines by the hydrogen atom on the α-carbon atom of PBN, thereby making a six-line spectrum *(3,36–38)*. However, the spectra derived from Aβ addition to PBN are reminiscent of alkyl nitroxides or alkyoxyinitroxides (three-line spectra) or hydronitroxides (four-line spectra). One way to account for this anomaly is if Aβ-derived free radicals cause decomposition of the PBN spin trap. In order to test this idea, PBN with a ^{13}C in the α-carbon was used *(16)*. Since ^{13}C has a nuclear spin (unlike ^{12}C), additional hyperfine lines should be observed. However, if the Aβ-derived free radicals caused decomposition of the PBN spin trap, then no ^{13}C coupling should be observed. Figure 2 shows that even with ^{13}C-PBN, only three EPR lines were found *(16)*, indicating that the Aβ-derived free radicals were capable of decomposing the spin traps used. In contrast to the toxic Aβ1–40 and Aβ25–35, the nontoxic reverse sequence of Aβ40–1 gave a traditional six-line EPR spectrum in the presence of PBN and metal chelators *(16)*. The four-line generating Aβ1–40 or Aβ25–35 peptide species were invariably less toxic than the respective three-line generating species *(15)*. That the four-line-generating species led to a trapped moiety that was a hydronitroxide was confirmed by use of D_2O *(16)*. In D_2O, deuterium-hydrogen exchange occurs, and the predicted nine-line EPR spectrum was observed *(16)* (since I = 1 for the N atom, three resonance lines are found, and since I = 1 for the D atom, each of these three lines is split into three lines by the D-nuclear magnetic moment, thereby yielding an EPR spectrum consisting of a triplet of triplets). The hyperfine coupling constants also matched those of known hydronitroxide, further confirming the identity of the four-line-generating species.

We generated several lines of evidence that the oxygen-dependent free radicals derived from Aβ-peptides were peroxyl in nature *(23,24)*. Incubation of Aβ-peptides from different lots with PBN in the presence of SOD did not affect the spectrum; i.e., three- or four-line EPR spectra were found. However, in the presence of catalase, the EPR signal was completely abrogated *(24)*. This latter result is unlikely the result of the presence in the incubate of a large protein that might serve as a "sponge" to capture free radicals, thereby preventing their reaction with PBN; otherwise, SOD should have done the same thing, but did not. PeroXOQuant™ is a commercially available, simple colorimetric assay for peroxyl species. We used this assay to find that Aβ-peptides gave a positive response, consistent with the catalase result, and consistent with peroxyl-type radical formation from Aβ peptides *(23)*. One possibility of reaction of Aβ-peptides with PBN to lead to its decomposition and formation of an alkoxyinitroxide (three-line-generating species) or hydronitroxide (four-line-generating species) involves a peroxyl radical (Fig. 3). Studies to determine this possibility more precisely are in progress.

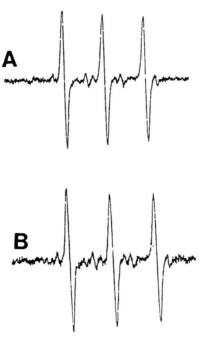

Fig. 2. (A) Reaction of highly toxic Aβ25–35 with ^{12}C-PBN to yield three EPR resonance lines. **(B)** Reaction of highly toxic Aβ25–35 with ^{13}C-PBN also to yield three EPR resonance lines, unequivocally demonstrating that the Aβ25–35-derived trapped free radical led to the decomposition of the PBN spin trap.

Aβ-peptide incubates generated ROS hydroxylation products (dihydroxybenzoic acids) when incubated with salicylate (13), consistent with the EPR results. Preincubation of the peptide in the absence of salicylate prevented this reaction, presumably because highly reactive Aβ-peptide free radicals were able to interact with nearby peptide molecules, perhaps not unlike what might occur in SP. If so, the resulting covalent bonds might account for the relative insolubility of plaque amyloid. The oxidatively sensitive enzymes GS and CK from rodent brain were inactivated by Aβ incubation (13,18). Both enzymes are decreased in activity in normal aging (41,42) and in the AD brain (7). In addition to rodent brain GS and CK, the Aβ-induced loss in enzyme activities was also found in sheep brain and astrocyte cell cultures as discussed below.

The precise chemical mechanism by which Aβ-peptides form free radical ROS in oxygenated buffers is still not clear. In order to determine if any compositional or structural changes were occurring with Aβ-peptides on incubation, amino acid analysis and circular dichroism studies were performed (15,24). The most obvious chemical change that occurs to Aβ25–35 during solution incubation is the conversion of C-terminal methionine (residue 35) to a species that coelutes on HPLC with methionine sulfoxide (Fig. 4) (15). This conversion occurs within 3 h at 37°C, in the absence of redox-active metals, and is completely prevented by millimolar levels of the free radical scavenger PBN (15). Dialkyl sulfides like methionine are known to participate in unusual free radical reaction chemistry (43). Methionine oxidation has been shown to affect dramatically secondary structure of model peptides: conversion to the sulfoxide leads to

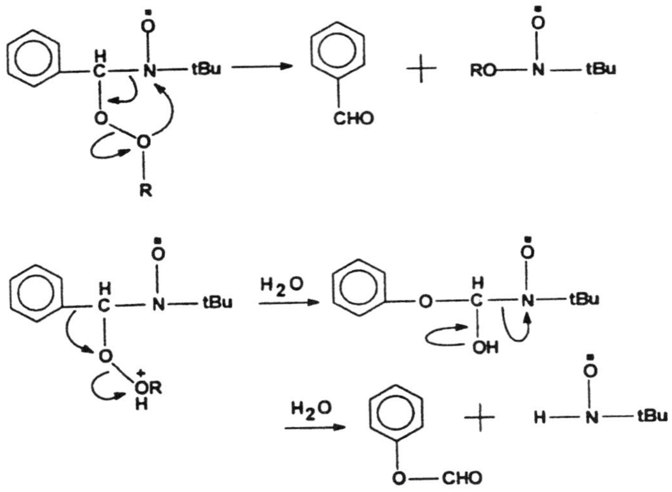

Fig. 3. Possible mechanism whereby a PBN-trapped putative peroxyl free radical leads to the decomposition of the PBN spin trap and formation of either an alkoxyinitroxide (three-line EPR spectrum generating species, top) or hydronitroxide (four-line EPR spectrum generating species, bottom).

predominately β-sheet conformation *(44)*, and it is well known that neurotoxic Aβ adopts a predominately β-sheet conformation in solution. In an attempt to determine if the C-terminal methionine might be important in the ability of Aβ25–35 to generate reactive free radicals, we obtained Aβ25–34, without terminal methionine. Initial studies of the incubation of this peptide with PBN suggest that no EPR spectrum is observed, consistent with the importance of methionine in these results and with the work of Pike et al. *(45)*. Also consistent with the potential importance of Met in Aβ chemistry and pathology, synthetic Aβ1–40 produced with a Met-sulfoxide in residue 35 reportedly formed fibrils at twice the rate of unmodified Aβ1–40 *(46)*, and others have shown that SP Aβ1–40 is rich in Met-sulfoxide *(47)*.

We undertook a circular dichroism study to determine if the solution structures of Aβ peptides were different in oxygenated or nitrogen-sparged buffers *(24)*, consistent with the notion that free radical reactivity and structure are related. The results indicated a pronounced oxygen dependence to the structure of the peptides in solution *(24)*. We have employed rudimentary molecular modeling of Aβ1–40 building in constraints of known distances of particular amino acids from solution NMR studies *(48)*. Although it is recognized that the resulting structure is not necessarily the structure with minimal energy, it was interesting to note that the methionine-35 residue was exposed to the outside of the peptide, where it could easily interact with Met residues of adjacent peptides or with lipid-localized free radicals in brain membranes (*see* Section 4.1.). The oxygen dependency to free radical generation, compositional changes, and solution structure alterations are consistent with an observation by Roses and coworkers, who found a dramatic increase in the rate of binding of Aβ1–40 to apolipoprotein E (ApoE) isoforms ApoE3 and ApoE4 in oxygenated buffer relative to nitrogen-sparged buffer *(49)*. Reducing agents prevented the Aβ/ApoE binding in oxygenated buffer.

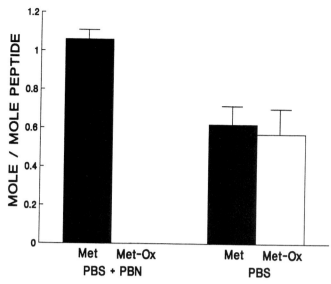

Fig. 4. Formation of a species that coelutes with Met-sulfoxide on HPLC traces following amino acid hydrolysis. No such species is seen in the presence of the free radical scavenger PBN. About one-half mole of the sulfoxide is formed per mole of starting material in PBS buffer.

Recently, Pike et al. *(45)* reported that the C-terminal region of Aβ25–35 was important in its neurotoxicity and that modifications of the 33-35 region of the amyloid peptide led to a loss of peptide aggregation. Based on this result and our own studies, we wondered whether the short, C-terminal fragment of Aβ25–35, i.e., Aβ32–35 (sequence Ile-Gly-Leu-Met, Table 1), would be capable of forming free radicals and demonstrating measures of toxicity *(22)*. We found that Aβ32–35 after 24 h of incubation with PBN would form a three-line EPR spectrum, similar to those of Aβ1–40 and Aβ25–35, but requiring a longer time period for detection *(22)*. Addition of the iron chelator, deferoxamine, to the buffer did not prevent the appearance of the signal, similar to other Aβ-peptides. Also similar to Aβ25–35, catalase abrogated the PBN spin adduct, consistent with a peroxyl radical *(22)*. Like Aβ1–40 and Aβ25–35, Aβ32–35 was neurotoxic to cultured hippocampal neurons and was able to inhibit GS, which was partially protected by the free radical antioxidant, vitamin E *(22)*. HPLC analysis of acid hydrolysates of Aβ32–35 showed, similar to Aβ25–35, a loss of methionine and an increase in a peak that coelutes with methionine sulfoxide. Somewhat disconcerting, samples were occasionally obtained from the supplier (Sigma, St. Louis, MO), which did not produce three-line EPR spectra with PBN; such samples were invariably nontoxic to GS, similar to the variable toxicity of other Aβ-peptides reported previously *(15,39,40)*.

These results demonstrate that Aβ-derived free radical chemistry is oxygen-dependent, and can be modulated by free radical scavengers and reducing agents, consistent with the idea that oxyradical redox chemistry may be significant in the role played by Aβ in the AD brain. Based on the oxygen dependency of Aβ-peptide free radical generation, the peroxyl nature of these free radicals, and apparent involvement of methionine in this process, we offer the following tentative mechanism by which these findings might be synthesized (Fig. 5). Following the chemistry of methionine-containing model

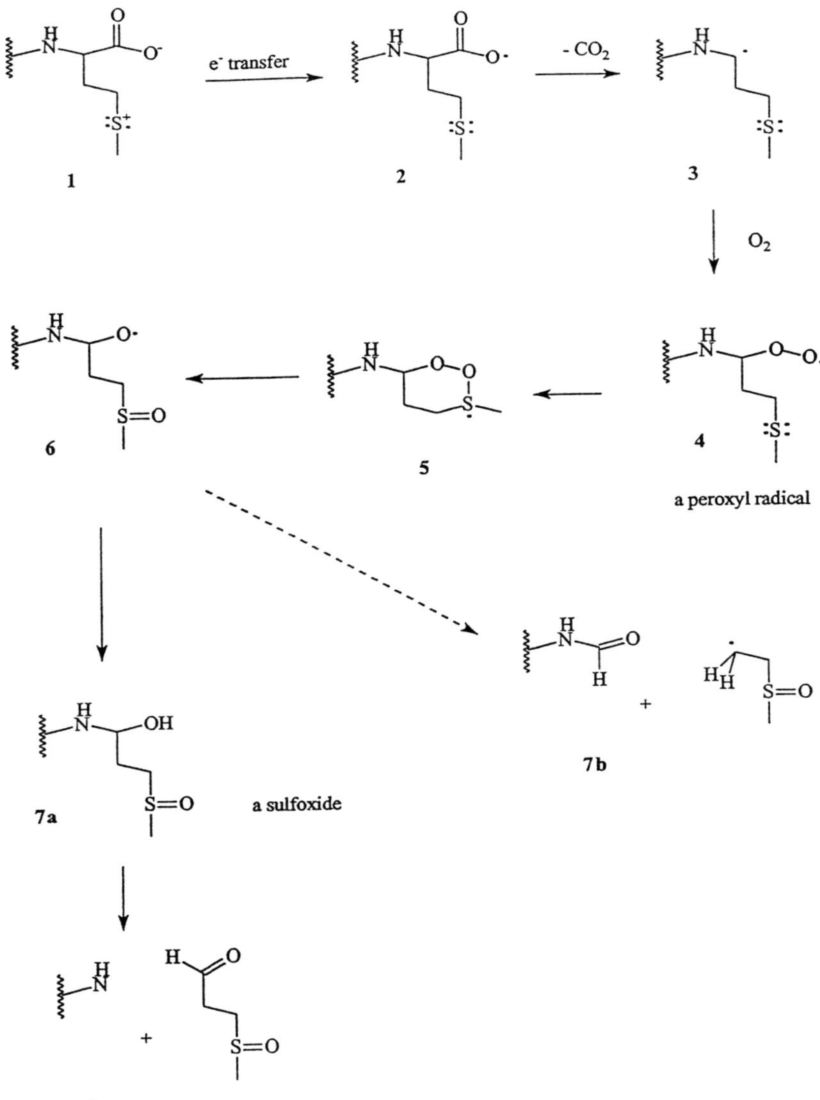

Fig. 5. Putative mechanism, based on known methionine free radical chemistry, to account for the involvement of methionine in the generation of an oxygen-dependent, Aβ-derived free radical and to account for both a peroxyl radical and formation of a sulfoxide. Bold numbers refer to intermediates or products discussed in the text.

peptide systems *(43)*, a sulfuramyl radical **(1)** can be formed from adjacent aligned peptides. This alignment of peptides might be facilitated in solution and in membrane systems by the hydrophobic nature of the C-terminus of Aβ-peptides, and is consistent with the molecular modeling studies noted above. Similar to known chemistry of methionine-containing model peptides *(43)*, electron transfer to the carboxylic acid oxygen of methionine forms an O-centered free radical intermediate **(2)**.

Subsequent electron redistribution can lead to loss of CO_2, resulting in a carbon-centered free radical adjacent to an N heteroatom (3). This carbon-centered free radical is favored, since the heteroatom can stabilize the radical. Addition of paramagnetic oxygen (O_2) to the carbon-centered free radical would lead to a peroxyl radical (4), consistent with our results enumerated above. Subsequent attack of this peroxyl radical on the sulfur atom would lead to a six-membered intermediate (5), which could decompose into an alkoxyl radical and a sulfoxide (6). As noted, we showed that Aβ peptides lose methionine and form a species that coelutes on HPLC with methionine sulfoxide. The alkoxyl radical could abstract an H atom from a nearby species resulting in a hydroxylated sulfoxide product (7a). Based on known methionine chemistry (43), such species can undergo subsequent fragmentation as indicated in Fig. 5. Similarly, the intermediate (6) can undergo fragmentation to form the C-centered free radical and the aldehyde (7b). Explicit tests of this tentative mechanism, which would account for the involvement of Met, the formation of peroxyl radicals, and the oxygen dependency of the process, are currently in progress.

3. THE Aβ-DERIVED FREE RADICAL MOLECULAR SHRAPNEL UNIFYING MODEL OF AD

Should the reactions of Aβ in solution be mimicked in AD brain, then a plausible unifying model for AD neurotoxicity and pathology can be developed. The results of explicit tests of this model are given in the following section of this chapter. In this model (Fig. 6), Aβ, formed outside the neuron by as yet unexplained mechanisms thought to involve thiol proteases (β-secretase), would generate oxygen-dependent free radicals that would rain down on the neuronal and glial cells like shrapnel, inserting into the membrane and binding to various proteins and lipids, thereby causing their dysfunction. Loss of Ca^{2+} homeostasis could occur, or removal of excitotoxic glutamate by glial cell glutamate transporter could be compromised. This could account for the reported synergy between Aβ and glutamate excitotoxicity in culture (35). Both mechanisms could then lead to subsequent neuronal death. Alternatively, Aβ-derived free radical attack on nearby peptides outside neurons could lead to their aggregation, forming the nucleus of the SP.

The merit of our free radical model for Aβ toxicity is its ability to unify existing AD data into a coherent theoretical framework. Our hypothesis is consistent with the many reports of altered membrane enzymes, transport proteins, structural and cytoskeletal proteins, lipids, and so forth, in AD (reviewed in refs. 2,3,50,51). It is highly unusual for a single disease to have so many different membrane components with altered function. However, if a "shower" of free radicals (shrapnel) generated by Aβ were to interact with whatever moiety was nearby, such a myriad of membrane alterations would be reasonable. Also, our hypothesis is consistent with the age-dependence of AD: younger persons may have greater antioxidant capacity (52–55) and can, therefore, withstand or combat amyloid-induced free radical stress; aging, possibly coupled to environmental insults that compromise antioxidant status, could encourage the phenomena reported in this chapter. Genetic factors contributing either to decreased antioxidant capacity or to altered binding to chaperon proteins, such as ApoE4, would also predispose a subject to these processes. In addition, our proposed scheme allows for the possibility of radical-promoted, protease-independent cleavage of APP at a protease-inaccessible site

Butterfield et al.

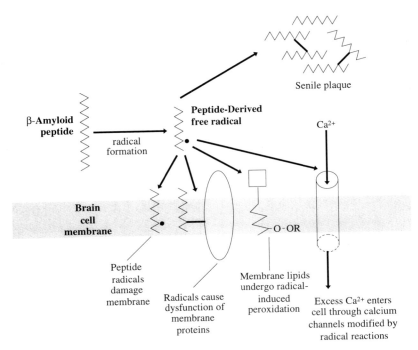

Fig. 6. Aβ-derived free radical shrapnel model of AD. Note that this model is consistent with reports of multiple membrane alterations of enzymes, proteins, transport proteins, and so forth, as well as lipid and protein oxidation and calcium ion accumulation in neurons and subsequent cell death in AD. *See text.*

within the lipid brayer. Moreover, our hypothesis of a free radical-based aggregation and neurotoxicity of Aβ offers possible therapeutic strategies in AD involving appropriate brain-accessible free radical scavengers, a possibility under active investigation in our laboratory. Finally, our model may help clarify the genesis of prion protein pathology, known to involve amyloid-like plaques and neurodegeneration *(56)*: it is reasonable that mechanisms similar to those developed in our studies of AD may be involved in prion disorders as well.

4. EVIDENCE SUPPORTING PREDICTIONS OF THE Aβ-DERIVED FREE RADICAL SHRAPNEL MODEL OF AD: LIPID AND PROTEIN OXIDATION, OTHER MEMBRANE DAMAGE, NEUROTOXICITY, PEPTIDE AGGREGATION, AND MODULATION OF THESE PHENOMENA BY FREE RADICAL SCAVENGERS

4.1. Lipid Oxidation by Aβ25–35

The lipid-specific spin-label derivatives of stearic acid, 5-nitroxide stearate (5-NS) or 12-NS, which differ only in the location of the paramagnetic center of the spin probe *(3,36)*, were added to gerbil neocortical synaptosomal membranes *(14)*. Such assays are useful EPR tools for the demonstration of peroxidation processes and their consequences *(3,36,57)*. Aβ25–35 was added to these spin-labeled membrane systems, and the kinetics of the loss of spin label signal intensity was monitored. If an Aβ-derived reactive free radical reduces the paramagnetic center of the nitroxide spin label, then the EPR signal intensity will decrease *(3,36)*. Aβ25–35, in accordance with the model, produces a free radical-mediated, 60% reduction of the 12-NS signal *(14)*. This spin label's paramagnetic center is located near the most common sites of unsaturation in membrane lipids. Also oxygen, being entirely nonpolar, is highly soluble deep in the hydrophobic portion of biological membranes. The paramagnetic center of 5-NS, located near the lipid/water interface, is hardly affected by Aβ25–35, and the nontoxic reverse sequence Aβ35–25, which, having a different primary amino acid sequence, presumably has a different secondary structure from Aβ25–35, causes little to no effect in either spin label *(14)*. Therefore, these results suggest that (1) Aβ25–35 interacts with and causes membrane lipid peroxidation damage in a selective manner, i.e., more damage deep within the bilayer than at the surface of the bilayer; and (2) the structure of the peptide radical is important in its ability to cause membrane damage, i.e., Aβ35–25 is nontoxic to synaptosomal membranes. The CD spectra discussed above also are consistent with the idea that structure and reactivity are related. Kang et al. *(58)*, using molecular modeling procedures, predicted that the Met 35 of Aβ25–35 would reside in membranes with this residue deep in the lipid bilayer. Our results *(14)* are in agreement with the prediction of Kang et al. *(58)*: if the Met-35 were located near the lipid/water interface, then there should have been loss of the 5-NS signal intensity, which does not occur. Confirming our observations consistent with lipid peroxidation caused by Aβ25–35, we spectroscopically measured levels of conjugated dienes, which are formed during lipid peroxidation, following exposure of gerbil neocortical synaptosomal membranes to Aβ25–35 (Fig. 7). An approx 70% increase in conjugated dienes over controls was found ($p < 0.02$, $N = 3$) (Fig. 7), consistent with the results of synaptosomal membrane lipid 12-NS spin labeling. In preliminary experiments, the lipophilic antioxidant, vitamin E, was able to inhibit greatly the Aβ-induced reduction of the 12-NS signal, consistent with a free radical process.

4.2. Synaptosomal Membrane Protein Oxidation by Aβ-Peptides

Free radical membrane damage deep within the lipid bilayer as inferred from the 12-NS reduction data above might also alter the structure and function of membrane proteins. To test this idea, we used protein-specific spin labeling. We previously developed and characterized a protein-specific spin-labeling procedure for synaptosomal membranes *(59)*. Using an Fe^{2+}/ascorbate free radical generating system, which generates protein carbonyl and inactivates enzymes of synaptosomal membranes *(60)*, we showed that the motion of the protein-specific spin label 2,2,6,6-tetramethyl-4-maleimidopiperidine-N-1-oxyl (MAL-6) covalently bound to neocortical synaptosomal membrane proteins was significantly reduced following free radical protein oxidation by Fenton chemistry *(60)*. Other free radical oxidative conditions studied in our laboratory, ischemia/reperfusion injury *(61–63)*, sepsis-released endotoxin *(64)*, or menadione *(65)*, also led to reduced motion of MAL-6. Using these results as a guide, we examined the effect of Aβ-peptides on brain synaptosomal membranes as monitored by MAL-6. The parameter used to assess protein-specific spin-label motion and membrane protein–protein interactions is the W/S ratio of MAL-6 *(3,36,59–65)*: lower values of the W/S ratio mean slower motion of the MAL-6 spin label bound to proteins, possibly because of increased steric hindrance, decreased segmental motion of spin-

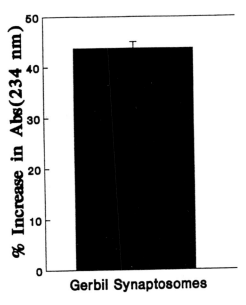

Fig. 7. Increase in conjugated dienes, a measure of lipid peroxidation, following treatment of gerbil neocortical synaptosomal membranes with highly toxic Aβ25–35 peptide. Conjugated dienes were monitored by the increase in absorbance at 234 nm.

label-binding sites on proteins, or increased protein–protein interactions *(3,36,59–65)*. A 30-min incubation of synaptosomes with Aβ25–35 significantly decreased the W/S ratio of subsequently added MAL-6, indicating that membrane proteins are also a target of Aβ25–35 free radical attack, consistent with the model proposed. In a related study, we added Aβ25–35 directly to MAL-6-labeled synaptosomal membranes *(23)*; the EPR signal intensity was reduced by peptide-derived free radicals, suggesting a direct oxidation of membrane proteins by the peptide.

Oxidation of hippocampal cultured neuronal cell membrane proteins was also demonstrated by means of a fluorescence staining technique *(18)*. In these experiments, oxidized proteins, rich in protein carbonyls *(52,53)*, are first treated with biotin-4-aminohydrazide, which reacts with membrane protein carbonyls to form the Schiff base. Biotinylated proteins are reacted with fluorescein isothiocynate-conjugated streptavidin. Fluorescence of the resulting complex can be visualized by confocal microscopy and the integrated fluorescence intensity of the micrographs quantified by computerized image analysis *(18)*. Figure 8 shows that Aβ-induced oxidative stress to rat cultured hippocampal neurons gave excellent responses ($p < 0.05$), confirming the EPR results. On "aging" of Aβ1–40 long enough to produce free radicals, fluorescence appears. As also shown in Fig. 8, the free radical scavenger propyl gallate inhibits Aβ-induced protein oxidation in cultured neurons, consistent with a free radical process.

Fluorescence was also used by us to demonstrate intracellular ROS production on exposure of cells to Aβ *(18)*. The redox-sensitive dye, 2',7'-dichlorofluorescin diacetate, is transported into hippocampal neuronal cultures, where it is converted to 2',7'-dichlorofluorescein (DCF). On reaction with ROS, fluorescence appears. Addition of Aβ (which in separate experiments had pre-aged to give maximal EPR signal intensity

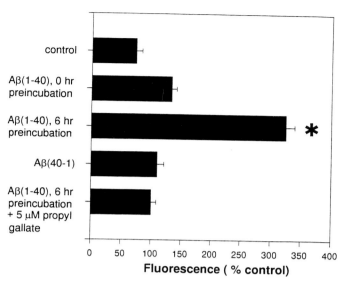

Fig. 8. Fluorescence intensity of FITC-labeled streptavidin following binding to biotin hydrazide, which in turn has been bound to oxidized proteins of cultured hippocampal neurons. Note that Aβ1–40, preincubated 6 h to give a strong free radical signal when incubated separately with PBN, yields a highly significant, approximate threefold increase in the fluorescence intensity compared to controls (no peptide; Aβ1–40 with no preincubation; nontoxic Aβ40–1). Note also that in the presence of a free radical scavenger, propyl gallate, no increase in fluorescence over controls is observed, consistent with a free radical process. *See text.*

in the presence of PBN) to neuronal cell cultures led to ROS production as monitored by the fluorescence. No significant increase in fluorescence was observed with fresh Aβ, consistent with the EPR spin-trapping studies described above. Subsequent to our publishing this result, Behl and coworkers *(25)* published similar findings on immortalized PC12 cells using the redox-sensitive dye 3-(4,5-dimethylthiazol-2-yl)-2,5-diphenyltetrazolium bromide (MTT). MTT is converted to a colored formazan product by reduction, apparently involving components of the mitochondrial cytochrome chain. Treatment of cells with H_2O_2 or Aβ diminished this conversion, indicative of a more oxidizing intracellular environment, consistent with our results. Although use of these transformed PC12 cells to gain insight into neurons has been criticized, these workers showed that numerous antioxidant compounds were able to inhibit this Aβ effect *(25)*, again consistent with our model of a free radical process associated with Aβ.

4.3. Multiple Transmembrane Protein Alterations

A prediction of the free radical shrapnel model for AD is that a shower of free radicals raining down on neuronal and glial membranes could alter the function of whatever moiety to which these free radicals bind. Lipid and protein oxidation clearly occurs as noted above. The membrane as a target for Aβ damage is supported by electron microscopic immunolocalization of Aβ to the neuronal plasma membrane of cultured cells *(35)*. A synergy between lipid and/or protein oxidation and localization of Aβ to plasma membranes may exist. We noted above that Aβ-peptides led to lipid peroxidation deep within the lipid brayer *(14)*. Such oxidation conceivably could lead to inactivation of transmembrane transport proteins. Since intracellular Ca^{2+} levels increase following Aβ administration *(35)*, we investigated the activity of several ion-motive ATPases in cultured neurons exposed to amyloid *(19)*. Neurons exposed to micromolar levels of Aβ25–35 or Aβ1–40 lose Na^+/K^+-ATPase activity (more than 50% loss in 3 h). However, Mg^{2+}-ATPase was affected after 10 h, whereas the Na^+/Ca^{2+}-exchanger was unaffected. Based on studies with ouabain, which affects K^+ flux, tetrodotoxin, a specific inhibitor of voltage-dependent Na^+ channels, or Na^+-deficient media, we suggested that increased intracellular Ca^{2+} levels were secondary to increased Na^+ influx. Aβ-induced impairment of Na^+/K^+-ATPase, Ca^{2+} influx, and cell death were all abrogated by incubation of the cells with the free radical scavengers vitamin E, propyl gallate, or PBN, consistent with the Aβ-derived free radical shrapnel model. Human autopsy Na^+/K^+-ATPase and Ca^{2+}-ATPase activities were also impaired by synthetic amyloid: 70 and 30% loss of activity, respectively, on exposure to 50 μM Aβ25–35 for 1 h *(19)*.

Amyloid, when added at low doses to mixed astrocyte and neuron cultures, predisposes the cells to subsequent glutamate-induced excitotoxic stress *(35)*. Astrocytes, located in the perisynaptic space, provide the principal mechanism for removal of excitotoxic glutamate following synaptic transmission. This is accomplished primarily by the action of the Na^+-dependent glutamate transport system. It has been reported recently that following Fenton chemistry oxyradical stress, Na^+-dependent glutamate transport is inhibited *(66)*. On transport to the astrocyte interior, glutamate is converted to glutamine by the oxidatively sensitive enzyme, GS; i.e., the glutamate transporter and GS systems represent the potential coupling of two oxidatively sensitive chemistries. Since Aβ-peptides disrupt membrane-bound ion transport systems, as already described *(19)*, we wondered if similar oxidative impairment to the astrocyte glutamate uptake system by Aβ-derived free radicals would occur. Such impairment might provide an explanation for the reported synergy between Aβ and excitotoxic glutamate *(35)*. Treatment of mixed neuronal/astrocyte cultures with 100 μM Aβ25–35 for 1 h significantly diminished Na^+-dependent glutamate uptake and GS activity *(24,67)*. Concomitant with Aβ treatment, we found significant elevation of intracellular ROS in astrocytes based on DCF fluorescence and a threefold increase in protein carbonyl *(24,67)*, a measure of protein oxidation as already discussed. Addition of ouabain indicated that this effect was not a simple result of Na^+/K^+-ATPase inhibition. Pretreatment of cultures with the more water-soluble vitamin E analog trolox prevented the damage to astrocytes *(24)*, consistent with Aβ-derived free radical damage and the shrapnel model.

Additional evidence for a confluence of GS and Aβ-induced cell neurotoxicity was produced in our laboratory *(21)*. We confirmed that Aβ-peptides decreased GS activity, and we showed that there was a simultaneous decrease in GS immunoreactivity *(21)*. Because GS can serve as a substrate for Aβ-induced oxyradicals, we expected that GS might serve to protect partially the Aβ-induced neurotoxicity. However, Aβ1–40-stimulated neurotoxicity was markedly exacerbated by addition of GS, indicating that interaction of GS with Aβ1–40 changed the properties of the peptide *(21)*. Gunnersen and Haley *(68)* reported a 42-kDa ATP-binding protein in AD CSF not present in controls. This protein was identified as GS, and was proposed as a diagnostic marker for AD. As noted, GS is normally found intracellularly in astrocytes. Free radical damage to membrane lipids and proteins could release GS that is subsequently observed in CSF in AD

(68). We wondered if oxidized GS would behave differently toward a protein-specific spin label directed at the 88 sulfhydryl groups per GS molecule than would unoxidized GS, and we wondered if highly purified control and AD human GS would show these differences. Using MTS (a methylthiosulfonate spin label specific for protein SH groups *[60,69–71]*), we measured the rate of uptake of MTS by sheep brain GS *(72)*. The results indicated that oxidized GS reacted with this SH group-specific spin label at a rate three times slower than unoxidized GS. Dr. Haley generously provided human control and AD GS highly purified from CSF. Similar studies with these systems showed that AD GS reacted with the MTS spin label between two and three times slower than did control GS. These results are consistent with oxidized GS in AD brain (*see* Section 4.5.), and suggest that free radical oxidation can dramatically alter the properties of both the target and amyloid itself.

As noted, we showed that GS interaction with Aβ1–40 leads to increased neurotoxicity *(21)*. This result is consistent with the notion that glial-derived proteins may play a role in Aβ aggregation and toxicity. We found that GS interaction with Aβ leads to abrogation of fibril formation with significantly increased Aβ-induced neurotoxicity *(73)*. A similar finding of increased Aβ toxicity with inhibition of fibril formation was reported for clusterin (apolipoprotein J) interaction with Aβ *(74)*. Recently, Mattson's group showed that interaction of thrombin, a protease found in SP, with Aβ1–40 also increased neurotoxicity, whereas protease nexin-1, also found in SP, protected neurons against Aβ-induced neurotoxicity *(75)*. Concomitant with increased neurotoxicity, thrombin was found to increase ROS production and accumulation of Ca^{2+}, whereas protease nexin-1 inhibited ROS production and Ca^{2+} accumulation *(75)*, consistent with free radical damage from Aβ.

4.4. Protection Against Aβ-Induced Damage and Peptide Aggregation by Free Radical Antioxidants

In several places throughout this chapter, mention has been made of one of the predictions of the shrapnel model, namely, the protective effects of free radical antioxidants against Aβ-peptide-derived membrane damage: PBN, vitamin E, or propyl gallate protect cells from Aβ-induced Na^+/K^+-ATPase impairment, Ca^{2+} influx, and cell death *(19)*; propyl gallate significantly attenuates Aβ-stimulated increased protein oxidation *(18)*; and trolox was effective in protecting astrocytes from Aβ-caused ROS and inhibition of Na^+-dependent glutamate uptake *(24)*. We have also found that the brain accessible free radical scavenger PBN protects GS from Aβ-stimulated loss of activity *(5)*: mean GS activity in a coincubate of 0.5 mg/mL gerbil brain cytosol extract and 1 mg/mL Aβ1–40 after 3 h in saline, pH 7.4, 37°C was decreased by 67% in the absence of PBN, but increased by 5% in the presence of 50 mM PBN compared to controls without Aβ or PBN *(5,72)*. Glutamine synthetase activity was also protected by PBN against Aβ25–35 as well *(5,72)*.

Amyloid is well known to aggregate in solution. We wondered if free radicals might be involved in this process. Figure 9A shows that 1 mg/mL Aβ1–40 forms fibrils as reported by others *(27,50)*. Addition of 5 mM PBN leads to a system of much less ordered and dense fibrils (Fig. 9B). No fibrils are found in the nontoxic reverse-sequence peptide, Aβ40–1 (Fig. 9C). A similar inhibition of fibril formation was reported by Tomiyama et al. on exposure of the potential antioxidant rifampicin to Aβ1–40 *(76)*.

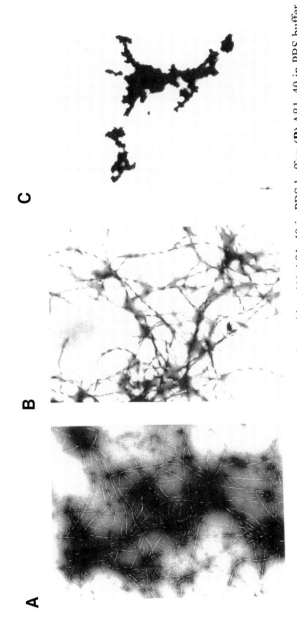

Fig. 9. Electron micrographs of fibril formation by Aβ peptides. **(A)** Aβ1–40 in PBS buffer; **(B)** Aβ1–40 in PBS buffer containing 5 m*M* of the free radical scavenger PBN; **(C)** Nontoxic Aβ40–1 showing no fibril formation.

Table 2
Summary of Demographics of Subjects Used in Rapid Postmortem Protocol

	Mean Age	Postmortem Interval	Duration of Illness
Control	78	4.6 h	12 yr
AD	80	4.4 h	—
P-value	0.9[a]	0.71[b]	—

[a]Student's two-sample *t*-test.
[b]Fisher's exact test.

Others have also reported protection by free radical antioxidants against Aβ-induced damage to PC12 and neuronal cells *(25,77–79)*. Our results, taken together with other reports of the efficacious effects of antioxidants against Aβ-induced ROS and cell damage *(18,19,24,76–79)*, are consistent with our free radical shrapnel model *(5,13,14)* and with our notion *(5,13,14)* that appropriate brain-accessible free radical scavengers may be a promising approach to therapeutic intervention in AD *(5,13,14)*.

4.5. Oxidative Damage in the AD Brain is Correlated to Regions of High Senile Plaque Density

As outlined, our research has provided ample evidence that synthetic Aβ is a source of membrane-damaging, neurotoxic free radicals. A prediction of our Aβ-derived free radical shrapnel model of AD is that AD brain regions high in SP should exhibit oxidative stress, whereas the cerebellum, poor in SP, should be relatively naive to oxidative stress. As a first test of this prediction, we investigated fresh autopsy material in AD and control brain *(7)*. Table 2 shows the demographic characteristics of the subjects used in the rapid postmortem protocol. Three different brain regions were examined: cerebellum (Cer), inferior parietal lobule (IPL), and hippocampus (Hip), the latter two rich in SP in AD, whereas Cer is poor in SP *(7)*. Four biomarkers of neuronal protein oxidation (W/S ratio of MAL-6-spin-labeled synaptosomes prepared and used immediately after autopsy, phenylhydrazine-reactive protein carbonyl content, glutamine synthetase activity, and CK activity) in three brain regions of AD-demented and age-matched control subjects were assessed. These end points indicate that AD brain protein may be more oxidized than that of control subjects. The W/S ratios of MAL-6 bound to membrane proteins in AD Hip and IPL synaptosomes were 30 and 46% lower, respectively, than corresponding values of tissue isolated from control brain; however, the difference between the W/S ratios of MAL-6 in AD and control synaptosomes from SP-poor Cer was not significant. As indicated, decreased W/S ratios of MAL-6 are associated with oxidized proteins *(23,59–65)*. Protein carbonyl content, a measure of protein oxidation, is increased 42 and 37% in the AD Hip and IPL regions, respectively, relative to AD Cer, whereas carbonyl content in control Hip and IPL is similar to that of control Cer. GS activity was decreased by an average of 27% in the AD brain; CK activity was decreased by 80%. The brain regional variation of these oxidation-sensitive biomarkers corresponds with established histopathological features of AD (SP and NFT densities). These results indicated that SP-dense regions of the AD brain may represent environments of elevated oxidative stress *(7)*, consistent with our Aβ-derived free radical shrapnel model.

5. β-AMYLOID-DERIVED FREE RADICAL OXIDATION: A FUNDAMENTAL PROCESS IN AD — SUMMARY AND FUTURE CONSIDERATIONS

Our research outlined in this chapter has demonstrated that Aβ is capable of producing free radical oxidation of membrane lipids and proteins from which, we assert, cell death eventually occurs. Based on these results, we have formulated an Aβ-derived free radical shrapnel unifying model that accounts for the three major observations for which any theory of AD would have to account:

1. Multiple membrane alterations of lipids, enzymes, transmembrane transport proteins, and so on, reported in the literature can be rationalized as discrete manifestations of Aβ-derived free radical shrapnel raining down on neuronal and glial cell membranes;
2. The age dependence of AD is consistent with this model based on the known loss of anti-oxidant capacity with age; and
3. The relative insolubility of SP may be related to Aβ-derived free radical attack of adjacent peptides, proteins, and other moieties.

Predictions of the Aβ-derived free radical shrapnel model, including lipid oxidation, protein oxidation, neurotoxicity, Ca^{2+} accumulation, inhibition of multiple transport proteins, abrogation of many of these effects by free radical scavengers, and correlation of protein oxidation in AD brain regions rich in SP, have all been borne out by experiment.

The precise molecular mechanisms by which Aβ-derived free radicals are produced are under investigation in our laboratory and remain to be elucidated. However, our studies, which led to the Aβ-derived free radical shrapnel model of AD, provide a strong basis for our notion that this is a fundamental process in AD. Our model provides a rational strategy for therapeutic intervention in AD, also under active investigation in our laboratory.

Paradigms involving transgenic mice and molecular biology will undoubtedly play a key role in future research into Aβ-derived free radicals and our understanding of AD.

Note Added in Proof

Others *(80)*, using EPR spin trapping with PBN, confirmed our findings that Aβ(1–40) yields 3-line EPR spectra, indicating Aβ free radical formation *(13)*. In addition, small angle X-ray studies unequivocally demonstrated that Aβ peptides insert into lipid bilayers *(81)*, consistent with the Aβ-associated free-radical model we developed and consistent with our Aβ-induced lipid peroxidation studies *(14)*.

ACKNOWLEDGMENTS

This work was supported in part by grants from the National Institutes of Health (AG-10836; AG-05119). We gratefully acknowledge Centaur Pharmaceuticals for their generous gift of ^{13}C-PBN. We thank Christian Schoneich for helpful discussions.

REFERENCES

1. Alzheimer, L. (1907) Uber eine eigenartige erkraankung der hirnrince. *Centralblatt Nervenheil Kunde Psychiat.* **30**, 177–179.
2. Katzman, R. and Saitoh, T. (1991) Advances in Alzheimer's Disease, *FASEB J.* **4**, 278–286.
3. Butterfield, D. A. (1986) Spectroscopic methods in degenerative neurological diseases, *Crit. Rev. Neurobiol.* **2**, 169–240.

4. Sheff, S. W. and Price, D. A. (1993) Synapse loss in temporal lobe in Alzheimer's disease, *Ann. Neurol.* **33**, 190–199.
5. Hensley, K., Butterfield, D. A., Hall, N., Cole, P., Subramaniam, R., Mark, R., Mattson, M. P., Markesbery, W. R., Harris, M. E., Aksenov, M., Aksenova, M., Wu, J. F., and Carney, J. M. (1995) Reactive oxygen species as casual agents in the neurotoxicity of the Alzheimer's disease-associated amyloid beta peptide, *Ann. NY Acad. Sci.* **786**, 120–124.
6. Halliwell, B. and Gutteridge, J. M. C. (1989) *Free Radicals in Biology and Medicine*, Clarendon, Oxford.
7. Hensley, K., Hall, N., Subramaniam, R., Cole, P., Harris, M., Aksenov, M., Aksenova, M., Gabbita, P., Wu, J. F., Carney, J. M., Lovell, M., Markesbery, W. R., and Butterfield, D. A. (1995) Brain regional correspondence between Alzheimer's disease histopathology and biomarkers of protein oxidation, *J. Neurochem.* **65**, 2146–2156.
8. Markesbery, W. R., Lovell, M. A., and Ehmann, W. D. (1994) Brain trace metals in Alzheimer disease, in *Alzheimer Disease* (Terry, R. D., Katzman, R., and Bick, K. L., eds.), Raven, New York, pp. 353–367.
9. Parker, W. D., Jr., Parks, J., Filley, C. M., and Kleinschmidt-Demasters, B. K. (1994) Electron transport chain defects in Alzheimer's disease brain, *Neurology* **44**, 1090–1096.
10. Nutisya, E. M., Bowling, A. C., and Beal, M. F. (1994) Cortical cytochrome oxidase activity is reduced in Alzheimer's disease, *J. Neurochem.* **63**, 2179–2184.
11. Smith, M. A., Taneda, S., Richey, P. L., Mikyata, S., Yan, S., Stern, D., Sayer, L., Monnier, V. M., and Perry, G. (1994) Advanced maillard reaction end products are associated with Alzheimer disease pathology, *Proc. Natl. Acad. Sci. USA* **91**, 5710–5714.
12. Colton, C. A., Snell, J., Chernyshev, O., and Gilbert, D. L. (1994) Induction of superoxide anion and nitric oxide production in cultured microglia, *Ann. NY Acad. Sci.* **738**, 54–63.
13. Hensley, K., Carney, J. M., Mattson, M. P., Aksenova, M., Harris, M., Wu, J. F., Floyd, R. A., and Butterfield, D. A. (1994) A model for β-amyloid aggregation and neurotoxicity based on free radical generation by the peptide: relevance to Alzheimer disease, *Proc. Natl. Acad. Sci. USA* **91**, 3270–3274.
14. Butterfield, D. A., Hensley, K., Harris, M., Mattson, M. P., and Carney, J. M. (1994) β–amyloid peptide free radical fragments initiate synaptosomal lipoperoxidation in a sequence-specific fashion: implications to Alzheimer's disease, *Biochem. Biophys. Res. Commun.* **200**, 710–715.
15. Hensley, K., Aksenova, M., Carney, J. M., and Butterfield, D. A. (1995) Amyloid β-peptide spin trapping I: enzyme toxicity is related to free radical spin trap reactivity, *NeuroReport* **6**, 489–493.
16. Hensley, K., Aksenova, M., Carney, J. M., and Butterfield, D. A. (1995) Amyloid β-peptide spin trapping II: Evidence for decomposition of the PBM spin adduct, *NeuroReport* **6**, 493–496.
17. Hensley, K., Butterfield, D. A., Aksenova, M., Harris, M., Wu, J., Floyd, R., Mattson, M., and Carney, J. M. (1995) A model for β-amyloid aggregation and neurotoxicity based on the free radical generating capacity of the peptide: implications of peptide-derived free radicals to Alzheimer's disease, *Proc. Western Pharmacol. Soc.* **38**, 113–120.
18. Harris, M. E., Hensley, K., Butterfield, D. A., Leedle, R. E., and Carney, J. M. (1995) Direct evidence of oxidative injury by the Alzheimer's amyloid β peptide in cultured hippocampal neurons, *Exp. Neurol.* **131**, 193–202.
19. Mark, R. J., Hensley, K., Butterfield, D. A., and Mattson, M. P. (1995) Amyloid β-peptide impairs ion-motive ATPase activities: evidence for a role in loss of neuronal Ca^{2+} homeostasis and cell death, *J. Neurosci.* **15**, 6239–6249.
20. Mattson, M. P., Carney, J. M., and Butterfield, D. A. (1995) Glycation: a tombstone in AD? *Nature* **373**, 481.
21. Aksenov, M. Y., Aksenova, M. V., Harris, M. E., Hensley, K., Butterfield, D. A., and Carney, J. M. (1995) Enhancement of Aβ(1-40) neurotoxicity by glutamine synthetase, *J. Neurochem.* **65**, 1899–1902.

22. Subramaniam, R., Howard, B. J., Hensley, K., Aksenova, M., Carney, J. M., and Butterfield, D. A. (1995) β-Amyloid (32-35) generates reactive free radicals that are toxic to biomolecules: implications to Alzheimer's disease, *Alzheimer's Res.* **1**, 141–144.

23. Butterfield, D. A., Martin, L., Carney, J. M., and Hensley, K. (1996) Aβ(25-35) peptide displays H_2O_2-like reactivity towards aqueous Fe^{2+}, nitroxide spin probes, and synaptosomal membrane proteins, *Life Sci.* **58**, 217–228.

24. Harris, M. E., Carney, J. M., Cole, P., Hensley, K., Howard, B. J., Martin, L., Bummer, P., Wang, Y., Pedigo, N., and Butterfield, D. A. (1995) β-amyloid peptide-derived, oxygen-dependent free radicals inhibit glutamate uptake in cultured astrocytes: implications to Alzheimer's disease, *NeuroReport* **6**, 1875–1879.

25. Behl, C., Davis, J. B., Lesley, R., and Shubert, D. (1994) Hydrogen peroxide medicates amyloid β protein toxicity, *Cell* **77**, 817–827.

26. Goodman, Y., Steiner, M. R., Steiner, S. M., and Mattson, M. P. (1994) Nordihydroguaiaretic acid protects hippocampal neurons against amyloid, β-peptide toxicity, and attentuates free radical and calcium accumulation, *Brain Res.* **654**, 171–176,

27. Selkoe, D. J. (1994) Alzheimer's disease: a central role for amyloid, *J. Neuropathol. Exp. Neurol.* **53**, 438–447.

28. Games, D., Adams, D., Alessandrini, R., Barbour, R., Berthelette, P., Blackwell, C., Carr, T., Clemens, J., Donaldson, T., Gillespie, F., Guido, T., Hagoplan, S., Johnson-Wood, K., Khan, K., Lee, M., Leibowitz, P., Lieberburg, I., Little, S., Masliah, E., McConlogue, L., Montoya-Zavala, M., Mucke, L., Paganini, L., Permiman, E., Power, M., Schenk, D., Seubert, P., Snyder, B., Soriano, F., Tan, F., Vital, J., Wadsworth, S., Wolozin, B., and Zhao, J. (1995) Alzheimer-type neuropathology in transgenic mice overexpressing V717F β-amyloid precursor protein, *Nature* **373**, 523–527.

29. Pike, C. J., Burdick, D., Walencewicz, A. J., Glabe, C. G., and Cotman, C. W. (1993) Neurodegeneration induced by β-amyloid peptides in vitro: role of peptide assembly state, *J. Neurosci.* **13**, 1676–1687.

30. Burdick, D., Soreghan, B., Kwon, M., Kosmoski, J., Knauer, M., Henshen, A., Yates, J., Cotman, C., and Glabe, C. (1992) Assembly and aggregation properties of synthetic Alzheimer's A4/β-amyloid peptide analogs, *J. Biol. Chem.* **267**, 546–554.

31. Yankner, B. A., Duffy, L. K., and Kirschnier, D. A. (1990) Neurotrophic and neurotoxic effects of amyloid β-protein: reversal by tachykinin neuropeptides, *Science* **250**, 279–282.

32. Jarrett, J. T., Berber, E. P., and Lansbury, P. T. (1992) The carboxy terminus of the β-amyloid protein is critical in the seeding of amyloid formation: implications for the pathogenesis of Alzheimer's disease, *Biochemistry* **32**, 4693–4697.

33. Jarrett, J. T. and Lansbury, P. T. (1993) "One-dimensional crystallization" of amyloid: a pathogenic mechanism in Alzheimer's disease? *Cell* **73**, 1053–1058.

34. Tomski, S. and Murphy, R. M. (1992) Kinetics of aggregation of synthetic β-amyloid peptides. *Arch. Biochem. Biophys.* **294**, 630–638.

35. Mattson, M. P., Barger, S. W., Cheng, B., Lieberburg, I., Smith-Swintosky, V. L., and Ryel, R. E. (1992) β-amyloid precursor protein metabolites and loss of neuronal Ca^{2+} homeostasis Alzheimer's disease, *Trends Neurosci.* **16**, 409–414.

36. Butterfield, D. A. (1982) Spin labeling in disease, *Biol. Magn. Reson.* **4**, 1–78.

37. Janzen, E. G. (1980) A Critical Review of Spin Trapping in biological systems, in *Free Radicals in Biology*, vol. 4 (Pryor, W. A., ed.), Academic, New York, pp. 115–154.

38. Chan, W. K. M., Decker, E. A., Lee, J., and Butterfield, D. A. (1994) EPR spin trapping studies of the hydroxyl radical scavenging activity of carnosine and related dipeptides, *J. Agricultural and Food Chemistry* **42**, 1407–1410.

39. May, P. C., Gitter, B. D., Waters, D. C., Simmons, L. K., Becker, G. W., Small, J. S., and Robinson, P. M. (1992) β-amyloid peptide in vitro toxicity: lot-to-lot variability, *Neurobiol. Aging* **13**, 605–607.

40. Simmons, L. K., May, P. C., Tomaselli, K. J., Ryel, R. E., Fuson, K. S., Brigham, E. F., Wright, S., Lieberburg, I., Becker, G. W., Brems, D. N., and Li, W. Y. (1994) Secondary structure of amyloid β peptide correlates with neurotoxic activity in vitro, *Mol. Pharmacol.* **45**, 373–379.

41. Smith, C. D., Carney, J. M., Tatsumo, T., Stadtman, E. R., Floyd, R. A., and Markesbery, W. R. (1992) Protein oxidation in aging brain, *Ann. NY Acad. Sci.* **663**, 110–119.

42. Oliver, C. N., Ahn, B. W., Moerman, E. J., Boldstein, S., and Stadtman, E. R. (1987) Age-related changes in oxidized proteins, *J. Biol. Chem.* **262**, 5488–5491.

43. Schoneich, C., Zhao, F., Madden, K. P., and Bobrowski, K. (1994) Side chain fragmentation of N-terminal threonine or serine residue induced through intramolecular protien transfer to hydioxy sulfuranyl radical formed at neighboring methionine in dipeptides, *J. Am. Chem. Soc.* **116**, 4641–4652.

44. Dado, G. P. and Gellman, S. H. (1994) Redox control of secondary structure in a designed peptide, *J. Am. Chem. Soc.* **115**, 12,609,12,610.

45. Pike, C. J., Walencewicz-Wasserman, A. J., Kosmoski, J., Cribbs, D. H., Glabe, C. G., and Cotman, C. W. (1995) Structure–activity analyses of β-amyloid peptides: contributions of the β25-35 region to aggregation and neurotoxicity, *J. Neurochem.* **64**, 253–265.

46. Synder, S. W., Ladror, U. S., Wade, W. S., Wang, G. T., Barrett, L. W., Matayoshi, E. D., Huffaker, J. H., Krafft, G. A., and Holzman, T. F. (1995) Amyloid-β aggregation: selective inhibition of aggregation in mixtures of amyloid with different chain lengths, *Biophys. J.* **67**, 1216–1228.

47. Naslund, J., Schierhorn, A., Hellman, U., Lanfelt, L., Roses, A. D., Tjernberg, L. O., Siberring, J., Gandy, S. E., Winblad, B., Greengard, P., Nordstedt, C., and Terenius, L. (1994) Relative abundance of alzheimer Aβ-amyloid peptide variants in Alzheimer disease and normal aging, *Proc. Natl. Acad. Sci. USA* **91**, 8378–8382.

48. Terzi, E., Holzemann, G., and Seelig, J. (1994) Alzheimer beta-amyloid peptide 25-35: electrostatic interactions with phospholipid membranes. *Biochemistry* **33**, 7434–7441.

49. Strittmatter, W. J., Weisgraber, K. H., Huang, D. Y., Dong, L. M., Salvesen, G. S., Pericak-Vance, M., Schmechel, D., Saunders, A. M., Goldgaber, D., and Roses, A. D. (1993) Binding of human Apolipoprotein E to synthetic amyloid β peptide: isofrom-specific effects and implications for late-onset Alzheimer disease, *Proc. Natl. Acad. Sci. USA* **90**, 8098–8102.

50. Selkoe, D. J. (1991) The molecular pathology of Alzheimer's disease, *Neuron* **6**, 487–498.

51. Corain, B., Iqbal, K., Nicolini, B., Wisniewshi, H., and Zatta, P., Winblad, B. (eds.) (1993) *Alzheimer's Disease: Advances in Clinical and Basic Research*, Wiley, New York.

52. Smith, C. D., Carney, J. M., Starke-Reed, P. E., Oliver, C. N., Stadtman, E. R., Floyd, R. A., and Markesbery, W. R. (1991) Excess brain protein oxidation and enzyme dysfunction in normal aging and Alzheimer disease, *Proc. Natl. Acad. Sci. USA* **88**, 10,540–10,543.

53. Carney, J. M., Starke-Reed, P. E., Oliver, C. N., Landrum, R. W., Cheng, M., Wu, J. F., and Floyd, R. A. (1991) reversal of age-related increase in brain protein oxidation, decrease in enzyme activity, and loss in temporal and spatial memory by chronic administration of the spin-trapping compound N-tert-butyl-α-phenylnitrone, *Proc. Nad. Acad. Sci. USA* **88**, 3633–3636.

54. Smith, C. D., Carney, J. M., Tatsumo, T., Stadtman, E. R., Floyd, R. A., and Markesbery, W. R. (1992) Protein oxidation in ageing brain, *Ann. NY Acad. Sci.* **663**, 110–119.

55. Starke-Reed, P. E. and Oliver, C. N. (1989) Protein oxidation and proteolysis during aging and oxidative stress, *Arch. Biochem. Biophys.* **275**, 559–567.

56. Prusiner, S. B. (1992) Biology and genetics of prion diseases, *Biochemistry* **31**, 12,277–12,288.

57. Minetti, M. and Scorza, G. (1991) Hypoxia-stimulated reduction of doxyl stearic acids in human red blood cells, *Biochim. Biophys. Acta.* **1074**, 112–117.

58. Kang, J., Lemair, H. G., Unterbeck, A., Salbaum, J. M., Masters, C. L., Grzeshik, K. H., Multhaup, G., Beyreuther, K., and Müller-Hill, B. (1987) The precursor of Alzheimer' disease A4 protein resembles a cell-surface receptor, *Nature* **325**, 733–736.

59. Umhauer, S. A., Isbell, B. I., and Butterfield, D. A. (1992) Spin labeling or membrane proteins in mammalian brain synaptic plasma membranes: partial characterization, *Anal. Lett.* **25,** 1201–1215.

60. Hensley, K., Hall, N., Shaw, W., Carney, J. M., and Butterfield, D. A. (1994) Electron paramagnetic resonance investigation of free radical induced alterations in neocortical synaptosomal membrane protein infrastructure, *Free Radical Biology & Medicine* **17,** 321–331.

61. Hall, N. C., Carney, J. M., Cheng, M. S., and Butterfield, D. A. (1995) Ischemica/reperfusion induced changes in membrane proteins and lipids of gerbil cortical synaptosomes, *Neuroscience* **64,** 81–89.

62. Hall, N. C., Carney, J. M., Cheng, M., and Butterfield, D. A. (1995) Prevention of ischemica/ reperfusion-induced alterations in synaptosomal membrane-associated proteins and lipids by *N-tert*-butyl-α-phenylnitrone and diflurormethylornithine, *Neuroscience* **69,** 591–600.

63. Hall, N. C., Dempsey, R. J., Carney, J. M., Donaldson, D. L., and Butterfield, D. A. (1995) Structural alterations in synaptosomal membrane-associated proteins and lipids by transient middle cerebral artery occulsion in the cat, *Neurochem. Res.* **20,** 1161–1169.

64. Bellary, S. S., Anderson, K. W., Arden, W. A., and Butterfield, D. A. (1995) Effect of lipopolysaccharide on the physical conformation of the erythrocyte cytoskeletal proteins, *Life Sci.* **56,** 91–98.

65. Trad, C. H. and Butterfield, D. A. (1994) Menadione induced cytotoxicity effects of human erythrocyte membranes studies by electron paramagnetic resonance, *Toxicol. Lett.* **73,** 145–155.

66. Volterra, A., Trotti, D., Tromba, C., Floridi, S., and Racagni, G. (1994) Glutamate uptake inhibition by oxygen free radicals in rat cortical astrocytes, *J. Neurosci.* **14,** 2924–2932.

67. Harris, M. E., Wang, Y., Pedigo, N. W., Jr., Hensley, K., Butterfield, D. A., and Carney, J. M. (1996) Aβ(25-35) inhibits Na$^+$-dependent glutamate uptake in rat hippocampal astrocyte cultures. *J. Neurochem.* **67,** 277–286.

68. Gunnersen, D. and Haley, B. (1992) Detection of glutamine synthetace in the cerebrospinal fluid of Alzheimer diseased patients: a potential diagnostic marker, *Proc. Natl. Acad. Sci. USA* **89,** 11,949–11,953.

69. Trad, C. H., James, W., Bhardwaj, A., and Butterfield, D. A. (1995) Selective labeling of membrane protein sulfhydryl groups with methanethisulfonate spin label, *J. Biochem. Biophys. Methods* **30,** 287–299.

70. Butterfield, D. A., Lee, J., Ganapathi, S., and Bhattacharyya, D. (1994) Biofunctional membranes IV. Active site structure and stability of an immobilized enzyme, papain, on modified polysulfone membranes studied by electron paramagnetic resonance and kinetics, *J. Membrane Sci.* **91,** 47–64.

71. Butterfield, D. A. and Lee, J. (1994) Active site structure and stability of the thiol protease, papain, studied by electron paramagnetic resonance employing a methanethiosulfonate spin label, *Arch. Biochem. Biophys.* **310,** 167–171.

72. Hensley, K. L. (1995) Magnetic Resonance Studies of Free Radical-Mediated Oxidative Stress in Brain: Relevance to Aging and Alzheimer's Disease and Other Neurological Disorders, Ph. D. Thesis, University of Kentucky.

73. Aksenov, M. Y., Aksenova, M. V., Butterfield, D. A., Hensley, K., Vigo-Pelfrey, C., and Carney, J. M. (1996) Glutamine synthetase-induced enhancement of Aβ(1-40) neurotoxicity accompanied by abrogation of fibril formation and amyloid β-peptide fragmentation, *J. Neurochem.* **66,** 2050–2056.

74. Oda, T., Wals, P., Osterburg, H., Johnson, S., Pasinetti, G., Morgan, T., Rozovsky, I., Stein, W. B., Synder, S., Holzman, T., Krafft, G., and Finch, C. (1995) Clusterin (apoJ) Alters the aggregation of amyloid β-peptide (Aβ1-42) and forms slowly sedimenting Aβ complexes that cause oxidative stress, *Exp. Neurol.* **136,** 22–31.

75. Smith-Swintosky, V. L., Zimmer, S., Fenton, J. W., and Mattson, M. P. (1995) Opposing actions of thrombin and protease nexin-1 on amyloid β-peptide toxicity and on accumulation of peroxides and calcium in hippocampal neurons, *J. Neurochem.* **65,** 1415–1418.

76. Tomiyama, T., Asano, S., Suwa, Y., Molia, T., Kataoka, K., Mori, H., and Endo, N. (1994) Rifampicin prevents the aggregation and neurotoxicity of amyloid β protein in vitro, *Biochem. Biophys. Res. Commun.* **204,** 76–83.

77. Goodman, Y. and Mattson, M. P. (1994) Staurosporine and K-252 compounds protect hippocampal neurons against amyloid β-peptide toxicity and oxidative injury, *Brain Res.* **650,** 170–174.

78. Goodman, Y. and Mattson, M. P. (1994) Secreted forms of β-amyloid precursor protein protect hippocampal neurons against amyloid β-peptide-induced oxidative injury, *Exp. Neurol.* **128,** 1–12.

79. Kumar, U., Dunlop, D. M., and Richardson, J. S. (1994) The acute neurotoxic effect of β-amyloid on mature cultures of rat hippocampal neurons is attenuated by the antioxidant U-78517F, *Intern. J. Neurosci.* **79,** 185–190.

80. Tomiyama, T., Shoji, A., Kataoka, K. I., Suwa, Y., Asano, S., Kaneko, H., and Endo, N. (1996) Inhibition of amyloid β-protein aggregation and neurotoxicity by rifampicin, *J. Biol. Chem.* **271,** 6839–6844.

81. Mason, R. P., Estermeier, J. D., Kelly, J. S., and Mason, P. E. (1996) Alzheimer's disease amyloid β-peptide 25-35 is localized in the membrane hydrocarbon core: X-ray diffraction analysis. *Biochem. Biophys. Res. Commun.* **222,** 78–82.

10

Inflammatory Pathways

Implications in Alzheimer's Disease

W. Sue T. Griffin, Jin G. Sheng, and Robert E. Mrak

1. INTRODUCTION

Alzheimer's disease (AD) is a dementing illness characterized clinically by global intellectual decline and pathologically by a profusion of microscopic brain lesions containing extracellular amyloid in a β-pleated sheet conformation (β-amyloid) associated with abnormal (dystrophic) neurites. These neuritic β-amyloid plaques are thought to originate as otherwise undistinguished deposits of amyloid protein—diffuse nonneuritic plaques. With condensation of this amyloid, accompanied by the appearance of dystrophic neurites, these amyloid deposits evolve into neuritic plaques containing both diffuse amyloid and β-amyloid (diffuse neuritic plaques). With further evolution, amyloid condenses into a central compact core of β-amyloid within the larger deposit of diffuse amyloid, yielding a dense core neuritic plaque. Continued condensation apparently is accompanied by a loss of associated diffuse amyloid as well as neuritic elements, yielding a dense core of β-amyloid. These dense core, nonneuritic plaques (sometimes referred to as burned-out plaques) are thought to represent an end stage of plaque evolution *(1)* (for schematic representation of plaque progression, please *see* Fig. 1A).

The pathophysiological mechanism driving this plaque progression (and presumably driving the clinical progression of the disease as well) has only recently begun to be investigated. It is now clear, however, that plaque-associated, activated glia—and the numerous inflammatory, trophic, and metabolic factors produced and secreted by them—are key mechanistic elements in this progression *(2,3)*. Each of the plaque types cited above (diffuse nonneuritic, diffuse neuritic, dense core neuritic, and dense core nonneuritic) has a distinct and characteristic profile of associated activated glia (microglia and astrocytes) *(4,5)*. These glia show a distinct topographical relationship to the amyloid deposits, a pattern of waxing and then waning numbers through the hypothesized sequence of plaque evolution, and a characteristic pattern of overexpression of glia-derived inflammatory neurotrophic and gliotrophic cytokines and other molecules potentially associated with the evolution of the plaques and of the disease (Fig. 1A). The complex interactions of these plaque-associated glial cells, their armamentarium of overexpressed cytokines and other molecules, and the known actions of these cytokines and molecules bear sufficient parallels to chronic, focal inflammatory pro-

From: Molecular Mechanisms of Dementia Edited by: W. Wasco and R. E. Tanzi Humana Press Inc., Totowa, NJ

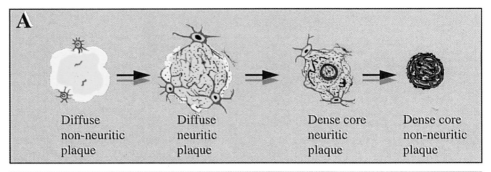

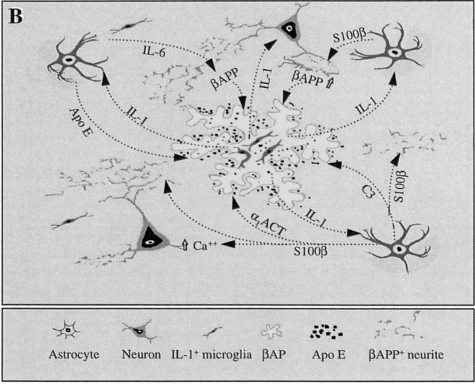

Fig. 1. Diagrammatic representation of proposed cellular and molecular events of plaque evolution. **(A)** Diagram of proposed evolutionary sequence of plaque types. The light yellow denotes diffuse amyloid, dark yellow denotes condensed β-amyloid, and dark brown denotes a dense β-amyloid core. **(B)** Pathogenic molecular interactions in a diffuse neuritic plaque. ACT, α₁-antichymotrypsin *(49)*; βAP, β-amyloid protein; βAPP, β-amyloid precursor protein; Apo E, apolipoprotein E; C3, complement protein C3 *(50)*; IL-1, interleukin-1; and IL-6, interleukin-6.

cesses found outside of the nervous system to suggest that the basic driving pathophysiological mechanism in AD is fundamentally an inflammatory one. In this chapter, we review the involvement of these glia and their actions in the evolution of the amyloid lesions in, and thus the clinical progression of, AD.

1. MICROGLIA AND INTERLEUKIN-1 (IL-1) IN PLAQUE EVOLUTION

Within the central nervous system, microglia are a resident population of cells that function much as monocytes and macrophages do in the periphery. They elaborate, among other factors, IL-1 *(6)*, a potent neurotrophic *(7)* and gliotrophic *(8)* cytokine. Their status as intrinsic CNS inflammatory cells is now well established *(9)*. Microglia overexpressing IL-1 are present, in small numbers, in more than 75% of the diffuse nonneuritic amyloid deposits of AD, the deposits thought to represent the earliest stages of plaque evolution and, thus, of disease progression *(4)*. With the appearance of neuritic elements (and therefore evolution of the amyloid deposit into a diffuse neuritic plaque), these plaque-associated microglia become further enlarged, more numerous, and contain more IL-1. With further amyloid condensation (forming a dense core neuritic plaque), this microglial response wanes, and it vanishes altogether in the end-stage dense-core, nonneuritic plaque.

IL-1 has several known functions relevant to plaque progression in AD. For instance, IL-1 upregulates expression of the β-amyloid precursor protein *(10,11)* (βAPP) through stimulation of the βAPP promoter *(12)* and also stimulates βAPP processing *(13)*. IL-1 has autocrine effects on microglia, including promotion of microglial proliferation in mixed neural cell cultures *(14)* and upregulation of microglial expression of IL-6, TNF-α, and of IL-1 itself *(15,16)*. IL-1 also has trophic effects on astrocytes, which are also integral components of the plaques of AD and participants in their evolution. In particular, IL-1 activates astrocytes *(8,17)* and upregulates astrocytic expression of NGF *(18)* and cytokines, including the neurite extension promoting factor S100β *(19)*. IL-1 may thus be responsible for many of the astrocytic actions and reactions that may contribute to the evolution of amyloid plaques in AD.

2. ASTROCYTES AND S100β IN PLAQUE EVOLUTION

Astrocytes have been slow to attract recognition as participants in inflammatory responses in the CNS, but it is now clear that they manifest many inflammatory-like actions *(20)*. In addition to their production of S100β, activated astrocytes express adhesion molecules and antigen presenting capabilities, including major histocompatibility complex antigens (for review *see* ref. *20*). IL-1-stimulated astrocytes also produce several proteins that accumulate in the β-amyloid deposits in AD, including α_1-antichymotrypsin *(21,22)*, the complement protein C3 *(23)*, and apolipoprotein E *(22)*. Activated astrocytes, overexpressing S100β, are near-constant components of amyloid-containing plaques in AD *(24,25)*, and their distribution and state of activation parallel that of microglia *(5)*. Like microglia, they are found in small numbers in most diffuse nonneuritic amyloid deposits, and are numerous and activated in diffuse neuritic plaques. Their numbers decrease in those neuritic plaques with dense cores, and they are only occasionally found in association with dense core nonneuritic plaques. Unlike microglia, plaque-associated astrocyte somas are found at the periphery of the plaque complex, forming an astrocytic shell encircling the neuritic, microglial, and proteinaceous deposit components of the plaque. In neuritic plaques, processes from these astrocytes infiltrate the interior of the plaque *(24)*.

Temporal lobe tissue from patients with AD contains elevated levels of biologically active S100β, and this S100β is immunohistochemically demonstrable in plaque-associated activated astrocytes and their processes *(5,24,25)*. S100β is now recognized as a secreted biological effector with autocrine and paracrine effects on glia and neurons *(26–28)*. Importantly for the evolution of amyloid deposits into neuritic β-amyloid plaques, S100β promotes the outgrowth of neurites *(29)*. Furthermore, S100β increases intracellular calcium concentration *(27)* and, in this way, may contribute to neuronal cell death in AD, a key event in promoting further inflammatory responses that include activation of microglia and astrocytes with the result being further overexpression of IL-1 and of S100β. This provides a mechanism for feedback amplification of this entire process and may thus explain the propagation of pathological changes in AD.

3. THE CYTOKINE CYCLE: A PATHOGENIC MECHANISM FOR PROPAGATION OF NEURODEGENERATION IN AD

These considerations suggest that a cascade or cycle of microglial activation with overexpression of IL-1, astrocyte activation with overexpression of S100β, neuronal cell injury and death, and consequent further overexpression of IL-1 and S100β is central to the evolution of amyloid deposits into the pathognomonic neuritic β-amyloid plaques of AD *(4,5)*. Based on the known functions of IL-1 and S100β and other pertinent molecules, a diagram of proposed cellular and molecular pathogenic interactions in diagnostic neuritic plaques is presented in Fig. 1B. In this scenario, a number of intrinsic or extrinsic factors, alone or in combination, lead to microglial activation with increased IL-1 expression. This, in turn, results in astrocyte activation, with upregulation of S100β expression, with consequent focal and inappropriate growth of neurites, and with increases in neuronal intracellular calcium levels and ultimately neuronal cell dysfunction and loss. Increased IL-1 levels would also, simultaneously, induce excessive synthesis and processing of βAPP, thus increasing the levels of both amyloidogenic βAPP fragments (favoring amyloid deposition) and neurotrophic βAPP fragments (contributing to further inappropriate growth of neurites).

The neuronal cell dysfunction or death resulting from these effects (i.e., the stress resulting from either elevated intracellular levels of calcium or abnormal growth of neurites), alone or in concert with β-amyloid activation of complement *(30)*, could then propagate such a cytokine-mediated cycle through further induction of glial activation with further cytokine elaboration. The elements of such a cytokine cycle, if operative in AD, should be evident early in the course of the disease and should also be evident in those conditions that increase the risk for later development of AD. Indeed, glial-based inflammatory pathways may be a common denominator of many diseases characterized by astrocyte and microglial activation (gliosis) and neuronal cell degeneration and loss. This proposed pathogenic cytokine cycle may thus be a generalizable concept in which glia-mediated inflammatory pathways drive a progressive downward spiral with continued neuron loss and neurological decline.

4. INFLAMMATORY PATHWAYS AND RISK FACTORS FOR AD

A number of conditions are known to be predisposing risk factors for AD. We have evidence for initiation of glia-mediated inflammatory pathways in several of these, including Down's syndrome, head trauma, and normal aging.

Patients with Down's syndrome (trisomy 21) inevitably show Alzheimer-like neuropathological changes at relatively early ages (the fourth and fifth decades) *(31)*.

Overexpression of IL-1, βAPP, and S100β is present in newborns and even fetuses with Down's syndrome *(2,32)*. Part of this overexpression may be attributable to gene triplication, since the gene encoding S100β *(33)*, like that of βAPP *(34,35)*, has been mapped to chromosome 21. However, the genes encoding the two isoforms of IL-1 do not map to chromosome 21, but rather to chromosome 2 *(36)*. This suggests some indirect effect (possibly involving a chromosome 21-encoded regulatory protein) of trisomy 21 on IL-1 expression.

Alzheimer patients more frequently have a history of head trauma than do aged patients without AD *(37–39)*. Following acute head trauma, there are diffuse cerebral increases in neuronal expression of βAPP *(40)* and microglial activation with overexpression of IL-1 *(41)*. Indeed, plaque-like associations of neuritic βAPP overexpression with activated microglia, overexpressing IL-1, can be found acutely following head trauma in patients as young as 11 yr of age *(41)*. This suggests that head trauma might prime basic inflammatory pathways that, with the passage of time and possibly additional insults, might predispose to the later development of AD.

In normal brain, aging is accompanied by various wear and tear processes and, presumably, associated reparative events. For instance, perhaps in response to wear and tear, there is increasing microglial activation with normal aging in monkeys *(42)*. In humans there is increasing astrocyte activation with normal aging accompanied by a progressive increase in S100β protein and mRNA expression *(43)*. S100β, because of its neurotrophic functions, has been implicated in repair responses to acute head injury *(44)*. Our results suggest that increased S100β expression with normal aging is a physiological response to normal wear and tear. This increased expression, however, might have the adverse effect of increasing one's susceptibility to pathological conditions, such as AD, that are driven in part by microglial and astrocytic activation and S100β overexpression.

In addition to these recognized risk factors for AD, it was recently shown that resected temporal lobe tissue from patients with intractable temporal lobe epilepsy has an increased incidence of Alzheimer-like neuritic plaques when compared with age-matched nondemented, nonepileptic autopsy controls *(45)*. This suggested "a direct influence of epileptic activity on [neuritic plaque] formation through some metabolic means" *(45)*. We have found overexpression of S100β, IL-1, and βAPP *(46,47)* in temporal lobe tissue resected from patients with intractable temporal lobe epilepsy. These findings, together with the known functions of these molecules and their proposed involvement in neuritic plaque evolution, provide a mechanism by which neuronal dysfunctions (e.g., those in epilepsy) may promote diffuse amyloid deposition and promote subsequent neuritic plaque formation.

5. THERAPEUTIC IMPLICATIONS

AD has traditionally been viewed as a degeneration of neurons. Previous therapeutic strategies have, therefore, concentrated on pharmacological replacement of lost neuronal function, using as a model L-dopa treatment for Parkinson's disease. The recognition of an inflammatory component in AD offers novel avenues for therapeutic intervention. Furthermore, the finding that inflammatory cytokine pathways are invoked early in predisposing conditions *(2,41)* suggests that therapeutic intervention might delay or even prevent the onset of AD in at-risk patients. Indeed, among siblings at high risk for AD, sustained use of nonsteroidal anti-inflammatory drugs is associated with delayed onset and reduced risk of AD *(48)*. Further elucidation of the molecular steps in inflammatory cytokine pathways involved in AD may provide substrates for development of additional novel therapeutic strategies.

ACKNOWLEDGMENTS

This work was supported in part by NIH AG 10208, AG 12411, and NS 27414. The authors appreciate the secretarial support of P. Free.

REFERENCES

1. Rozemuller, J. M., Eikelenboom, P., Stam, F. C., Beyreuther, K., and Masters, C. L. (1989) A4 protein in Alzheimer's disease: primary and secondary cellular events in extracellular amyloid deposition, *J. Neuropathol. Exp. Neurol.* **48,** 674–691.
2. Griffin, W. S. T., Stanley, L. C., Ling, C., White, L., Macleod, V., Perrot, L. J., White, C. L., III, and Araoz, C. (1989) Brain interleukin 1 and S–100 immunoreactivity are elevated in Down syndrome and Alzheimer disease, *Proc. Natl. Acad. Sci. USA.* **86,** 7611–7615.
3. Rozemuller, J. M., Stam, F. C., and Eikelenboom, P. (1990) Acute phase proteins are present in amorphous plaques in the cerebral but not cerebellar cortex of patients with Alzheimer's disease, *Neurosci. Lett.* **119,** 75–78.
4. Griffin, W. S. T., Sheng, J. G., Roberts, G. W., and Mrak, R. E. (1995) Interleukin–1 expression in different plaque types in Alzheimer's disease, *J. Neuropathol. Exp. Neurol.* **54,** 276–281.
5. Mrak, R. E., Sheng, J. G., and Griffin, W. S. T. (1996) Correlation of astrocytic S100β expression with dystrophic neurites in amyloid plaques of Alzheimer's disease, *J. Neuropathol. Exp. Neurol.* **55,** 273–279.
6. Righi, M., Mori, L., De Libero, G., Sironi, M., Biondi, A., Mantovani, A., Donini, S. D., and Ricciardi-Castagonoli, P. (1989) Monokine production by microglial cell clones, *Eur. J. Immunol.* **19,** 1443–1448.
7. Brenneman, D. E., Schultzberg, M., Bartfai, T., and Gozes, I. (1992) Cytokine regulation of neuronal survival, *J. Neurochem.* **58,** 454–460.
8. Giulian, D. and Lachman, L. B. (1985) Interleukin-1 stimulation of astroglial proliferation after brain injury, *Science* **228,** 497–499.
9. Thomas, W. E. (1992) Brain macrophages: evaluation of microglia and their functions, *Brain Res. Rev.* **17,** 61–74.
10. Goldgaber, D., Harris, H. W., Hla, T., Maciag, T., Donnelly, R. G., Jacobsen, J. S., Vitek, M. P., and Gajdusek, D. C. (1989) Interleukin 1 regulates synthesis of amyloid beta-protein precursor mRNA in human endothelial cells, *Proc. Natl. Acad. Sci. USA* **86,** 7606–7610.
11. Forloni, G., Demicheli, F., Giorgi, S., Bendotti, C., and Angeretti, N. (1992) Expression of amyloid precursor protein mRNAs in endothelial, neuronal and glial cells: modulation by interleukin-1, *Brain Res. Mol. Brain Res.* **16,** 128–134.
12. Donnelly, R. J., Freidhoff, A. J., Beer, B., Blume, A. J., and Vitek, M. P. (1990) Interleukin-1 stimulates the beta-amyloid precursor protein promoter, *Cell. Mol. Neurobiol.* **10,** 485–495.
13. Buxbaum, J. D., Oishi, M., Chen, H. I., Pinkas-Kramarski, R., Jaffe, E. A., Gandy, S. E., and Greengard, P. (1992) Cholinergic agonists and interleukin 1 regulate processing and secretion of the Alzheimer/A4 amyloid protein precursor, *Proc. Natl. Acad. Sci. USA.* **89,** 10,075–10,078.
14. Ganter, S., Northoff, H., Mannel, D., and Gebicke-Harter, P. J. (1992) Growth control of cultured microglia, *J. Neurosci. Res.* **33,** 218–230.
15. Sebire, G., Emilie, D., Wallon, C., Hery, C., Devergne, O., Delfraissy, J. F., Galanaud, P., and Tardieu, M. (1993) In vitro production of IL-6, IL-1 beta, and tumor necrosis factor-alpha by human embryonic microglial and neural cells, *J. Immunol.* **150,** 1517–1523.

16. Lee, S. C., Liu, W., Dickson, D. W., Brosnan, C. F., and Berman, J. W. (1993) Cytokine production by human fetal microglia and astrocytes. Differential induction by lipopolysaccharide and IL-1 beta, *J. Immunol.* **150**, 2659–2667.

17. Giulian, D., Woodward, J., Young, D. G., Krebs, J. F., and Lachman, L. B. (1988) Interleukin-1 injected into mammalian brain stimulates astrogliosis and neovascularization, *J. Neurosci.* **8**, 2485–2490.

18. Berkenbosch, F., Robakin, N., and Blum, M. (1991) Interleukin–1 in the central nervous system: a role in the acute phase response and in brain injury, brain development and the pathogenesis of Alzheimer's disease, in *Peripheral Signaling of the Brain. Role in Neural-Immune Interactions, Learning and Memory* (Frederickson, R. C. A., McGaugh, J. L., and Felten, D. L., eds.), Hogrefe and Huber, Toronto, pp. 131–145.

19. Sheng, J. G., Ito, K., Skinner, R. D., Mrak, R. E., Rovnaghi, C. R., Van Eldik, L. J., and Griffin, W. S. T. (1996) In vivo and in vitro evidence supporting a role for the inflammatory cytokine interleukin-1 as a driving force in Alzheimer pathogenesis, *Neurobiol. Aging* in press.

20. Frohman, E. M., van den Noort, S., and Gupta, S. (1989) Astrocytes and intracerebral immune responses, *J. Clin. Immunol.* **9**, 1–9.

21. Perlmutter, D. H., Dinarello, C. A., Punsal, P. I., and Colten, H. R. (1986) Cachectin/tumor necrosis factor regulates hepatic acute-phase gene expression, *J. Clin. Invest.* **78**, 1349–1354.

22. Das, S., Geller, L., Niethammer, M., and Potter, H. (1994) Expression of the Alzheimer amyloid-promoting factors α_1-antichymotrypsin and apolipoprotein E is induced in astrocytes by IL–1, *Neurobiol. Aging* **15**, S17.

23. Rus, H. G., Kim, L. M., Niculescu, F. I., and Shin, M. L. (1992) Induction of C3 expression in astrocytes is regulated by cytokines and Newcastle disease virus, *J. Immunol.* **148**, 928–933.

24. Marshak, D. R., Pesce, S. A., Stanley, L. C., and Griffin, W. S. T. (1992) Increased S100β neurotrophic activity in Alzheimer disease temporal lobe, *Neurobiol. Aging* **13**, 1–7.

25. Sheng, J. G., Mrak, R. E., and Griffin, W. S. T. (1994) S100β protein expression in Alzheimer's disease: potential role in the pathogenesis of neuritic plaques, *J. Neurosci. Res.* **39**, 398–404.

26. Marshak, D. R. (1990) S100β as a neurotrophic factor, *Prog. Brain Res.* **86**, 169–181.

27. Barger, S. W. and Van Eldik, L. J. (1992) S100β stimulates calcium fluxes in glial and neuronal cells, *J. Biol. Chem.* **267**, 9689–9694.

28. Selinfreund, R. H., Barger, S. W., Pledger, W. J., and Van Eldik, L. J. (1991) Neurotrophic protein S100β stimulates glial cell proliferation, *Proc. Natl. Acad. Sci. USA.* **88**, 3554–3558.

29. Kligman, D. and Marshak, D. R. (1985) Purification and characterization of a neurite extension factor from bovine brain, *Proc. Natl. Acad. Sci. USA* **82**, 7136–7139.

30. Rogers, J., Cooper, N. R., Webster, S., Schultz, J., McGeer, P. L., Styren, S. D., Civin, W. H., Brachova, L., Bradt, B., and Ward, P. (1992) Complement activation by beta-amyloid in Alzheimer disease, *Proc. Natl. Acad. Sci. USA.* **89**, 10,016–10,020.

31. Wisniewski, K. E., Wisniewski, H. M., and Wen, G. Y. (1985) Occurrence of neuropathological changes and dementia of Alzheimer's disease in Down's syndrome, *Ann. Neurol.* **17**, 278–282.

32. Baggott, P. J., Sheng, J. G., Cork, L., Del Biggio, M. R., Brumback, R., Roberts, G. W., Mrak, R. E., and Griffin, W. S. T. (1993) Expression of Alzheimer's disease (AD)-related proteins during development in Down's syndrome (DS), *Soc. Neurosci. Abstract* **19 (part 1)**, 182.

33. Allore, R., O'Hanlon, D., Price, R., Neilson, K., Willard, H. F., Cox, D. R., Marks, A., and Dunn, R. J. (1988) Gene encoding the β subunit of S100 protein is on chromosome 21: implications for Down syndrome, *Science* **239**, 1311–1313.

34. Tanzi, R. E., Gusella, J. F., Watkins, P. C., Bruns, G. A., St. George-Hyslop, P., Van Keuren, M. L., Patterson, D., Pagan, S., Kurnit, D. M., and Neve, R. L. (1987) Amyloid β protein gene: cDNA, mRNA distribution, and genetic linkage near the Alzheimer locus, *Science* **235**, 880–884.

35. Goldgaber, D., Lerman, M. L., McBride, W. O., Saffiotti, U., and Gajdusek, D. C. (1987) Isolation, characterization, and chromosomal localization of human brain cDNA clones coding for the precursor of the amyloid of brain in Alzheimer's disease, Down's syndrome and aging, *J. Neural Transm.* **24(Suppl.),** 23–28.

36. Boultwood, J., Breckon, G., Birch, D., and Cox, R. (1989) Chromosomal localization of murine interleukin–1 alpha and beta genes, *Genomics* **5,** 481–485.

37. Gautrin, D. and Gauthier, S. (1989) Alzheimer's disease: environmental factors and etiologic hypotheses, *Can. J. Neurol. Sci.* **16,** 375–387.

38. Graves, A. B., White, E., Koepsell, T. D., Reifler, B. V., van Belle, G., Larson, E. B., and Raskind, M. (1990) The association between head trauma and Alzheimer's disease, *Am. J. Epidemiol.* **131,** 491–501.

39. Mayeux, R., Ottman, R., Tang, M. X., Noboa-Bauza, L., Marder, K., Gurland, B., and Stern, Y. (1993) Genetic susceptibility and head injury as risk factors for Alzheimer's disease among community-dwelling elderly persons and their first-degree relatives, *Ann. Neurol.* **33,** 494–501.

40. Gentleman, S. M., Nash, M. J., Sweeting, C. J., Graham, D. I., and Roberts, G. W. (1993) β-amyloid precursor protein (β-APP) as a marker for axonal injury after head injury, *Neurosci. Lett.* **160,** 139–144.

41. Griffin, W. S. T., Sheng, J. G., Gentleman, S. M., Graham, D. I., Mrak, R. E., and Roberts, G. W. (1995) Microglial interleukin-1α expression in human head injury: correlations with neuronal and neuritic β-amyloid precursor protein expression, *Neurosci. Lett.* **176,** 133–136.

42. Sheffield, L. G., Purcell, J. A., and Berman, N. E. J. (1995) Microglial activation in monkeys increases with age, *Soc. Neurosci. Abstract* **21 (part 1),** 470.

43. Sheng, J. G., Mrak, R. E., Rovnaghi, C. R., Kozlowska, E., Van Eldik, L. J., and Griffin, W. S. T. (1996) Human brain S100β and S100β mRNA expression increases with age: pathogenic implications for Alzheimer's disease, *Neurobiol. Aging* **17,** 359–363.

44. Kato, K., Suzuki, F., Morishita, R., Asano, T., and Sato, T. (1990) Selective increase in S-100β protein by aging in rat cerebral cortex, *J. Neurochem.* **54,** 1269–1274.

45. Mackenzie, I. R. A. and Miller, L. A. (1994) Senile plaques in temporal lobe epilepsy, *Acta Neuropathol.* **87,** 504–510.

46. Sheng, J. G., Boop, F. A., Mrak, R. E., and Griffin, W. S. T. (1994) Increased neuronal beta-amyloid precursor protein expression in human temporal lobe epilepsy: association with interleukin-1 alpha immunoreactivity, *J. Neurochem.* **63,** 1872–1879.

47. Griffin, W. S. T., Yeralan, O., Sheng, J. G., Boop, F. A., Mrak, R. E., Rovnaghi, C. R., Burnett, B. A., Feoktistova, A., and Van Eldik, L. J. (1995) Overexpression of the neurotrophic cytokine S100β in human temporal lobe epilepsy, *J. Neurochem.* **65,** 228–233.

48. Breitner, J. C. S., Welsh, K. A., Helms, M. J., Gaskell, P. C., Gau, B. A., Roses, A. D., Pericak-Vance, M. A., and Saunders, A. M. (1995) Delayed onset of Alzheimer's disease with non-steroidal anti-inflammatory and histamine H2 blocking drugs, *Neurobiol. Aging* **16,** 523–530.

49. Pasternack, J. M., Abraham, C. R., Van Dijcke, B. J., Potter, H., and Younkin, S. G. (1989) Astrocytes in Alzheimer's disease grey matter express alpha1-antichymotrypsin mRNA, *Am. J. Pathol.* **135,** 827–834.

50. Levi-Strauss, M. and Mallat, M. (1987) Primary cultures of murine astrocytes produce C3 and factor B, two components of the alternative pathway of complement activation, *J. Immunol.* **139,** 2361–2366.

11

Inflammatory Mediators in Alzheimer's Disease

Joseph Rogers and Stephen O'Barr

In 1984, when our laboratory first began conducting research on inflammation and Alzheimer's disease (AD) *(1)*, the brain was still widely considered to be immunologically privileged (reviewed in ref. *2*). Now, a virtual textbook of inflammatory mediators have been shown to be present in the central nervous system (CNS) or expressed by CNS cells in culture (Table 1). Most of these molecules are known to be increased in expression in AD limbic and neocortex compared to similar samples from nondemented elderly (ND) patients. By understanding the functions of inflammatory mediators in general, and their interactions with AD pathology in particular, a better appreciation of their pathogenic potential may be fostered.

1. MAJOR HISTOCOMPATIBILITY COMPLEX (MHC)

MHC type I and type II cell-surface glycoproteins are profusely expressed by AD microglia (Table 1), especially in gray matter and in the context of cross-β-pleated amyloid β peptide (Aβ) deposits. Although expression of the MHC is generally taken to connote antigen-presenting capability, such a function is not well established for AD microglia. B-lymphocytes, antibody-producing cells, are not evident in AD brain, nor is there, as yet, unequivocal evidence for any brain-specific autoantibody production in AD *(112)*. Thus, MHC expression by AD microglia is more likely an index of the high reactivity of this cell type, the brain's resident tissue phagocyte *(3,9,11)*, particularly in the context of innate immune responses. In this non-Ig-mediated context, activated microglia can bring to bear numerous destructive mechanisms, including the respiratory burst *(81)*, secretion of inflammatory mediators, such as cytokines *(34,46,109)*, and direct phagocytosis of opsonized targets *(34)*.

2. ACUTE-PHASE REACTANTS

Many of the acute-phase reactants have been found to be upregulated in the AD brain (Table 1). These molecules play multiple roles in conventional inflammatory responses, from initiating to halting them, and may have additional significance in AD through unique interactions with AD pathology. For example, both α1-antichymotrypsin and serum amyloid P bind Aβ and may alter its propensity to aggregate into the more toxic cross-β-pleated configuration *(113–116)*. As will be seen, this ability to interact with AD through both conventional and AD-idiosyncratic mechanisms is a common theme for many inflammatory mediators that are upregulated in AD.

From: Molecular Mechanisms of Dementia *Edited by: W. Wasco and R. E. Tanzi Humana Press Inc., Totowa, NJ*

Table 1
Inflammatory Markers in Brain

Marker	Ref.	Method	Δ in AD	Comments
MHC I				
	3	IHC	↑	Microglia
	4	IHC	↔	Microglia
MHC II				
HLA-DR	*5*	IHC	↑	Microglia
	6	IHC	↑	Microglia
	7	IHC	↑	Microglia
	8	IHC	↑	2–3X in microglia
	4	IHC	↑	Microglia
	9	IHC	↑	12X in microglia
	10	IHC	↑	Microglia
	1	IHC	↑	Astrocytes, microglia
	11	WB/IHC/EM	↑	Microglia
HLA-DP	*7*	IHC	↑	Microglia
HLA-DQ	*7*	IHC	↑	Microglia
Acute-Phase Reactants				
α1-Antichymotrypsin	*12*	IHC/WB	↑	Glia
	13	IHC	↑	Only in grey matter astrocytes
	14	IHC	↑	Tangles, plaques
	15	IHC	↑	Hippocampus
	16	IHC	↑	Plaque cores; not seen in vascular amyloid
	17	ELISA	↑	Serum
	18	ELISA	↑	CSF and serum
	19	Immunodiffuse	↑	1.5X in serum
	15	IHC	↔	Cerebral cortex
	20	NB		Human microglial cultures (↑ with dexamethasone)
α2-Macroglobulin	*21*	IHC	↑	2–6X in neocortex
	21	IHC	↑	1–2X in hippocampus
	22	IHC	↑	Only in neuritic plaques
	23	ELISA	↑	2X
	24	WB/IHC		Rat primary astrocyte cultures
Serum amyloid P	*25*	IHC/WB	↑	Plaques
	26	IHC	↑	Plaques, tangles, vasculature
	27	IHC	↑	Tangles
	28	IHC	↑	Plaques
α1-antitrypsin	*14*	IHC	↑	Plaques, tangles
	29	IHC	↑	Plaques
C-reactive protein	*30*	IHC	↑	Plaques
	23	ELISA	↑	3X
	31	IHC	↑	0.3–1.5X in neocortex and hippocampus

continued

Table 1
Inflammatory Markers in Brain (*continued*)

Cytokines				
IL-1α	*32*	IHC	↑	Microglia
	33	IHC	↑	Microglia
	34	ELISA		Human microglia cultures (↑ with LPS/Aβ)
	35	NB		Rat astrocyte cultures (↑ with LPS)
IL-1β	*36*	ELISA	↑	3.7X
	23	ELISA	↔	
	37	ELISA		Human astrocyte cultures (↑ with LPS)
IL-3	*34*	PCR	↑	Microglia
	38	ELISA		Astrocyte/microglia cultures (↑ with LPS)
IL-5	*39*	ELISA/NB		Mouse astrocytes
IL-6	*21*	IHC	↑	Plaques
	40	ELISA	↑	1.5X
	34	PCR	↑	Microglia
	23	ELISA		50 fg/mg in AD; not determined in ND
	41	ELISA		2.8X in culture with LPS
IL-8	*41*	ELISA		Increase with LPS
GMCSF	*41*	Bioassay		Increase with LPS
TNF-α	*42*	ELISA	↑	10X in serum
	43	ELISA	↑	4X in serum
	44	IHC		PD glia (↑ compared to control)
	45	ELISA		PD (↑ 3.7X compared to control)
	46	PCR		Human glial cultures (↑ 2–3X with measles virus)
	37	ELISA		Human astrocyte cultures (↑ with LPS)
CSF-1	*41*	ELISA		Human astrocyte cultures (↑ with LPS)
TGF-α	*47*	ELISA		PD (↑ 2X compared to control)
TGF-β1	*48*	ELISA		PD CSF and serum
	49	ELISA		PD (↑ 2X in brain and CSF compared to control)
MoAP	*50*	NB/ELISA		Fetal astrocyte cultures (↑ 4.4X with TGFβ or TNF-α)
MIP-1α	*51*			Mouse astrocyte cultures (↑ 20X with LPS, ↔ with IL-1β, TNF-α)
Complement proteins				
C1q	*52*	WB	↑	3.6X in superior frontal gyrus
	53	IHC	↑	Plaques

continued

Table 1
Inflammatory Markers in Brain *(continued)*

	5	IHC	↑	Plaques
	54	IHC	↑	Plaques
	55	IHC	↑	Plaques
	56	IHC	↑	Plaques
	57	IHC	↑	Plaques
	4	IHC	↑	Plaques
	58	IHC	↑	Plaques
	59	IHC	↑	Plaques
C4	54	IHC	↑	Plaques
	55	IHC	↑	Plaques
	56	IHC	↑	Plaques
	59	IHC	↑	Plaques
C4d	60	IHC	↑	Plaques
	57	IHC	↑	Plaques
	4	IHC	↑	Plaques
	58	IHC	↑	Plaques
C3	5	IHC	↑	Plaques
	55	IHC	↑	Plaques
	56	IHC	↑	Plaques
	59	IHC	↑	Plaques
	61	IHC	↑	Microglia
	53	IHC		
	54	IHC		
	62	WB		Mouse microglia cultures (↑ with LPS)
C3b	54	IHC	↑	Plaques
C3c	53	IHC	↑	Plaques
	54	IHC	↑	Plaques
	4	IHC	↑	Plaques
C3d	53	IHC	↑	Plaques
	54	IHC	↑	Plaques
	57	IHC	↑	Plaques
	4	IHC	↑	Plaques
C7	4	IHC	↑	Plaques
	59	IHC		
C9	4	IHC	↑	Plaques
	59	IHC		
C5b-9	63	IHC/EM	↑	Tangles, neurons
	57	IHC	↑	Tangles
	4	IHC	↑	Plaques
	64	IHC	↑	Plaques
	58	IHC	↑	Plaques
	65	EM	↑	Myelinated and unmyelinated neurons (endocytotic vesicles)
	59	IHC		

continued

Table 1
Inflammatory Markers in Brain *(continued)*

Complement mRNAs				
C1q	66	*In situ* hybrid	↑	2.5X
	67	PCR	↑	
	68	NB	↑	3.5X
	69	NB		Human microglia cultures (↑ with LPS)
C4	66	*In situ* hybrid	↑	3.0X
	67	PCR	↑	3.27X
	34	NB		Human microglia cultures (↑ with LPS)
C3	68	NB	↔	
	67	PCR	↑	3.01X
	70	NB		Human glial cultures (↑ with IL-1β, TNF-α)
	34	PCR		Microglia cultures (↑ with LPS)
Complement defense proteins				
Protectin (CD59)	64	IHC	↑	Plaques
	71	IHC	↑	Tangles
Clusterin (APOJ)	72	IHC	↑	Plaques, CSF
	73	NB	↑	2X in hippocampus
	64	IHC	↑	Plaques
Vitronectin (S-protein)	74	IP/IHC	↑	Reactive microglia
C4BP	27	IHC	↑	Plaques
	75	IHC/WB	↑	
C1-INH	53	IHC	↑	Plaques
	76	IHC/PCR/WB	↑	Plaques
Complement defense protein mRNAs				
Protectin (CDS9)	71	PCR	↑	
Clusterin	73	NB	↑	2X in hippocampus
C1-INH	77	PCR	↑	Plaques
Eicosanoids				
Prostaglandin D2	78	Bioassay	↓	Frontal cortex
	79	Bioassay		Rat cortex endothelium (↑ with IL-1, IL-6)
	80	HPLC		Rat microglia
Leukotriene C4	80	HPLC		Rat microglia
Reactive oxygen intermediates				
Superoxide ions	81	Bioassay		Rat microglia cultures (↑ 2X with PMA, IFN-γ, Aβ)
Nitric oxide	82	Bioassay		Rat brain cultures (↑ with arginine)
Thrombin and plasmin systems				
Thrombin	83	IHC	↑	Plaques, tangles
Thrombin receptor	84	IHC		Rat astrocytes and neurons
Antithrombin III	85	IHC/WB	↑	6X
Tissue factor	86	IHC	↑	Plaques

continued

Table 1
Inflammatory Markers in Brain (*continued*)

Hageman factor	87	WB/IHC	↑	Plaques
TPA	88	IHC	↑	Plaques
	88	IHC	↑	Plaques
	69			Brain cell culture (↑ with growth factor)
	89	WB		Rat microglia culture (↑ with IL-1, bFGF, ↓ with LPS)
PAI I	90	IHC		Astrocytes (↑ after axotomy)
PAI II	91	IHC	↑	reactive microglia
Protease nexin-1	92	IHC		
	93	WB	↓	7X
Protease nexin-1/ thrombin complex	93	WB	↑	
Plasminogen	94	IHC		Cultured microglia
Thrombin and plasmin system mRNAs				
Prothrombin	95	PCR		Human brain
	84	*In situ* hybrid		Rat neurons
Thrombin receptor	84	*In situ* hybrid		Rat astrocytes and neurons
Antithrombin III	85	NB	↑	6X
PAI I	90	NB	↔	
	96	*In situ* hybrid	↔	
Protease nexin-1	93	NB	↔	
Hageman factor	87	PCR	↔	
UPA	97	*In situ* hybrid		Rat brain
Adhesion molecules				
ICAM-1	5	IHC	↑	Plaques
	61	IHC	↑	Plaques
	98	IHC	↑	Plaques
	99	IHC	↑	Plaques
	100	Bioassay		Mouse astrocyte cultures (↑ 3.5X with INF-γ)
NCAM	101	WB/ELISA	↔	
LFA-1 (CD1 la)	102	IHC	↑	Microglia
	103	IHC		Rat brain (↑ with kianate)
VCAM-l	104	NB		Human astrocyte cultures (↑ with TNF-α, IFN-γ, IL-1β)
ICAM	103	IHC		Rat brain (↑ with kianate)
Cytokine receptors				
IL-1RA	23	ELISA	↔	
IL-2R	7	IHC	↑	Microglia
	105	IHC		PD microglia
CSFR-1	106	IHC	↑	Microglia
Cytokine receptor mRNAs				
IL-lR	107	NB		Rat astrocytes
IL-2R	108	NB		Human brain, rat astrocytes
	109	NB/PCR		Mouse microglia cultures (↑ with LPS)

continued

Table 1
Inflammatory Markers in Brain *(continued)*

Complement receptors				
CR3	*110*	IHC	↑	Plaques
	53	IHC	↑	Plaques
	61	IHC	↑	Plaques
CR4	*110*	IHC	↑	Microglia
	5	IHC	↑	Microglia
Other receptors				
CSF-1 receptor	*106*	IHC	↑	Microglia
FcγR1	*4*	IHC	↑	Microglia
	110	IHC	↑	Microglia
Other				
LCA	*4*	IHC	↑	Microglia
	102	IHC	↑	Microglia
	111	IHC	↑	Microglia

EM, electron microscopy; IP, immunoprecipitation; HPLC, high pressure liquid chromatography; TPA, tissue plasminogen activator; PAI, plasminogen activator inhibitor; UPA, urokinase plasminogen activator; LCA, leukocyte common antigen; IHC, immunohistochemistry; NB, Northern blot; WB, Western blot; PCR, polymerase chain reaction; ELISA, enzyme-linked immunoabsorption assay; ↑, increase in AD compared to ND; ↓, decrease in AD compared to ND; ↔, no significant or detectable difference between AD and ND; ↑, increase; ↓, decrease. Absence of a symbol in the "Δ in AD" column indicates experiments that did not apply to AD (e.g., rat cultures) or experiments wherein only presence of a marker was established.

3. CYTOKINES

Cytokines are autocrine and paracrine messengers of immune and inflammatory responses, amplifying, sustaining, and in some cases dampening them. Produced by glia (Table 1), those cytokines that have been identified as increased in expression in AD are proinflammatory, particularly interleukin- (IL-) 1, IL-6, and tumor necrosis factor-α (TNF-α). These latter three molecules are, in fact, the primary cytokine mediators of inflammation and tend to induce each other, so that their levels are most often correlated in various organs and under various conditions *(1,32,37,40)*.

Pathogenic mechanisms of the proinflammatory cytokines are well known, and include stimulation of increased acute-phase protein synthesis, vascular permeability, cell adhesion molecule expression, T- and B-cell activation, and colony-stimulating factor synthesis. TNF-α, which is reportedly upregulated not only in AD brain, but also in AD serum *(42,43)*, is particularly damaging to tissue and is a major pathogenic player in such inflammatory conditions as bacterial toxic shock and toxic shock syndrome *(117)*.

In addition to these conventional mechanisms, certain cytokines interact uniquely with AD pathology. IL-1β, for example, appears to influence amyloid precursor protein (APP) production *(118–121)*, potentially increasing secretion of Aβ. Aβ, in turn, may influence the synthesis of IL-1 and other cytokines *(36,120,122,156)*.

4. COMPLEMENT

Complement is a series of more than 20 proteins, many of them serine proteases, which interact to form two converging cascades. The classical pathway is invoked by the activation of Clq, which activates Clr and Cls, which in turn activate C4, C2, and

C3. The alternative pathway converges at the C3 step, with both pathways going on to C5 activation and formation of the membrane attack complex. The latter is made up of an activation fragment of C5, C5b, complexed with C6, C7, C8, and multiple C9 moieties, hence the designation C5b-9. The C5b-9 complex forms a ring-like structure that binds to cellular membranes, displaces membrane phospholipids, and opens a transmembrane channel permitting Ca^{2+} influx. If a sufficient number of C5b-9 complexes bind to a cell, it may be lysed. Notably, the membrane-binding step, which occurs when C7 is linked to C5b6, requires a membrane. If activation has occurred on a noncellular surface, the C5b67 complex is released and can bind to adjacent cells, resulting in the phenomenon of bystander lysis. As will be seen, this process most likely accounts for the colocalization of C5b-9 immunoreactivity with neuronal membranes in AD.

In addition to formation of the membrane attack complex, complement provides several other pathogenic mechanisms. The C4b, C3b, and C3bi activation fragments of C4 and C3, for example, can bind to cellular membranes to serve as opsonins. Tissue phagocytes that express receptors to the opsonins are thereby directed to the opsonized surface for attack. The anaphylotoxins, C4a, C3a, and C5a, are additional fragments that diffuse away from the activation site, broadening its scope and chemotactically signaling to inflammatory cells.

With the exception of the alternative pathway *(58)*, virtually all the complement proteins, activation fragments, and complement receptors described above have been reported in the AD brain (Table 1). In several cases, mRNAs for complement-related molecules have also been demonstrated (Table 1). These proteins and mRNAs are significantly increased in expression in AD compared to ND samples, and are often not detected in the latter. They colocalize precisely with sites of AD neurodegeneration: compacted (cross-β-pleated) Aβ deposits, neurofibrillary tangles, and neuropil threads (Table 1). Ultrastructural studies *(63,65)* show C5b-9 fixation on neurites coursing through compacted Aβ plaques. In some instances, these neurites can be observed to endocytose and bleb the complement that has bound to their membranes. This phenomenon, well documented to occur in the periphery, is especially important to note in AD, because it demonstrates that inflammation is doing more than removing the detritus of already existent AD damage. That is, detritus does not bleb or endocytose; living cells under complement attack do.

Where they have been assayed, distributions of complement proteins have followed patterns of AD vulnerability. Therefore, for example, the cerebellum is largely unaffected in AD and has some sevenfold less Clq than the severely impacted superior frontal gyrus from the same AD patients *(52)*. C5b-9 is not detectable in the AD cerebellum *(60)*, but is profuse in the AD limbic and frontal cortex *(11,57,58,63)*. Further, in a subset of six elderly patients presenting without history of dementia, but with sufficient entorhinal cortex plaques and tangles to otherwise qualify for the diagnosis of AD, C5b-9 immunoreactivity is slightly elevated above the undetectable levels observed in ND patients without AD pathology, but is 10-fold or more decreased compared to AD patients *(123)*.

In addition to the conventional means of complement assault, unique interactions between Clq and Aβ have been documented *(124–126)*. Clq binds Aβ at a 10 amino acid site located on the A chain of its collagen tail *(127)*. This site is the locus for antibody-independent Clq activation by several molecules, including C-reactive protein *(128)*, and is replicated six times per molecule because of the hexamer structure of Clq. The Aβ site for binding to Clq has not been as precisely defined, but is likely to reside somewhere between the 1st and 16th N-terminal amino acids of Aβ *(58)*. These binding sites and properties provide for two interactive mechanisms by which complement reactions may be uniquely sustained in AD. The first is suggested by calculations of the distances between adjacent Aβ-binding sites on Clq and their excellent fit with putative distances between Aβ residues in models of the Aβ cross-β-pleat *(124)*. By binding multiple Aβ molecules in close physical proximity to each other, the propensity of Aβ to aggregate into the cross-β-pleat configuration may be facilitated. Alternatively, Clq may simply stabilize or nucleate nascent chains of cross-β-pleated Aβ. Regardless of which mechanism is operative, in vitro studies show that Clq enhances Aβ aggregation by as much as an order of magnitude *(125,126)*. This enhancement is preserved at nanomolar concentrations of the reactants, whereas it tends to drop out for other molecules that have been reported to have a similar effect on Aβ aggregation, the "pathological chaperones" (e.g., α1-antichymotrypsin) *(113,126)*. In the presence of Clq, the resistance of aggregated Aβ to resolubilization (e.g., by dilution) is also increased *(125)*. These phenomena would be expected to enhance Aβ toxicity because the latter is correlated with increased Aβ aggregation *(129–131)*.

In addition to effects on Aβ, Clq/Aβ binding has potentially important effects on Clq as well. Clq is activated in an antibody-independent fashion *(58,127,128)*, leading to full activation of the classical pathway. This can be shown directly in vitro by incubating serum with Aβ and measuring production of C3b *(58)* or C5b-9, the terminal complement component *(123)*, or indirectly *in situ* by demonstrating highly colocalized immunoreactivity for each of the complement components, including C5b-9, in the proximity of aggregated Aβ deposits. Interestingly, the more aggregated the Aβ, the better activator of Clq it becomes *(123)*, providing yet another level of tandem interaction between these molecules. That is, Clq facilitates Aβ aggregation, and Aβ aggregation facilitates Clq activation.

The potency of complement activation by Aβ appears to compare favorably with that caused by other known antibody-independent activators, such as coat proteins of certain RNA tumor viruses *(132)*. It is almost certainly less than that provided by Ig, however, and this is wholly consistent with the chronic, progressive nature of AD: if Aβ were as potent a complement activator as Ig, then the inflammation resulting in the AD brain would probably be lethal in a matter of days. As it is, the presence of Aβ throughout the course of AD provides a modest, but chronic stimulus that may sustain inflammation at low, but consistent levels for a decade or more. Cumulated over such a time span, it is difficult to imagine that inflammation would not ultimately become a significant source of tissue damage to the AD brain.

Finally, it may be worth noting another potentially unique interaction of inflammation and other putative pathogenic processes in AD. C5b-9, as discussed earlier, essentially uses calcium dysregulation as a pathogenic mechanism. Such attack can be lethal to a cell or not, depending on the number of membrane attack complex molecules fixed at any given time to the cell's membrane. There may exist, therefore, the potential for synergistic interactions between complement fixation and other calcium dysregulatory mechanisms that have been proposed to occur in AD (cf *60*). To date, such interactions have apparently not been studied, but may warrant exploration in the future.

5. COMPLEMENT DEFENSE PROTEINS

Inactivation of complement occurs at several steps in the cascade by different regulators. The first is the glycoprotein C1-inhibitor (C1-INH), which inhibits C1qr2s2 complex formation by binding activated C1r2s2 and causing its disassociation from C1q. Since formation of the C1 complex is the primary step in classical complement-mediated cell lysis, its inhibition by C1-INH is crucial in stopping spontaneous complement activation before the cascade can amplify. Both C1-INH *(53,76)* and C1-INH mRNA *(76)* are upregulated in AD.

C3, the convergence point of the classical and alternative pathways, is regulated by several molecules collectively known as the regulators of complement activation (RCA). C4-binding protein (C4bp), for example, is a soluble RCA protein that binds C4, allowing it to be cleaved into two inert fragments. It is also increased in expression in AD *(27,75)*.

Formation of the membrane attack complex, C5b-9, is a further site for complement regulation. The secreted proteins vitronectin (S-protein) and clusterin (APOJ, SP40, 40) inactivate C5b-9 formation by binding C5b-7 and converting it from a hydrophobic to a hydrophilic complex. This hinders membrane attack complex insertion into the target membrane. Both proteins are elevated in AD *(64,73,74)*. Protectin (CD59, MIRL, HRF20) also binds C5b-7, but is associated with the external membrane surface where it may be mobile, actively targeting invading C5b-9 complexes *(133)*. This protein, too, is increased in AD *(71)* and increases Aβ aggregation *(134)*.

Elevated expression of the complement defense molecules in AD goes to the heart of the question of how functionally relevant AD inflammation may be. In the periphery, cells under and in the vicinity of complement attack secrete these proteins to protect themselves from both targeted and bystander lysis. Nature is not so wasteful as to upregulate complement defense molecules in the absence of a physiologically relevant attack. Therefore, as in the periphery, we take the AD increase in complement defense molecules (Table 1) as evidence of an ongoing and significant inflammatory attack on the tissue there. Moreover, as in the periphery, we should expect areas of complement defense to colocalize with areas of inflammatory attack, which in turn should colocalize with areas of degeneration. This is precisely the case. Complement defense proteins colocalize with markers off inflammation, which in turn colocalize with those brain regions known to be vulnerable in AD. Aβ deposits, neurofibrillary tangles, and neuropil threads are especially consistent loci for inflammatory mediators in general and complement defense proteins in particular. Finally, it has been said that inflammation may only exist in the AD brain to clear up the detritis of already existing damage from other causes. However, a dead cell, detritis, does not make complement defense proteins. Living cells threatened by pathogenic inflammatory mechanisms do.

6. ADHESION MOLECULES AND RECEPTORS

As part of the acute-phase inflammatory response, altered expression of the intercellular adhesion molecules ICAM-1 and VCAM-1 occurs. In AD brain, these adhesion molecules are produced by astrocytes associated with amyloid-rich plaques *(5,64,99,100)*. In astrocyte cultures, ICAM-1 and VCAM-1 expression is upregulated by TNF-α, interferon-γ (IFN-γ), and IL-1β *(43,104)*, cytokines that induce many localized and systemic changes observed in the acute-phase response and two of which, TNF-α and IL-1β, are known to be upregulated in AD *(36,42,43)*. Expression of LFA-1, the ICAM-1 receptor, is increased in AD microglia, providing another potential mechanism for microglial recruitment to inflammatory sites of Aβ deposition *(102)*.

7. COMPLEMENT, CYTOKINE, AND OTHER RECEPTORS

Complement, cytokine, and other receptors are upregulated in AD brain (Table 1). This is most often in the context of microglia, the brain's resident tissue phagocyte, and may subserve multiple pathogenic functions. Inflammatory chemoattractant signaling, for example, is likely to account for the clustering of microglia at sites of AD pathology, such as aggregated Aβ deposits. This follows because Aβ activates complement and AD microglia possess receptors to complement activation fragments. We would then expect, and find *(10,11)*, microglial migration to sites of Aβ-mediated complement activation.

Complement and cytokine receptors have the additional role of amplifying inflammation by inducing other inflammatory processes. IL-1, IL-6, and TNF, for example, all induce each other through such mechanisms *(1)*.

Still another function of the complement receptors is the triggering of phagocytosis when C3 activation fragments are bound to scavenger cells carrying CR3 or CR4 receptors. CR4 is expressed by AD microglia *(5,110)*. Like LFA-1 (which binds to ICAM-1) *(135)*, the complement receptors may also assist in the recruitment of glial cells to inflammatory sites.

The roles of other receptors that have been identified in AD are presently less clear. Leukocyte and Fc receptors, for example, have been demonstrated *(4,102,136)*, but a role for leukocytes or Ig in AD is not well established.

8. EICOSANOIDS

The eicosanoids leukotriene A4 and prostaglandin D2 are produced from arachidonic acid metabolism and elicit secondary immune responses, such as increased vascular permeability and vasodilation. In brain, eicosanoids are secreted by cerebral endothelial cells *(79)* and are upregulated by IL-1 and IL-6. Increased permeability of the blood–brain barrier may increase blood monocyte infiltration and further elevate the inflammatory response seen in AD. In culture, eicosanoids are secreted by mixed glia *(80)*. Anti-inflammatory drugs that block the eicosanoid cascade in glial cultures also appear to alter APP secretion *(137)*. In particular, metabolites of the leukotriene pathway may promote APP secretion, whereas prostaglandin metabolites, which are decreased in AD brain *(78)*, may inhibit its release.

9. THROMBIN AND PLASMIN SYSTEMS

The thrombin and plasmin systems are proteolytic cascades involved in cell migration and remodeling at inflammatory sites. Thrombin, which initiates the coagulation cascade, is associated with Aβ deposits in the AD brain *(83)*. Its inhibitor, protease nexin-1, is downregulated 14% when compared with control brain *(93)*. In culture, thrombin inhibits growth of neuronal processes *(138)*. It would be of interest, therefore, to evaluate whether or not thrombin might play a role in the "aberrant sprouting" that has been documented in AD *(139)*.

Plasminogen is secreted by astrocytes *(94)* and, with plasmin, stimulates neurite outgrowth *(140)*. Both plasminogen activators and plasminogen activation inhibitors exhibit increased expression in AD brain *(88,90,91)*.

10. CLINICAL STUDIES

There are now some 14 clinical studies that suggest in one way or another that anti-inflammatory therapy may be beneficial in AD *(136,141–153)*. Some of this research points to the possibility that common anti-inflammatory drugs may prevent or delay the onset of AD. For example, we found that arthritis patients over age 65, a population where many would be expected to be taking anti-inflammatory medication on a chronic basis, have a significantly reduced risk of AD *(151)*. Similar findings have since been widely reported *(136,144,145,147–149)*, and are more directly addressed by the work of Breitner and colleagues *(142)* in elderly identical twins with apparently different susceptibilities to AD. The latter appears in part to be explained by different histories of anti-inflammatory drug use.

The inexorable cognitive decline of AD may also be significantly affected by anti-inflammatory drug therapy. For example, in a recent retrospective study conducted at The Johns Hopkins Medical School *(152)*, disease progression was checked on a yearly basis in some 200 probable AD patients. Nearly 40 of these were subsequently found to have been taking nonsteroidal anti-inflammatory agents throughout much of the trial. Cognitive decline in these patients was significantly less than that of the other patients. Similarly, in a very small ($N = 28$ probable AD patients) but prospective clinical trial, we observed a significant therapeutic benefit of the nonsteroidal anti-inflammatory in-domethacin compared to placebo, as measured by the Alzheimer's Disease Assessment Scale, the Boston Naming Test, and the Min-Mental Status Examination *(153)*.

11. CONTROVERSIAL ISSUES

As reviewed here, there is substantial evidence at both basic and clinical science levels of an important role for inflammation in AD. Several issues and common misconceptions, however, continue to require attention.

The first of these is whether inflammation is primary or secondary in AD. The presumptive answer is almost certainly the latter. Inflammation most likely arises as a secondary response to other pathophysiologic events in the AD brain, just as it most often does in the periphery in other disorders. It would be remarkably naive, however, to take this as evidence that AD inflammation has no pathogenic significance. The inflammatory response to head injury may be a secondary event, but it is equally or more likely to kill the patient than the primary event. Toxic shock syndrome is a potentially lethal, secondary, inflammatory response to a generally innocuous primary stimulus. In the same way, AD inflammation may arise from multiple neurodegenerative sources: amyloid burden, neurofibrillary tangle formation, prior head trauma, failure of apolipoprotein E- (ApoE)-mediated or other repair mechanisms, defects in the presenilins, or even aging itself. The important point is that, taken over the course of a decade or more, the inflammatory response has a high potential to do as much or more damage than any or all of these more primary pathogens.

It is also possible, although less likely, that inflammation may be one of the primary pathogenic sources in AD. Investigations to date have tended to focus on colocalization of inflammatory mediators with the pathology that already exists in AD brain. The spaces in between, where subsequent pathology will arise, have not been so closely examined. Presumably, it is there that one would expect to see a primary pathogen at work; in this regard, it may be worth noting that neuropil threads (paired helical filament [PHF]-positive axons coursing through the neuropil) do exhibit numerous signs of inflammatory activity. Likewise, although reactive microglia tend to cluster at sites of Aβ deposition, they are also far more densely packed throughout the neuropil in AD compared to ND patients. The difficulty, of course, is that the presence of a putative primary pathogen at an unimpaired neuropil site could equally be taken as evidence that the pathogen is innocuous. In postmortem tissue, one can never know. Perhaps tissue-culture *(154)* or transgenic animal *(155)* approaches will prove amenable to resolving these questions.

The time scale of AD pathogenesis is another issue that may commonly be ill considered in AD research generally and AD inflammation research in particular. Is it reasonable, for example, to criticize Aβ neurotoxicity experiments for their typically nonphysiologic doses when one is trying to obtain a significant effect over a few days' exposure? The time scale of AD pathogenesis is more likely to be decades than days. Likewise, there appear to be some who expect the same vigorous inflammatory reaction in AD brain as in toxic shock syndrome. Clearly this cannot be the case, or else AD would be a lethal disorder lasting only a few hours. In sum, AD inflammation is not only a secondary response, but it is likely to be a weak secondary response. Nonetheless, the basic science and clinical evidence make clear that it is also an important response.

Finally, the research so far indicates that AD inflammation incorporates more of the innate than the humoral immune response. This is regrettable, since it leaves us largely unable to take advantage of the great strides that have been made through development and utilization of such experimental models as experimental allergic encephalitis. It also leads to misunderstanding. Since brain-specific autoantibodies, B-cells, T-cell anomalies, and other characteristics of abnormal humoral immune responses have been the most prominent objects of research in mainstream neuroimmunology (e.g., multiple sclerosis research), and since these mechanisms have proven difficult to demonstrate convincingly in AD, there may be a tendency to view AD inflammation research as somewhat more primitive and less completely formed. On the contrary, much that has been demonstrated concerning the innate immune response, particularly with respect to complement and the roles of microglia, has been at a very sophisticated level that has attracted leading immunologists to the field (cf *58,127*) and might be explored to advantage in areas that have heretofore been viewed mostly in the context of the humoral response. Moreover, the innate immune response is a very potent arm of the system, and there is precedent in certain disorders for its being a dominant source of pathology compared to the humoral response. Perhaps the cytokines, which play prominent roles in both innate and humoral immune mechanisms, will serve as a middle ground through which these presently isolated research directions will meet.

12. SUMMARY AND CONCLUSIONS

Indirect and direct evidence from both basic and clinical research supports the importance of inflammation as one of the pathogenic mechanisms operative in AD. Beginning at the simplest level, the following points have been reviewed here:

1. Inflammatory mediators are widely observed in the CNS (Table 1).
2. They are most often substantially elevated in expression in the AD compared to the ND brain (Table 1).
3. In addition to their known cytopathic actions, many of the inflammatory mediators exhibit unique, idiosyncratic interactions with AD pathology. Complement, for example, is activated by aggregated Aβ in the absence of antibody *(7,130)*. Thus, a chronic stimulus for the activation of complement is present throughout the course of AD. Complement also accelerates the aggregation of Aβ *(124–126)*. Cytokine expression may alter APP metabolism *(42,118,120,121)*.
4. Inflammation may be a necessary component of AD pathogenesis. For example, brain areas, such as cerebellum, may show widespread Aβ deposition, yet there is little or no AD neurodegeneration in this structure. Cerebellar Aβ is only rarely aggregated into the cross-β-pleat configuration, however, and would therefore not be expected to activate complement strongly, a result that has been confirmed *(60)*. Likewise, we have studied a subset of patients without clinical history of dementia, but with profuse entorhinal cortex Aβ deposition and neurofibrillary tangle formation. These patients have levels of reactive microglia and inflammatory mediators that are more comparable to ND than AD patients *(123)*.
5. Inflammation may be sufficient to cause AD neurotoxicity. The membrane attack complex and other complement components can be observed on dystrophic neurites within the AD brain *(63,65)*. This is not simply a mopping up of dead tissue from other AD causes, as evidenced by the fact that the cells are actively defending themselves by blebbing, endocytosis *(65)*, and the secretion of complement defense molecules *(27,64,71–76,143)*. In culture, inflammatory mechanisms mediated by Aβ enhance the toxicity of Aβ by some 100-fold or more *(130)*.
6. Anti-inflammatory drugs delay the onset and slow the progression of AD *(136,141–153)*.

Taken together, these data strongly support the notion that inflammation plays an important role in AD pathogenesis. Certainly, it is not the only AD pathogenic mechanism. However, as reviewed here, inflammation encompasses a wide range of phenomena, just as AD pathogenesis may encompass a wide range of phenomena. The intereactions between the two that have already been demonstrated may only be the first view of a very large, therapeutically relevant resource in the fight against AD.

REFERENCES

1. Rogers, J., Singer, R. H., Luber-Narod, J., and Bassell, G. J. (1986) Neurovirologic and neuroimmunologic considerations in Alzheimer's disease, *Neurosci. Abstr.* **12**, 944.
2. Hickey, W. F., Hsu, B. L., and Kimura, H. (1991) T-lymphocyte entry into the central nervous system, *J. Neurosci. Res.* **28**, 254–260.
3. Tooyama, I., Kimura, H., Akiyama, H., and McGeer, P. L. (1990) Reactive microglia express class and class II major histocompatibility antigens in Alzheimer disease, *Brain Res.* **23**, 273–280.
4. McGeer, P. L., Akiyama, H., Itagaki, S., and McGeer, E. G. (1989) Immune system response in Alzheimer's disease, *Can. J. Neurol. Sci.* **16**, 516–527.
5. Eikelenboom, P., Rozemuller, J. M., Kraal, G., Stam, F. C., McBride, P. A., Bruce, M. E., and Fraser, H. (1991) Cerebral amyloid plaques in Alzheimer's disease but not in scrapie-affected mice are closely associated with a local inflammatory process, *Virchows Archives B Cell Pathol.* **60**, 329–336.
6. Itagaki, S., McGeer, P. L., and Akiyama, H. (1989) Relationship of microglia and astrocytes to amyloid deposits of Alzheimer's disease, *J. Neuroimmunol.* **24**, 173–182.
7. Luber-Narod, J. and Rogers, J. (1988) Immune system associated antigens expressed by cells of the human central nervous system, *Neurosci. Lett.* **94**, 17–22.

8. Mattiace, L. A., Davies, P., and Dickson, D. W. (1990) Detection of HLA-DR on microglia in postmortem human brain is a function of clinical and technical factors, *Am. J. Pathol.* **136,** 1101–1114.

9. McGeer, P. L., Itagaki, S., Tago, H., and McGeer, E. G. (1987) Reactive microglia in patients with senile dementia of the Alzheimer type are positive for histocompatibility glycoprotein HLA-DR, *Neurosci. Lett.* **79,** 195–200.

10. Rogers, J., Luber-Narod, J., Styren S. D., and Civin, W. H. (1988) Expression of immune systemassociated antigen by cells of the human central nervous system. Relationship to the pathology of Alzheimer disease, *Neurobiol. Aging* **9,** 339–349.

11. Styren, S. D., Civin, W. H., and Rogers, J. (1990) Molecular, cellular, and pathologic characterization of HLA-DR immunoreactivity in normal elderly and Alzheimer disease brain, *Exp. Neurol.* **110,** 93–104.

12. Abraham, C. R., Selkoe, D. J., and Potter, H. (1988) Immunochemical identification of the serine protease inhibitor, α_1-antichymotrypsin in the brain amyloid deposits of Alzheimer's disease, *Cell* **52,** 487–501.

13. Abraham, C. R., Shirahama, T., and Potter, H. (1990) α_1-Antichymotrypsin is associated solely with amyloid deposits containing the β-protein, *Neurobiol. Aging* **11,** 123–129.

14. Gollin, P. A., Kalaria, R. N., Eikelenboom, P., Rozemuller, A., and Perry, G. (1992) a_1-Antitrypsin and a_1-antichymotrypsin are in the lesions of Alzheimer's disease, *Neuroreport* **3,** 201–203.

15. Rozemuller, J. M., Stam, F. C., and Eikelenboom, P. (1990) Acute phase proteins are present in amorphous plaques in the cerebral but not in the cerebellar cortex of patients with Alzheimer's disease, *Neurosci. Lett.* **119,** 75–78.

16. Rozemuller, J. M., Abbink, J. J., Kamp, A. M., Stam, F. C., Hack, C. E., and Eikelenboom, P. (1991) Distribution pattern and fuctional state of alpha 1-antichymotrypsin in plaques and vascular amyloid in Alzheimer's disease, *Acta Neuropathol.* **82,** 200–207.

17. Licastro, F., Morini, M. C., Polazzi, E., and Davis, L. J. (1995) Increased serum alpha 1-antichymotrypsin in patients with probable Alzheimer's disease: an acute phase reaction without the peripheral acute phase response, *J. Neuroimmunol.* **57,** 71–75.

18. Licastro, F., Parnetti, L., Morini, M. C., Davis, L. J., Cucinotta, D., Gaiti, A., and Senin, U. (1995) Acute phase reactant alpha 1-antichymotrypsin is increased in cerebrospinal fluid and serum of patients with probable Azlheimer disease, *Alzheimer's Disease and Associated Disorders* **9,** 112–118.

19. Lieberman, J., Schleissner, L., Tachiki, K. H., and Kling, A. S. (1995) Serum alpha 1-antichymotrypsin level as a marker for Alzheimer-type dementia, *Neruobiol. Aging* **16,** 747–753.

20. Das, S. and Potter, H. (1995) Expression of the Alzheimer amyloid-promoting factor anitchymotrypsin is induced in human astrocytes by IL-1, *Neuron* **14,** 447–456.

21. Bauer, J., Strauss, S., Schreiter-Gasser, U., Ganter, U., Schlegel, P., Witt, I., Volk, B., and Berger, M. (1991) Interleukin-6 and α_2-macroglobulin indicate an acute-phase state in Alzheimer's disease cortices, *FEBS Lett.* **285,** 111–114.

22. Van Gool, D., De Strooper, B., Van Leuven, F., Triau, E., and Dom, R. (1993) α_2-macroglobulin expression in neuritic-type plaques in patients with Alzheimer's disease, *Neurobiol. Aging* **14,** 233–237.

23. Wood, J. A., Wood, P. L., Ryan, R., Graff-Radford, N. R., Pilapil, C., Robitaille, Y., and Quirion, R. (1993) Cytokine indices in Alzheimer's temporal cortex: no changes in mature IL-1b or IL-1RA but increases in the associated acute phase proteins IL-6, a_2-macroglobulin and C-reactive protein, *Brain Res.* **629,** 245–252.

24. Gebicke-Haerter, P. J., Bauer, J., Brenner, A., Gerok, W. (1987) Alpha 2-macroglobulin synthesis in an astrocyte subpopulation, *J. Neurochem.* **49,** 1139–1145.

25. Coria, F., Castano, E., Prelli, F., Larrondo-Lillo, M., van Duinen, S., Shelanski, M. L., and Frangione, B. (1988) Isolation and characterization of amyloid P component from Alzheimer's disease and other types of cerebral amyloidosis, *Lab. Invest.* **58,** 454–458.

26. Duong, T., Pommier, E. C., and Schiebel, A. B. (1989) Immunodetection of the amyloid P component in Alzheimer's disease, *Acta Neuropathol.* **78**, 429–437.

27. Kalaria, R. N. and Kroon, S. N. (1992) Complement inhibitor C4-binding protein in amyloid deposits containing serum amyloid P in Alzheimer's disease, *Biochem. Biophys. Res. Commun.* **186**, 461–466.

28. Akiyama, H., Yamada, T., Dawamata, T., and McGeer, P. L. (1991) Association of amyloid P component with complement proteins in neurologically diseased tissue, *Brain Res.* **548**, 349–352.

29. Smith, M. A., Kalaria, R. N., and Perry, G. (1993) Alpha 1-trypsin immunoreactivity in Alzheimer disease, *Biochem. Biophys. Res. Commun.* **193**, 579–584.

30. Iwamoto, N., Nishiyama, E., Ohwada, J., and Arai, H. (1994) Demonstration of CRP immunoreactivity in brains of Alzheimer's disease: immunohistochemical study using formic acid pretreatment of tissue sections, *Neurosci. Lett.* **177**, 23–26.

31. Strauss, S., Bauer, J., Ganter, U., Jonas, U., Berger, M., and Volk, B. (1992) Detection of interleukin-6 and a_2-macroglobulin immunoreactivity in cortex and hippocampus of Alzheimer's disease patients, *Lab. Invest.* **66**, 223–230.

32. Sheng, J. G., Mrak, R. E., and Griffin, W. S. (1995) Microglial interleukin-1 alpha expression in brain regions in Alzheimer's disease: correlation with neuritic plaque distribution, *Neuropathol. Appl. Neurobiol.* **21**, 290–301.

33. Griffin, W. S., Sheng, J. G., Roberts, G. W., and Mrak, R. E. (1995) Interleukin-1 expression in different plaque types in Alzheimer's disease: significance in plaque evolution, *J. Neuropathol. Exp. Neurol.* **54**, 276–281.

34. Walker, D. G., Kim, S. U., and McGeer, P. L. (1995) Complement and cytokine gene expression in cultured microglia derived from post-mortem human brains, *J. Neurosci. Res.* **40**, 478–493.

35. Lieberman, A. P., Pitha, P. M., Shin, H. S., and Shin, M. L. (1989) Production of tumor necrosis factor and other cytokines by astrocytes stimulated with lipopolysaccharide or a neurotropic virus, *Proc. Natl. Acad. Sci. USA* **86**, 6348–6352.

36. Cacabelos, R., Alvarez, X. A., Fernandez-Novoa, L., Franco A., Mangues, R., Pellicer, A., and Nishimura, T. (1994) Brain interleukin-1 beta in Alzheimer's disease and vascular dementia, *Methods Findings Exp. Clin. Pharmacol.* **16**, 141–145.

37. Sharif, S. F., Hariri, R. J., Chang, V. A., Barie, P. S., Wang, R. S., and Ghajar, J. B. (1993) Human astrocyte production of tumour necrosis factor-alpha, interleukin-1 beta and interleukin-6 following exposure to lipopolysaccharide endotoxin, *Neurol. Res.* **15**, 109–112.

38. Gebicke-Haerter, P. J., Appel, K., Taylor, G. D., Schobert, A., Rich, I. N., Northoff, H., and Berger, M. (1994) Rat microglial interleukin-3, *J. Neuroimmunol.* **50**, 203–214.

39. Swada, N., Suzumura, A., Itoh, Y., and Marunouchi, T. (1993) Production of interleukin-5 by mouse astrocytes and microglia in culture, *Neurosci. Lett.* **155**, 175–178.

40. Shalit, F., Sredni, B., Stern, L., Kott, E., and Huberman, M. (1994) Elevated interleukin-6 secretion levels by mononuclear cells of Alzheimer's patients, *Neurosci. Lett.* **174**, 130–132.

41. Aloisi, F., Care, A., Borsellino, G., Gallo, P., Rosa, S., Bassani, A., Cabibbo, A., Testa, U., Levi, G., and Peschle, C. (1992) Production of hemolymphopoietic cytokines (IL-6, IL 8, colony-stimulating factors) by normal human astrocytes in response to IL-1 beta and tumor necrosis factor-alpha, *J. Immunol.* **149**, 2358–2366.

42. Fillit, H., Ding, W., Buee, L., Kalman, J., Altstiel, L., Lawlor, B., and Wolf-Klein, G. (1991) Elevated circulating tumor necrosis factor levels in Alzheimer's disease, *Neurosci. Lett.* **129**, 318–320.

43. Cacabelos, R., Alverez, X. A., Franco-Maside, A., Fernandez-Novao, L., and Caamano, J. (1994) Serum tumor necrosis factor (TNF) in Alzheimer's disease and multi-infarct dementia, *Methods Findings Exp. Clin. Pharmacol.* **16**, 29–35.

44. Boka, G., Anglade, P., WallachL, D., Javoy-Agrid, G., Agid, Y., and Hirsch, E. C. (1994) Immunocytochemical analysis of tumor necrosis factor and its receptors in Parkinson's disease, *Neurosci. Lett.* **172**, 151–l54.

45. Mogi, M., Harada, M., Riederer, P., Narabayashi, H., Fujita, K., and Nagatsu, T. (1994) Tumor necrosis factor-α (TNF-α) increases both in the brain and in the cerebrospinal fluid from parkinsonian patients, *Neurosci. Lett.* **165**, 208–210.

46. Yamabe, T., Dhir, G., Cowan, E. P., Wolf, A. L., Bergey, G. K., Krumholz, A., Barry, E., Hoffman, P. M., and Dhib-Jalbut, S. (1994) Cytokine-gene expression in measles-infected adult human glial cells, *J. Neuroimmunol.* **49**, 171–179.

47. Mogi, M., Harada, M., Kondo, T., Riederer, P., Inagaki, H., Minami, M., and Nagatsu, T. (1994) Interleukin-1β, interleukin-6, epidermal growth factor and transforming growth factor-α are elevated in the brain from parkinsonian patients, *Neurosci. Lett.* **180**, 147–150.

48. Chao, C. C., Hu, S., Frey, W. H., II, Ala, T. A., Tourtelotte, W. W., and Peterson, P. K. (1994) Transforming growth factor beta in Alzheimer's disease, *Clin. Diagn. Lab. Immunol.* **1**, 109,110.

49. Mogi, M., Harada, M., Kondo, T., Narabayashi, H., Riederer, P., and Nagatsu, T. (1995) Transforming growth fator-beta 1 levels are elevated in the striatum and in the ventricular cerebrospinal fluid in Parkinson's disease, *Neurosci. Lett.* **193**, 129–132.

50. Hurwitz, A. A., Lyman, W. D., and Berman, J. W. (1995) Tumor necrosis factor alpha and transforming growth factor beta upregulate astrocyte expression of monocyte chemoattractant protein-1, *J. Neuroimmunol.* **57**, 193–198.

51. Murphy, G. M., Jr., Jia, X. C., Song, Y., Ong, E., Shrivastava, R., Bocchini, V., Lee, Y. L., and Eng, L. F. (1995) Macrophage inflammatory protein 1-alpha mRNA expression in an immortalized microglial cell line and cortical astrocyte cultures, *J. Neurosci. Res.* **40**, 755–763.

52. Brachova, L., Lue, L.-F., Schultz., J., El Rashidy, T., and Rogers, J. (1993) Association cortex, cerebellum, and serum concentrations of Clq and factor B in Alzheimer's disease, *Mol. Brain Res.* **18**, 329–334.

53. Eikelenboom, P., Hack, C. E., Rozemuller, J. M., and Stam, F. C. (1989) Complement activation in amyloid plaques in Alzheimer's dementia, *Virchows Archives B Cell Pathol.* **56**, 259–262.

54. Eikelenboom, P. and Stam, F. C. (1984) An immunohistochemical study on cerebral vascular and senile plaque amyloid in Alzheimer's dementia, *Virchows Archives B Cell Pathol.* **47**, 17–25.

55. Ishii, T. and Haga, S. (1984) Immuno-electron-microscopic localization of complements in amyloid fibrils of senile plaques, *Acta Neuropathol. (Berl.)* **63**, 296–300.

56. Ishii, T., Haga, S., and Kametani, F. (1988) Presence of immunoglobulins and complements in the amyloid plaques in the brain of patients with Alzheimer's disease, in *Immunology and Alzheimer's Disease* (Pouplard-Barthelaix, A., Emile, J., and Christen, Y., eds.), Springer-Verlag, Berlin, pp. 17–29.

57. McGeer, P. L., Akiyama, H., Itagaki, S., and McGeer, E. G. (1989) Activation of the classical complement pathway in brain tissue of Alzheimer patients, *Neurosci. Lett.* **107**, 341–346.

58. Rogers, J., Cooper, N. R., Webster, S., Schultz, J., McGeer, P. L., Styren, S. D., Civin, W. H., Brachova, L., Bradt, B., Warcl, P., and Lieberburg, I. (1992) Complement activation by β-amyloid in Alzheimer disease, *Proc. Nat. Acad. Sci. USA* **89**, 10,016–10,020.

59. Veerhuis, R., van der Valk, P., Janssen, I., Zhan, S. S., Van Nostrand, W. E., and Eikelenboom, P. (1995) Complement activation in amyloid plaques in Alzheimer's disease brains does not proceed further than C3, *Virchows Archives* **426**, 603–610.

60. Lue, L.-F. and Rogers, J. (1992) Full complement activation fails in diffuse plaques of the Alzheimer's disease cerebellum, *Dementia* **3**, 308–313.

61. Eikelenboom, P., Zhan, S. S., Kamphorst, W., van der Valk, P., and Rozemuller, J. M. (1994) Cellular and substrate adhesion molecules (integrins) and their ligands in cerebral amyloid plaques in Alzheimer's disease, *Virchows Archives* **424**, 421–427.

62. Haga, S., Ikeda, K., Sato, M., and Ishii, T. (1993) Synthetic Alzheimer amyloid beta/A4 peptides enhance production of complement 3 component by cultured microglial cells, *Brain Res.* **601**, 88–94.

63. Itagaki, S., Akiyama, H., Saito, H., and McGeer, P. L. (1994) Ultrastructural localization of complement membrane attack complex (MAC)-like immunoreactivity in brains of patients with Alzheimer's disease, *Brain Res.* **645,** 78–84.

64. McGeer, P. L., Kawamata, T., and Walker, D. G. (1992) Distribution of clusterin in Alzheimer brain tissue, *Brain Res.* **579,** 337–341.

65. Webster, S. D., Lue, L.-F., McKinley, M., and Rogers, J. (1992) Ultrastructural localization of complement proteins to neuronal membranes and β-amyloid peptide containing Alzheimer's disease pathology, *Neurosci. Abstr.* **18,** 765.

66. Johnson, S. A., Lampert-Etchells, M., Pasinetti, G. M., Rozovsky, I., and Finch, C. E. (1992) Complement mRNA in the mammalian brain: responses to Alzheimer's disease and experimental brain lesioning, *Neurobiol. Aging* **13,** 641–648.

67. Walker, D. G. and McGeer, P. L. (1992) Complement gene expression in human brain: comparison between normal and Alzheimer disease cases, *Mol. Brain Res.* **14,** 106–109.

68. Fischer, B., Schmol, H., Riederer, P., Bauer, J., Platt, D., and Popa-Wagner, A. (1995) Complement Clq and C3 mRNA expression in the frontal cortex of Alzheimer's patients, *J. Mol. Med.* **73,** 465–471.

69. Tranque, P., Naftolin, F., and Robbins, R. (1994) Differential regulation of astrocyte plasminogen activators by insulin-like growth factor-I and epidermal growth factor, *Endocrinology* **134,** 2606–2613.

70. Barnum, S. R., Jones, J. L., and Benveniste, E. N. (1993) Interleukin-1 and tumor necrosis factor mediated regulation of C3 gene expression in human astroglioma cells, *Glia* **7,** 225–236.

71. McGeer, P. L., Walker, D. G., Akiyama, H., Kawamata, T., Guan, A. L., Parker, C. J., Okada, N., and McGeer, E. G. (1991) Detection of the membrane inhibitor of reactive lysis (CD59) in diseased neurons of Alzheimer brain, *Brain Res.* **544,** 315–319.

72. Choi-Miura, N.-H., Ihara, Y., Fukuchi, K., Takeda, M., Nakano, Y., Tobe, T., and Tomita, M. (1992) SP-40, 40 is a constituent of Alzheimer's amyloid, *Acta Neuropathol.* **83,** 260–264.

73. May, P. C., Lampert-Etchells, M., Johnson, S. A., Poirier, J., Masters, J. N., and Finch, C. E. (1990) Dynamics of gene expression for a hippocampal glycoprotein elevated in Alzheimer's disease and in response to experimental lesions in rat, *Neuron* **5,** 831–839.

74. Akiyama, H., Kawamata, T., Dedhar, S., and McGeer, P. L. (1991) Immunohistochemical localization of vitronectin, its receptor and beta-3 integrin in Alzheimer brain tissue, *J. Neuroimmunol.* **32,** 19–28.

75. Tuohy, J. M., Schultz, J. J., Brachova, L., Lue, L.-F., and Rogers, J. (1993) Evidence of increased levels of C4 binding protein in Alzheimer's disease, *Neurosci. Abstr.* **19,** 834.

76. Walker, D. G., Yasuhara, O., Patston, P. A., McGeer, E. G., and McGeer, P. L. (1995) Complement C1 inhibitor is produced by brain tissue and is cleaved in Alzheimer disease, *Brain Res.* **675,** 75–82.

77. May, P. C. and Finch, C. E. (1992) Sulfated glycoprotein 2: new relationships of this multifunctional protein to neurodegeneration, *Trends Neurosci.* **15,** 391–396.

78. Wong, P. T., McGeer, P. L., and McGeer, E. G. (1992) Decreased prostaglandin synthesis in postmortem cerebral cortex from patients with Azleheimer's disease, *Neurochem. Int.* **21,** 197–202.

79. de Vries, H. E., Hoogendoorn, K. H., van Dijk, J., Zijlstra, F. J., van Dam, A. M., Breimer, D. D., van Verkel, T. J., de Boer, A. G., and Kuiper, J. (1995) Eicosanoid production by rat cerebral endothelial cells: stimulation by lipopolysaccharide, interleukin-1 and interleukin-6, *J. Neuroimmunol.* **59,** 1–8.

80. Matsuo, M., Hamasaki, Y., Fujiyama, F., and Miyazaki, S. (1995) Eicosanoids are produced by microglia, not by astrocytes, in rat glial cell cultures, *Brain Res.* **685,** 201–204.

81. Colton, C. A. and Gilbert, D. L. (1993) Microglia, an in vivo souce of reactive oxygen species in the brain, *Adv. Neurol.* **59,** 321–326.

82. Brown, G. C., Bolanos, J. P., Heales, S. J. R., and Clark, J. B. (1995) Nitric oxide produced by activated astrocytes rapidly and reversibly inhibits cellular respiration, *Neurosci. Lett.* **193,** 201–104.

83. Akiyama, H., Ikeda, K., Kondo, H., and McGeer, P. L. (1992) Thrombin accumulation in brains of patients with Alzheimer's disease, *Neurosci. Lett.* **146,** 152–154.

84. Weinstein, J. R., Gold, S. J. Cunningham, D. D., and Gall, C. M. (1995) Cellular localization of thrombin receptor mRNA in rat brain: expression by mesencephalic dopaminergic neurons and codistribution with prothrombin mRNA, *J. Neurosci.* **15,** 2906–2919.

85. Kalaria, R. N., Golde, T., Kroon, S. N., and Perry, G. (1993) Serine protease inhibitor antithrombin III and its messenger RNA in the pathogenesis of Alzheimer's disease, *Am. J. Pathol.* **143,** 886–893.

86. McComb, R. D., Miller, K. A., and Carson, S. D. (1991) Tissue factor antigen in senile plaques of Alzheimer's disease, *Am. J. Pathol.* **139,** 491–494.

87. Yasuhara, O., Walker, D. G., and McGeer, P. L. (1994) Hageman factor and its binding sites are present in senile plaques of Alzheimer's disease, *Brain Res.* **654,** 234–240.

88. Rebeck, G. W., Harr, S. D., Strickland, D. K., and Hyman, B. T. (1995) Multiple, diverse senile plaque-associated proteins are ligands of an apolipoprotein E receptor, the alpha 2-macroglobulin receptor/low-density-lipoprotein receptor-related protein, *Ann. Neurol.* **37,** 211–217.

89. Nakajima, K., Tsuzaki, N., Shimojo, M., Hamanoue, M., and Kohsaka, S. (1992) Microglia isolated from rat brain secrete a urokinase-type plasminogen activator, *Brain Res.* **577,** 285–292.

90. Reddington, M., Hass, C., and Kreutzlberg, G. W. (1994) The plasminogen activator system in neurons and glia during motoneuron regeneration, *Neuropathol. Appl. Neurobiol.* **20,** 188–190.

91. Akiyama, H., Ideda, K., Kondo, H., Kato, M., McGeer, E. G., and McGeer, P. L. (1993) Microglia express the type 2 plasminogen activator inhibitor in the brain of control subjects and patients with Alzheimer's disease, *Neurosci. Lett.* **164,** 233–235.

92. Choi, B. H., Suzuki, M., Kim, T., Wagner, S. L., and Cunningham, D. D. (1990) Protease nexin-1. Localization in the human brain suggests a protective role against extravasated serine proteases, *Am. J. Pathol.* **137,** 741–747.

93. Wagner, S. L., Geddes, J. W., Cobnan, C. W., Lau, A. L., Gurwitz, D., Isackson, P. J., and Cunningham, D. D. (1989) Protease nexin-1 an antithrombin with neurite outgrowth activity, is reduced in Alzheimer's disease, *Proc. Natl. Acad. Sci. USA* **86,** 8284–8288.

94. Nakajima, K., Tsuzaki, N., Takemoto, N., and Kohsaka, S. (1992) Production and secretion of plasminogen in cultured rat brain rnicroglia, *FEBS Lett.* **308,** 179–182.

95. Dihanich, M., Kaser, M., Reinhard, E., Cunningham, D. D., and Monard, D. (1991) Prothrombin mRNA is expressed by cells of the nervous system, *Neuron* **6,** 575–581.

96. Yamamoto, M., Sawaya, R., Mohanam, S., Loskutoff, D. J., Bruner, J. M., Rao, V. H., Oka, K., Tomonaga, M., Nicolson, G. L., and Rao, J. S. (1994) Expression and cellular localization of messenger RNA for plasminogen activator inhibitor type I in human astrocytomas in vivo, *Cancer Res.* **54,** 3329–3332.

97. Dent, M. A., Sumi, Y., Morris, R. J., and Seeley, P. J. (1993) Urokinase-type plasminogen activator expression by neurons and oligodendrocytes during process outgrowth in developing rat brain, *Eur. J. Neurosci.* **5,** 633–647.

98. Frohman, E. M., Frohman, T. C., Gupta, S., de Fougerolles, A., and van den Noort, E. (1991) Expression of intercellular adhesion molecule-1 (ICAM-1) in Alzheimer's disease, *J. Neurol. Sci.* **106,** 105–111.

99. Verbeek, M. M., Otte-Holler, I., Westphal, J. R., Wesseling, P., Ruiter, D. J., and de Waal, R. M. W. (1994) Accumulation of intercellular adhesion molecule-1 in senile plaques in brain tissue of patients with Alzheimer's disease, *Am. J. Pathol.* **144,** 104–116.

100. Satoh, J., Kim, S. U., Kastrukoff, L. F., and Takei, F. (1991) Expression and induction of intercellular adhesion molecules (ICAMs) and major histocompatibility complex (MHC) antigens on cultured murine oligodendrocytes and astrocytes, *J. Neurosci. Res.* **29,** 1–12.

101. Gillian, A. M., Brion, J.-P., and Breen, K. C. (1994) Expression of the neural cell adhesion molecule (NCAM) in Alzheimer's disease, *Neurodegen.* **3,** 283–291.

102. Rozemuller, J. M., Eikelenboom, P., Pals, S. T., and Stam, F. C. (1989) Microglial cells around amyloid plaques in Alzheimer's disease express leucocyte adhesion molecules of the LFA-1 family, *Neurosci. Lett.* **101,** 228–292.

103. Akiyama, H., Tooyama, I., Kondo, H., Ideda, K., Kimura, H., McGeer, E. G., and McGeer, P. L. (1994) Early response of brain resident microglia to kainic acid-induced hippocampal lesions, *Brain Res.* **635,** 257–268.

104. Rosenman, S. J., Shrikant, P., Dubb, L., Benveniste, E. N., and Ransohoff, R. M. (1995) Cytokine-induced gene expression of vascular cell adhesion molecule-1 (VCAM-1) in astrocytes and astrocytoma cell lines, *J. Immunol.* **154,** 1888–1899.

105. McGeer, P. L., McGeer, E. G., Itagaki, S., and Mizukawa, K. (1987) Anatomy and pathology of the basal ganglia, *Can. J. Neurol. Sci.* **12,** 363–372.

106. Akiyama, H., Nishimura, T., Kondo, H., Ikeda, K., Hayashi, V., and McGeer, P. L. (1994) Expression of the receptor for macrophage colony stimulating factor by brain microglia and its upregulation in brains of patients with Alzheimer's disease and amyotrophic lateral sclerosis, *Brain Res.* **639,** 171–174.

107. Tomozawa, Y., Inoue, T., and Satoh, M. (1995) Expression of type I interleukin-1 receptor mRNA and its regulation in cultured astrocytes, *Neurosci. Lett.* **195,** 57–60.

108. Eizenberg, O., Faberelman, A., Lotan, M., and Schwartz, M. (1995) Interleukin-2 transcripts in human and rodent brains—possible expression by astrocytes, *J. Neurochem.* **64,** 1928–1936.

109. Sawada, M., Suzumura, A., and Marunouchi, T. (1995) Induction of functional interleukin-2 receptor in mouse microglia, *J. Neurochem.* **64,** 1973–1979.

110. Akiyama, H. and McGeer, P. L. (1990) Brain microglia constituvely express b-2 integrins, *J. Neuroimmunol.* **30,** 81–93.

111. Akiyama, H., Ikeda, K., Katoh, M., McGeer, E. G., and McGeer, P. L. (1994) Expression of MRP14, 27E10, interferon-alpha and leucocyte common antigen by reactive microglia in postmortem human brain tissue, *J. Neuroimmunol.* **50,** 195–201.

112. Rogers, J. and Rovigatti, U. (1988) Immunologic and tissue culture approaches to the neurobiology of aging, *Neurobiol. Aging* **9,** 759–762.

113. Fraser, P. E., Nguyen, J. T., McLachlan, D. R., Abraham, C. R., and Kirschner, D. A. (1993) α_1-Antichymotrypsin binding to Alzheimer Ab peptides is sequence specific and induces fibril disaggregation in vitro, *J. Neurochem.* **61,** 298–305.

114. Ma, J., Yee, A., Brewer, H. B., Das, S., and Potter, H. (1994) Amyloid-associated proteins α_1-antichymotrypsin and apolipoprotein E promote assembly of Alzheimer β-protein into filaments, *Nature* **372,** 92–94.

115. Hamazaki, H. (1995) Amyloid P component promotes aggregation of Alzheimer's beta-amyloid peptide, *Biochem. Biophys. Res. Commun.* **211,** 349–353.

116. Tennent, G. A., Loval, L. B., and Pepys, M. B. (1995) Serum amyloid P component prevents proteolysis of the amyloid fibrils of Alzheimer disease and systemic amyloidosis, *Proc. Natl. Acad. Sci. USA* **92,** 4299–4303.

117. Koller, M., Hensler, T., Konig, B., Prevost, G., Alouf, J., and Konig, W. (1993) Induction of heat-shock proteins by bacterial toxins, lipid mediators and cytokines in human leukocytes, *Infect. Dis.* **278,** 365–376.

118. Buxbaum, J. D., Oishi, M., Chen, H. I., Pinkas-Kramarski, R., Jaffe, E. A., Gandy, S. E., and Greengard, P. (1992) Cholinergic agonists and interleukin-1 regulate processing and secretion of the Alzheimer b/A4 amyloid protein precursor, *Proc. Natl. Acad. Sci. USA* **89,** 10,075–10,078.

119. Forloni, G., Demicheli, F., Giorgi, S., Bendotti, C., and Angeretti, N. (1992) Expression of amyloid precursor protein mRNAs in endothelial, neuronal and glial cells: modulation by interleukin-1, *Mol. Brain Res.* **16,** 128–134.

120. Goldgaber, D., Harris, H. W., Hla, T., Maciag, T., Donnelly, R. J., Jacobsen, J. S., Vitek, M. P., and Gajdusek, C. (1989) Interleukin-1 regulates synthesis of amyloid β-protein precursor mRNA in human endothelial cells, *Proc. Natl. Acad. Sci. USA* **86,** 7606–7610.

121. Gray, C. W. and Patel, A. J. (1993) Regulation of β-amyloid precursor protein isoform mRNAs by transforming growth factor-bl and interleukin-lb in astrocytes, *Mol. Brain Res.* **19,** 251–256.

122. Araujo, D. M. and Cotman, C. W. (1992) β-Amyloid stimulates glial cells in vitro to produce growth factors that accumulate in senile plaques in Alzheimer's disease, *Brain Res.* **569,** 141–145.

123. Brachova, L., Lue, L.-F., Byttner, S., Sue, L., Civin, W. H., Schultz, J., Tuohy, J., and Rogers, J. (1993) Reduced complement activation in nondemented patients with excessive β-amyloid peptide deposition, *Neurosci. Abst.* **19,** 833.

124. Webster, S., Glabe, C., and Rogers, J. (1995) Multivalent binding of complement protein Clq to the amyloid β-peptide promotes the nucleation phase of Ab aggregation, *Biochem. Biophys. Res. Commun.* **217,** 869–875.

125. Webster, S., O'Barr, S., and Rogers, J. (1994) Enhanced aggregation and β structure of amyloid b peptide after co-incubation with Clq, *J. Neurosci. Res.* **39,** 448–456.

126. Webster, S. and Rogers, J. (1996) Relative efficacies of amyloid b peptide (Ab) binding proteins in Ab aggregation, *J. Neurosci. Res.* submitted for publication.

127. Jiang, H., Burdick, D., Glabe, C. G., Cotman, C. W., and Tenner, A. J. (1994) β-amyloid activates complement by binding to a specific region of the collagen-like domain of the Clq chain, *J. Immunol.* **152,** 5050–5059.

128. Jiang, H., Robey, F. A., and Gewurz, H. (1992) Localization of sites through which C-reactive protein binds and activates compleme:nt to residues 14-26 and 76-92 of the human Clq A chain, *J. Exp. Med.* **175,** 1373–1379.

129. Pike, C. J., Walencewicz, A. J., Glabe, C. G., and Cotman, C. W. (1991) In vitro aging of β-amyloid protein causes peptide aggregation and neurotoxicity, *Brain Res.* **56,** 311–314.

130. Schultz, J., Schaller, J., McKinley, M., Bradt, B., Cooper, N., May, P., and Rogers, J. (1994) Enhanced cytotoxicity of amyloid b-peptide by a complement dependent mechanism, *Neurosci. Lett.* **175,** 99–102.

131. Yankner, B. A., Duffy, L. K., and Kirschner, D. A. (1990) Neurotrophic and neurotoxic effects of amyloid-beta protein: Reversal by tachykinin neuropeptides, *Science* **250,** 279–282.

132. Cooper, N. R. (1985) The classical comp]ement pathway: activation and regulation of the first complement component, *Adv. Immunol.* **37,** 151–157.

133. Meri, S., Morgan, B. P., Davies, A., Daniels, R. H., Olavesen, M. G., Waldman, H., and Lachmann, P. J. (1990) Human protectin (CD59), an 18,000–20,000 MW complement lysis restricting factor, inhibits C5b-8 catalysed insertion of C9 into lipid bylayers, *Immunology* **71,** 1–9.

134. Oda, T., Wals, P., Osterburg, H. H., Johnson, S. A., Pasinetti, G. M., Morgan, T. E., Rozovsky, I., Stine, W. B., Snyder, S. W., and Holzman, T. F. (1995) Clusterin (apoJ) alters the aggregation of amyloid beta-peptide (A beta 1-42) and forms slowly sedimenting A beta complexes that cause oxidative stress, *Exp. Neurol.* **136,** 22–31.

135. Ross, G. D. and Vetvicka, V. (1993) CR3 (CD11b, CD18) a phagocyte and NK cell membrane receptor with multiple ligand specificities and functions, *Clin. Exp. Immunol.* **92,** 181–184.

136. Myllykangas-Luosujarvi, R., and Isomaki, H. (1994) Alzheimer's disease and rheumatoid arthritis, *Br. J. Rheumatol.* **33,** 501,502.

137. Kinouchi, T., Ono, Y., Sorimachi, H., Ishiura, S., and Suzuki, K. (1995) Arachidonate metablites affect the secretion of an N-termal fragment of Alzheimer's disease amyloid percursor protein, *Biochem. Biophys. Res. Comm.* **209,** 841–849.

138. Jalink, K. and Moolenaar, W. H. (1992) Thrombin receptor activation causes rapid neural cell rounding and neurite retraction independent of classic second messengers, *J. Cell. Biol.* **118,** 411–419.

139. Masliah, E., Mallory, M., Hansen, L., Alford, M., Albright, T., DeTeresa, R., Terry, R., Baudier, J., and Saitoh, T. (1991) Patterns of aberrant sprouting in Alzheimer's Disease, *Neuron* **6,** 729–739.

140. Nagata, K., Nakajima, K., Takemoto, N., Saito, H., and Kohsaka, S. (1993) Microglia-derived plasminogen enhances neurite outgrowth from explant cultures of rat brain, *Int. J. Dev. Neurosci.* **11**, 227–237.
141. Andersen, K., Launer, L. J., Ott, A., Hoes, A. W., Breteler, M. M. B., and Hofman, A. (1995) Do nonsteroidal antiinflammatory drugs decrease the risk for Alzheimer's disease? *Neurology* **45**, 1441–1445.
142. Breitner, J. C. S., Gau, B. A., Welsh, K. A., Plassman, B. L., McDonald, W. M., Helmas, M. J., and Anthony, J. C. (1994) Inverse association of anti-inflammatory treatments and Alzheimer's disease, *Neurology* **44**, 227–232.
143. Breitner, J. C. S., Welsh, K. A., Helms, M. J., Gaskell, P. C., Gau, B. A., Roses, A. D., Pericak-Vance, M. A., and Saunders, A. M. (1995) Delayed onset of Alzheimer's disease with nonsteroidal anti-inflammatory ancl histamine H2 blocking drugs, *Neurobiol. Aging* **16**, 520–523.
144. Broe, G. A., Henderson, A. S., Creasey, H., McCusker, E., Korten, H. E., Jorm, A. F., Longley, W., and Anthony, J. C. (1990) A case-control study of Alzheimer's disease in Australia, *Neurology* **40**, 1698–1707.
145. Canadian Study of Health and Aging (1994) Risk factors for Alzheimer's disease in Canada, *Neurology* **44**, 2073–2080.
146. Graves, A. B., White, E., Koepsell, T. D., Reifler, B. V., van Belle, G., Larson, E. B., and Raskind, M. (1990) A case-control study of Alzheimer's disease, *Ann. Neurol.* **28**, 766–774.
147. Jenkinson, M. I., Bliss, M. R., Brain, A. T., and Scott, D. L. (1989) Rheumatoid arthritis and senile dementia of the Alzheimer's type, *Br. J. Rheumatol.* **28**, 86,87.
148. Li, G., Shen, Y. C., Chen, C. H., Zhau, Y. W., and Silverman, J. M. (1992) A case-control study of Alzheimer's disease in China, *Neurology* **42**, 1481,1482.
149. Lucca, U., Tettamanti, M., Forloni, G., and Spagnoli, A. (1994) Nonsteroidal antiinflammatory drug use in Alzheimer's disease, *Biol. Psychiatry* **36**, 854–856.
150. McGeer, P. L., Harada, N., Kimura, H., McGeer, E. G., and Schulzer, M. (1992) Prevalence of dementia amongst elderly Japanese with leprosy: apparent effect of chronic drug therapy, *Dementia* **3**, 146–149.
151. McGeer, P. L., McGeer, E. G., Rogers, J., and Sibley, J. (1990) Anti-inflammatory drugs and Alzheimer's disease, *Lancet* **335**, 10–37.
152. Rich, J. B., Rasmusson, D. X., Folstein, M. F., Carson, K. A., Kawas, C., and Brandt, J. (1995) Nonsteroidal anti-inflammatory drugs in Alzheimer's disease, *Neurology* **45**, 51–55.
153. Rogers, J., Kirby, L. C., Hempelman, S. R., Berry, D. L., McGeer, P. L., Kaszniak, A. W., Zalinski, J., Cofield, M., Mansukhani, L., Willson, P., and Kogan, F. (1993) Clinical trial of indomethacin in Alzheimer's disease, *Neurology* **43**, 1609–1611.
154. Lue, L.-F., Brachova, L., Walker, D. G., and Rogers, J. (1996) Characterization of glial cultures from rapid autopsies of Alzheimer's and control patients, *Neurobiol. Aging*, **17**, 421–429.
155. Games, D., Adams, D., Alessandrini, R., Barbour, R., Berthelette, P., Blackwell, C., Carr, T., Clemens, J., Donaldson, T., Gillespie, F., et al. (1995) Alzheimer-type neuropathology in transgenic mice overexpressing V717F beta-amyloid precursor protein, *Nature* **373**, 523–527.
156. Gitter, B. D., Cox, L. M., Keith, P. T., Rydel, R. E., and May, P. C. (1993) Amyloid beta peptide (Aβ) potentiates cytokine secretion by interleukin-1β activated human astrocytoma cells, *Neurosci. Abstr.* **19**, 832.

τ Protein and the Neurofibrillary Pathology of Alzheimer's Disease

Michel Goedert, John Q. Trojanowski, and Virginia M.-Y. Lee

1. INTRODUCTION

Alzheimer's disease is characterized clinically by a progressive loss of memory and other cognitive functions, resulting in a profound dementia. The intellectual decline is accompanied by the progressive accumulation in the brain of insoluble fibrous material, extracellularly in the form of senile plaques, and intracellularly in the form of neurofibrillary lesions. Alzheimer's disease is genetically heterogenous, with different primary causes leading to the same phenotype and neuropathology. It is therefore possible that the activation of several distinct pathological pathways can lead to the disease, with neuritic plaques and neurofibrillary lesions representing the points of convergence of these events. It follows that a study of the mechanisms that lead to the formation of plaques and neurofibrillary lesions is essential for an understanding of the pathogenesis of all forms of Alzheimer's disease. The formation of neurofibrillary lesions is believed to lead to the symptoms of the disease, which result most probably from the degeneration of nerve cells in cerebral cortex and hippocampal formation, with ensuing neuronal cell loss and reduction in synapse numbers.

Neurofibrillary lesions are found in nerve cell bodies and apical dendrites as neurofibrillary tangles, in distal dendrites as neuropil threads, and in abnormal neurites associated with some amyloid plaques (reviewed in refs. *1* and *2*) (Fig. 1). Ultrastructurally, all three lesions contain abnormal paired helical filaments (PHFs) as their major fibrous components and straight filaments (SFs) as their minor fibrous components *(3)* (Fig. 2). Neurofibrillary lesions develop in the vast majority of nerve cells that undergo degeneration in Alzheimer's disease. Their relative insolubility enables them to survive after the death of the affected nerve cells as extracellular tangles (or ghost tangles) that accumulate in the neuropil. These are then engulfed by astrocytes and microglial cells and are probably slowly degraded.

In the recent past, significant progress has been made in unravelling the molecular composition of PHFs and in deducing possible mechanisms that may lead to their assembly. Current evidence suggests that they are made of microtubule-associated protein τ in a hyperphosphorylated state. Moreover, earlier results indicating that the extent and topographical distribution of neurofibrillary lesions provide a reliable pathological

From: Molecular Mechanisms of Dementia *Edited by: W. Wasco and R. E. Tanzi Humana Press Inc., Totowa, NJ*

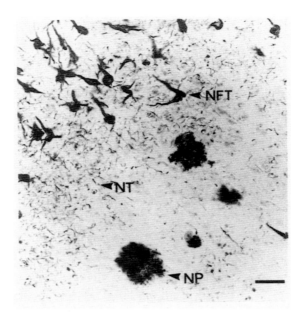

Fig. 1. Neurofibrillary pathology in the entorhinal cortex. The section was stained with an anti-τ serum. NFT, neurofibrillary tangle; NT, neuropil thread; NP, neuritic plaque. Scale bar, 100 μm.

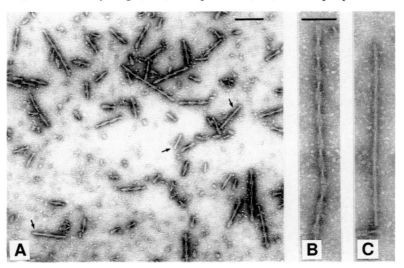

Fig. 2. Electron micrographs of negatively stained abnormal filaments from the brain of an Alzheimer's disease patient. **(A)** Low-power view showing predominantly paired helical filaments, but with a few straight filaments (arrows). **(B,C)** High-power view of a paired helical filament (B) and a straight filament (C). Scale bars: (A) 200 nm; (B,C) 100 nm.

correlate of the degree of dementia have been confirmed and extended *(4,5)*. The finding of large numbers of amyloid deposits in some cognitively normal individuals (also known as "pathological ageing") has shown that amyloid deposits are not sufficient for dementia *(6)* (Fig. 3). By contrast, large numbers of neurofibrillary lesions in hippocampus and/or cerebral cortex are accompanied by dementia (Fig. 3).

**Pathological   Alzheimer's
ageing   disease**

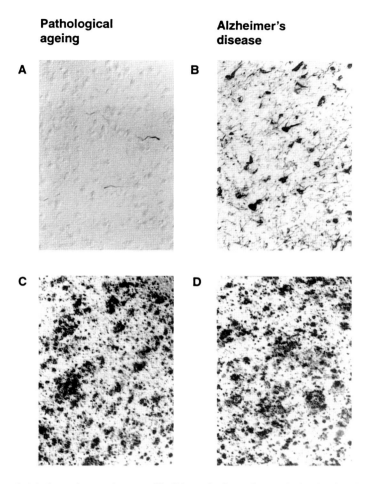

Fig. 3. Amyloid deposits and neurofibrillary lesions in pathological aging **(A,C)** and Alzheimer's disease **(B,D)**. Sections through frontal cerebral cortex were stained with an anti-τ antibody (A,B) or an anti-Aβ antibody (C,D). Note the similar density of Aβ deposits in both pathological aging and Alzheimer's disease. Note also the large number of neurofibrillary lesions in Alzheimer's disease, as well as their absence in pathological aging.

2. NEUROPATHOLOGICAL STAGES OF ALZHEIMER'S DISEASE

The development of the neurofibrillary lesions is not random, but follows a stereotyped pattern with regard to affected nerve cell types, cellular layers, and brain regions, with little individual variation. This has been used to define six neuropathological stages of Alzheimer's disease *(4)*. The very first nerve cells in the brain to develop neurofibrillary lesions are located in layer pre-α of the transentorhinal region, thus defining stage I. Stage II shows a more severe involvement of this region, as well as a mild involvement of the pre-α layer of the entorhinal cortex. Patients with this pathology are cognitively unimpaired, indicating that stages I and II may represent clinically silent stages of Alzheimer's disease. Mild impairments of cognitive function become apparent in stages III and IV. Stage III is characterized by severe neurofibrillary lesions in the pre-α layers of both entorhinal and transentorhinal regions. The vast majority of nerve cells show neurofibrillary tangles and dendritic neuropil threads. The first extracellular tangles also appear during stage III. In stage IV, the deep pre-α layer develops extensive neurofibrillary lesions. During stages III and IV, mild changes are also seen in layer I of Ammon's horn of the hippocampus and in a number of subcortical nuclei, such as the basal forebrain magnocellular nuclei and the anterodorsal thalamic nucleus. The major feature of stages V and VI is the massive development of neurofibrillary lesions in isocortical association areas. They meet the criteria for the neuropathological diagnosis of Alzheimer's disease and are found in patients who were severely demented at the time of death.

The stereotyped nature of the temporal and spatial development of neurofibrillary lesions contrasts with the development of Aβ deposits. They show a density and distribution pattern subject to great individual variation, precluding their use for the neuropathological staging of Alzheimer's disease. In general, the first Aβ deposits occur in isocortical areas of the frontal, temporal, and occipital lobes. This contrasts with the neurofibrillary lesions, which first appear in the transentorhinal region. Moreover, Aβ deposits develop relatively late in the fascia dentata of the hippocampus, the major termination area of the pre-α layer cells of the entorhinal cortex. It follows that neurofibrillary lesions in the pre-α layer can develop with no parts of these cells or their processes in contact with Aβ deposits. These findings are inconsistent with the view that the neurofibrillary pathology develops as a mere consequence of the neurotoxic action of Aβ *(7)*.

3. STRUCTURE OF THE PHF

The PHF, as its name suggests, consists of two strands of subunits that twist around one another in a helical fashion (Fig. 3). When viewed in the electron microscope, the helical twist and relative disposition of the two strands give rise to images in which the width alternates between 8 and 20 nm, with an apparent period of 80 nm *(8)*.

PHFs can be isolated either in the form of tangle fragments *(9,10)* or in the form of dispersed filaments *(11,12)*. The two types of PHFs have τ epitopes in common, but differ in their solubility in strong denaturing agents. Although a majority of dispersed PHFs are soluble in guanidine or sodium dodecyl sulfate, a majority of tangle fragment PHFs are insoluble in these reagents. Both types of PHFs differ also in their sensitivity to proteases. Pronase treatment of tangle preparations removes a fuzzy coat from the PHF and leaves behind a pronase-resistant core. The morphology of the core is similar to that of untreated PHFs, but structural details are seen more clearly because the disordered coat has been removed. From electron micrographs, it is possible to compute a map of the cross-sectional density in the core. Such maps show two C-shaped morphological units, corresponding to the two strands of the PHF, arranged in a base-to-base manner *(8)*. When dispersed filaments are treated with pronase under the same conditions, they are completely degraded *(13)*, illustrating the differing protease sensitivities of tangle fragment PHFs and of dispersed PHFs.

Straight filaments represent a minority species, both in tangle fragment and dispersed filament preparations. Images of SFs show approximately the same periodicity as PHFs, but a much less marked modulation in width *(14)* (Fig. 3). Straight filaments and PHFs share τ epitopes and behave in a similar manner when treated with pronase. Rarely, hybrid filaments are observed that show a sharp transition from a segment of

PHF into a segment of SF. This indicates that PHFs and SFs contain identical or closely related subunits that are arranged differently in the two types of filament. This is supported by the computed cross-section of the SF, which shows two C-shaped subunits very similar to those seen in the PHF, but arranged back-to-back rather than base-to-base *(14)*. The SF is thus a structural variant of the PHF in that both contain two strands of closely related or possibly identical subunits, but the relative arrangement of the two strands differs in the two kinds of filaments.

4. τ PROTEIN

τ is an abundant protein in both central and peripheral nervous systems (reviewed in ref. *15*). In brain, it is found predominantly in nerve cells, where it is concentrated in nerve cell axons *(16)*. This contrasts with the distribution of the neurofibrillary lesions in Alzheimer's disease, which are found in nerve cell bodies, dendrites, and axons. Molecular cloning has shown that multiple τ isoforms are produced from a single gene through alternative mRNA splicing *(17–19)*. In adult human brain, six isoforms are found, ranging from 352 to 441 amino acids, and differing from each other by the presence or absence of three inserts *(19,20)* (Fig. 4). The most striking feature of the τ sequences is the presence of three or four tandem repeats of 31 or 32 amino acids located in the carboxy-terminal half *(19,21)*. Experiments with recombinant τ proteins show that the repeats constitute microtubule-binding domains *(22,23)*. Microtubules assembled in the presence of τ show arms projecting from the surface *(24)*. τ thus consists of a carboxy-terminal microtubule-binding domain and an amino-terminal projection domain. In addition to being distinguished by the presence of three or four tandem repeats, some τ isoforms contain 29 or 58 amino acid inserts located near the amino-terminus (Fig. 4). Isoforms with a large additional insert in the amino-terminal half have been described in the peripheral nervous system *(25,26)*. τ is subject to developmentally regulated alternative mRNA splicing in that, in immature brain, only the transcript encoding the shortest isoform with three repeats is expressed *(19)*. The developmental shift of τ bands from a simple fetal pattern to a more complex adult pattern thus involves the transition from the expression of the isoform with three repeats and no inserts to the expression of all six isoforms.

τ is a phosphoprotein *(27)*, and phosphorylation is also developmentally regulated. Thus, τ from immature brain is phosphorylated at more sites than τ from adult brain, implying selective dephosphorylation of the shortest isoform during brain maturation. Moreover, experiments with rat brain slices have shown that τ phosphorylation in developing brain is more dynamic than in adult brain *(28)*. τ from newborn brain is phosphorylated at 13 known sites in the shortest isoform, whereas, in adult brain, it is phosphorylated at at least nine sites in all six isoforms (Fig. 5). Phosphorylation sites have been identified through the use of mass spectrometry *(29,30)* and of phosphorylation-dependent anti-τ antibodies *(1,13,31–40)*. Thus, in fetal brain, τ is phosphorylated at serine residues 198, 199, 202, 235, 262, 396, 400, 404, and 422, and at threonine residues 181, 205, 217, and 231 (according to the numbering of the longest human brain τ isoform) (Fig. 5). In adult brain, τ is phosphorylated at serine residues 199, 202, 235, 262, 396, and 404, and at threonine residues 181, 205, and 231 (Fig. 5). With the exception of Ser262, all known phosphorylation sites in τ are located outside the microtubule-binding repeat region. Phosphorylation is heterogenous, implying that a given τ

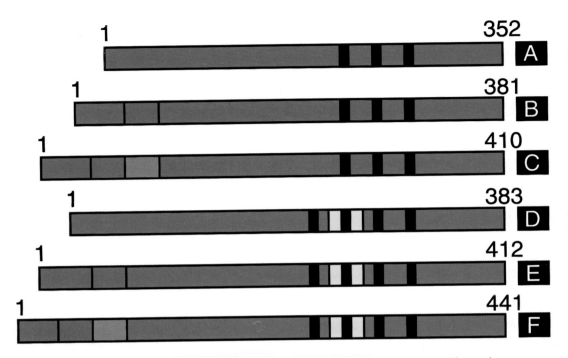

Fig. 4. Schematic representation of the six human brain τ isoforms **(A–F)**. The region common to all isoforms is shown in blue, and the inserts that distinguish them are shown in red, green, or yellow. The three (in isoforms A–C) or four (in isoforms D–F) tandem repeats are shown by black bars. The number of amino acids is indicated. The 352 amino acid isoform (A) is expressed in fetal brain, whereas all six isoforms (A–F) are expressed in adult brain.

molecule is phosphorylated at some, but not all, of these sites. Many of these sites are serine or threonine residues that are followed by a proline, suggesting that protein kinases with a specificity for seryl-proline and threonyl-proline phosphorylate τ in normal brain. Accordingly, mitogen-activated protein (MAP) kinase, glycogen synthase kinase-3 (GSK3), and cyclin-dependent kinase-5 (CDK5) phosphorylate τ at a number of the above serine/threonine-proline residues in vitro *(41–48)*. In addition, GSK3, as well as cAMP-dependent protein kinase and Ca^{2+}/calmodulin-dependent protein kinase II, phosphorylate serine residue 262 of τ in vitro, as does a 110-kDa protein kinase from brain *(41,49–51)*.

The phosphorylation state of a protein is the result of a balance between protein kinase and protein phosphatase activities. Of the major phosphatase activities present in a crude brain extract, τ phosphorylated by MAP kinase, GSK3, CDK5, or cAMP-dependent protein kinase is dephosphorylated predominantly by the trimeric form of protein phosphatase 2A *(52,53)*. The same has been shown for τ from adult human brain *(54)*. Protein phosphatase 2A has also been shown to play an important role in the dephosphorylation of τ in primary cultures of rat nerve cells, postmitotic neuron-like cells derived from a human teratocarcinoma cell line, and human neuronal cell lines *(55–58)*. Treatment of cultured rat nerve cells and postmitotic neuron-like cells with microtubule-depolymerizing agents leads to a dephosphorylation of τ *(58,59)* that is effected by protein phosphatase 2A *(58)*. The finding that a substantial proportion of

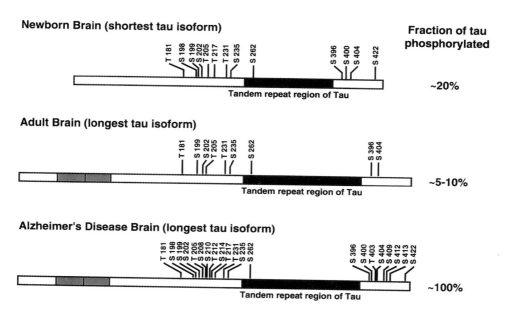

Fig. 5. Identified phosphorylation sites in τ from newborn brain, adult brain, and Alzheimer's disease brain. In newborn brain, only the shortest τ isoform is expressed, whereas six isoforms are expressed in adult human brain. In adult brain and Alzheimer's disease brain, all six τ isoforms are phosphorylated on the residues shown here for the longest isoform. The approximate fraction of τ that is phosphorylated at the sites shared between newborn brain, adult brain, and Alzheimer's disease brain is shown on the right.

the cytosolic pool of protein phosphatase 2A from a number of neuronal and nonneuronal cell lines is associated with microtubules *(60)* indicates that it is well positioned to regulate τ phosphorylation in vivo. On treatment of cultured nerve cells and postmitotic neuron-like cells with a Ca^{2+} ionophore, protein phosphatase 2B has also been shown to participate in the dephosphorylation of τ *(55,56)*. Moreover, a recent study in adult rat using chronic intraventricular infusion of okadaic acid sufficient to inhibit protein phosphatase 2A activity has shown a marked hyperphosphorylation of τ, as well as its somatodendritic localization *(59a)*. Interestingly, this treatment also led to the formation of Aβ-containing extracellular deposits *(59a)*.

5. τ FUNCTIONS

Ever since its discovery *(60a)*, τ has been known to be a potent promoter of tubulin polymerization in vitro. The binding of τ to microtubules reduces their dynamic instability *(61)*. Analysis of the dynamics of the growth of individual microtubules indicates that τ increases the rate of association and decreases the rate of dissociation of tubulin molecules at the growing end; it also inhibits the transition to the catastrophic shortening phase. Binding studies have indicated that the affinity of the 31 or 32 amino acid repeat region for microtubules is concentrated in 18 amino acid-binding elements that are separated by flexible linker sequences *(22)*. However, recent results have shown that the picture is more complex, with at least one linker region contributing significantly toward microtubule binding *(23)*. This is in keeping with the highly conserved nature of the whole repeat region between species (reviewed in ref. *15*).

τ has a similar function in vivo; when microinjected into fibroblasts, it produces an increase in microtubule mass and an increased resistance of microtubules to depolymerizing agents *(62)*. Several laboratories have transfected various τ constructs into cells that do not normally express τ. In the transfected cells, τ binds to microtubules, enhances microtubule stability and, in some cases, induces microtubule bundling *(32,63–68)*. The bundle thickness is 10–100 times that of normal microtubules, with an average distance of ~20 nm between adjacent microtubules. Bundling is probably a consequence of the microtubule stabilization effected by τ. At present, it is unclear whether microtubule bundling has a physiological correlate or whether it results from the nonphysiological overexpression of τ in some cell types. Experiments with truncated τ proteins have confirmed the critical role played by the tandem repeat region in microtubule binding; however, the inclusion of sequences flanking the repeats appears to be essential for optimal binding and bundling. In particular, the proline-rich region upstream of the repeats appears to be essential for tubulin binding in vivo; this region contains a cluster of serine/threonine-proline phosphorylation sites.

In Sf9 cells infected with a baculovirus construct, the overexpression of τ results in the extension of long and thin neurite-like extensions *(64)*. However, overexpression of τ does not invariably lead to the extension of neurite-like processes. This might be owing to different levels of expression and phosphorylation in the various cell types. Tensile forces exerted by the cortical actin network are likely to represent another factor. Thus, cells transfected with the microtubule-associated protein MAP2c only grow processes when treated with the actin depolymerizing drug cytochalasin B *(69)*.

The introduction into cultured developing cerebellar nerve cells of antisense oligonucleotides to block τ expression prevents the differentiation of the short neurites, one of which would otherwise have developed into an axon *(70)*. Similarly, τ antisense oligonucleotides produce a retraction of neurites in PC12 cells treated with nerve growth factor *(71)*. By contrast, mice with an inactivating mutation in the τ gene show normal brain development *(72)*; moreover, cultured developing cerebellar nerve cells from these animals grow a normal complement of axons and dendrites, demonstrating that τ protein is not essential for process outgrowth and axonal morphology *(72)*.

Phosphorylation negatively regulates the ability of τ to bind to microtubules. τ phosphorylated by MAP kinase has one-tenth the ability of nonphosphorylated τ to bind to microtubules *(61)*. Little is known about the relative contributions made by individual phosphorylated residues. A study using transfected cells has shown that phosphoserine 396 makes a significant contribution toward the reduced ability of τ to bind to microtubules *(32)*. This and similar approaches should permit identification of the other sites involved.

6. τ PROTEIN AND THE PHF

Protein chemistry and molecular cloning established directly that τ forms an integral component of the PHF *(9,10,18)*, thereby putting more indirect immunohistochemical studies on a solid basis *(73)*. The τ sequences obtained from pronase-treated PHFs have shown not only that both three and four repeats contribute to the core of the PHF, but that a length of protein containing only three repeats is protected *(74)*. This indicates that the amino-terminal half of τ is lost by proteolysis either *in situ* because of endog-

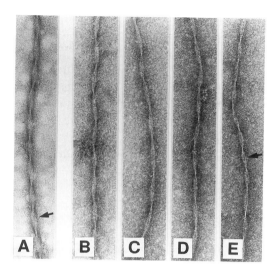

Fig. 6. PHF from the brain of an Alzheimer's disease patient and filaments assembled in vitro from a nonphosphorylated 99 amino acid fragment of τ encompassing three tandem repeats. **(A)** Pronase-treated Alzheimer's disease PHF. **(B–E)** Filaments resembling PHFs assembled from expressed τ protein. The arrows indicate regions of filament where the characteristic pattern of four white stain-excluding lines parallel to the filament axis can be seen. Scale bar, 100 nm.

enous proteases or during tangle purification because of added proteases. In Alzheimer's disease brain, the amino-terminal half and part of the carboxy-terminus of τ are lost during the transition from intra- to extracellular tangles *(75)*.

The above results were obtained using PHFs extracted from tangle fragments. Because of the insolubility of these filaments, it was not possible to conclude that τ is the only component of the PHF or to show whether there are other components. This situation changed with the development of extraction techniques for dispersed PHFs *(11)*. A study involving purification of these filaments to apparent homogeneity has provided strong evidence that τ forms the PHF *(12)*.

In addition, it has been shown that paired helical-like filaments can be assembled in vitro from bacterially expressed nonphosphorylated three-repeat fragments of τ *(76,77)* (Fig. 6). Filaments similar to PHFs were produced by dialysis or by hanging drop equilibration of the fragments against high concentrations of Tris at acidic pH. A series of filaments made from three repeats of τ are shown in Fig. 6B–E, compared with a pronase-treated PHF from an Alzheimer tangle preparation (Fig. 6A). The dimensions of the artificial filaments are very much like those of Alzheimer PHFs (Fig. 6B–E). A characteristic pattern of four longitudinal white, stain-excluding lines can also be seen. The production of artificial paired helical-like filaments lends strong support to the view that τ is the only component necessary to form the PHF. However, these results do not provide any information regarding filament formation in vivo, since they were obtained with partial τ sequences and required nonphysiological buffer conditions.

Unlike tangle fragment PHFs, a large proportion of dispersed PHFs contains the whole of τ *(12,13,78,79)*. This indicates that dispersed filaments constitute an earlier

stage of PHFs than the bulk of filaments isolated from tangle fragments. A further difference between tangle fragment and dispersed PHFs is that the majority of tangle fragment
PHFs are ubiquitinated *(80,81)*. Several lysine residues in the repeat region of τ that
ubiquitin becomes attached to have been identified, indicating that these residues are
located on the surface of the PHF *(82)*. The natural history of the PHF after assembly thus
leads from an initial guanidine-soluble intracellular form to a very insoluble, proteolyzed,
ubiquitinated, and crosslinked extracellular form, with a multitude of intermediates.

τ protein extracted from PHFs runs as three major bands of 60, 64, and 68 kDa
apparent molecular mass, with a variable amount of background smear *(11,12,83)*. The
latter results from partially proteolyzed and crosslinked PHFs. These PHF-τ bands run
more slowly on gels than normal or recombinant τ. They contain the whole of τ, as they
stain with antibodies directed against the amino- and carboxy-termini of τ. After treatment with alkaline phosphatase at high temperature, the three PHF-τ bands become six
bands that align with the recombinant τ isoforms *(13,84,85)*. The relative proportions
of the six bands are similar to those of soluble τ from adult brain. Thus, PHFs contain
all six adult brain τ isoforms in a hyperphosphorylated state. PHF-τ has a greatly reduced
ability to bind to microtubules; this functional impairment results entirely from
hyperphosphorylation, since dephosphorylated PHF-τ binds as well to microtubules,
as does normal τ *(32,86)*. The reduced binding of PHF-τ to microtubules, coupled with
reduced levels of normal τ, probably destabilizes microtubules in Alzheimer's disease,
resulting in the impairment of vital cellular processes, such as rapid axonal transport,
and leading to the degeneration of affected nerve cells

PHF-τ is both abnormally phosphorylated and hyperphosphorylated (Fig. 5). Abnormal phosphorylation means that more residues are phosphorylated in PHF-τ than in
normal brain τ, whereas hyperphosphorylation means that for a given site, a higher
proportion of τ molecules is phosphorylated in PHF-τ than in normal brain τ. To date,
a large number of these sites have been identified by mass spectrometry *(87,89)* and
through the use of phosphorylation-dependent anti-τ antibodies *(12,35–40,88)*. They
include serines 198, 199, 202, 208, 210, 214, 231, 235, 262, 396, 400, 404, 409, 412,
413, and 422 and threonines 181, 205, 212, 217, and 403 (Fig. 5). Some of these sites
are also phosphorylated in τ from developing rat brain. Although similar sites of phosphorylation were not detected in τ from adult human autopsy brain, studies of adult
human brain τ obtained from fresh cortical biopsy samples suggest that the majority of
these sites are also phosphorylated in adult human brain, but to a smaller extent than in
fetal brain *(37)*. However, a number of additional sites have been identified as phosphorylation sites in PHF-τ by mass spectrometry that have so far not been found in rapidly
isolated fetal rat τ or in biopsy-derived adult human brain τ *(89)*. It remains to be seen
whether these sites are truly abnormally phosphorylated in PHF-τ. This will depend on
the production of novel phosphorylation-dependent anti-τ antibodies and on future mass
spectrometric studies performed on rapidly isolated fetal and adult human brain τ.
AP422, which is specific for phosphoserine 422 in τ, is such a novel antibody; it
strongly recognizes PHF-τ, but is virtually unreactive with biopsy-derived adult human
brain τ, implying that Ser422 is abnormally phosphorylated in PHF-τ *(40)*. About half
of the known phosphorylation sites in PHF-τ are serine or threonine residues followed
by a proline. With the exception of Ser262, all known sites are located outside the
microtubule-binding repeat region.

These findings imply the deregulation of phosphorylation–dephosphorylation mechanisms in Alzheimer's disease. MAP kinase, GSK3, and CDK5 phosphorylate many of the hyperphosphorylated Ser/Thr-Pro sites of τ in vitro *(36,42–48,52,90)*. In the presence of heparin, GSK3 also phosphorylates the non-Ser/Thr-Pro site Ser262 *(49,50,91)*. Interestingly, MAP kinase is the only known enzyme that phosphorylates τ at Ser422, suggesting that MAP kinase or a MAP kinase-like enzyme may be involved in the abnormal phosphorylation of τ *(40)*. Cyclic AMP-dependent protein kinase phosphorylates three of the non-Ser/Thr-Pro sites (Ser214, Ser262, and Ser409), and it also phosphorylates another three sites (Ser324, Ser356, and Ser416) that have not been reported to be phosphorylated in PHF-τ *(51,92)*. Calcium/calmodulin-dependent protein kinase II phosphorylates one non-Ser/Thr-Pro site (Ser262) that is phosphorylated in PHF-τ and one site (Ser416) that has not been reported to be phosphorylated *(51,93)*. However, it is unclear whether the underlying defect results from an increased protein kinase activity, a decreased protein phosphatase activity, or a combination of both. The finding that nonassembled soluble τ is more prone to postmortem dephosphorylation than assembled PHF-τ has led to the suggestion that a reduced activity of protein phosphatases may be responsible for the hyperphosphorylation of τ in Alzheimer's disease *(37,94,95)*.

Whatever the mechanisms involved, it appears unlikely that τ is the only hyperphosphorylated protein. In affected nerve cells, PHFs probably constitute the most visible manifestation of the deregulation of phosphorylation/dephosphorylation mechanisms at Ser/Thr-Pro sites and at non-Ser/Thr-Pro sites. Normal brain function might be disrupted by the hyperphosphorylation of proteins that are not normally phosphorylated to such an extent in vivo. The degree of phosphorylation is the only known difference between PHF-τ and normal adult τ, with almost all of the hyperphosphorylated sites located outside the tandem repeat region. As a consequence, τ is prevented from binding to microtubules and is believed to self-assemble through the tandem repeat region into the PHF.

Studies demonstrating a correlation between the abundance of neurofibrillary lesions and dementia in Alzheimer's disease have prompted recent efforts to measure cerebrospinal fluid (CSF) levels of τ by enzyme-linked immunosorbant assay (ELISA) in Alzheimer's disease patients and controls *(96–101)*. The overwhelming consensus that has emerged from these studies is that the levels of CSF-τ are significantly elevated in Alzheimer's disease patients when compared with normal elderly controls. Although elevated CSF-τ levels were also detected in some patients with acute neurological conditions (such as encephalitis and stroke), these diseases can be readily distinguished from Alzheimer's disease on clinical grounds. It remains to be seen whether CSF-τ levels will permit a distinction between Alzheimer's disease and other disorders with τ pathology. Although additional research is needed to confirm and extend these findings, the results reported to date suggest that CSF-τ levels may provide an objective antemortem diagnostic test for Alzheimer's disease. Thus, measurement of τ levels (alone or in conjunction with other CSF proteins, such as Aβ, secreted APP, certain proteases, protein kinases, protein phosphatases, and so forth) in multiple CSF samples from the same patient at periodic intervals may yield powerful new strategies for monitoring the progression of Alzheimer's disease and the response to novel therapeutic agents.

7. OUTLOOK

Over the recent past, the molecular nature of the PHF has been largely understood, with some hints regarding what may lead to its formation. However, at present, we have only a very partial understanding of the mechanisms that lead to the phosphorylation of τ in normal brain and to its hyperphosphorylation in Alzheimer's disease. We also fail to understand the mechanisms that govern filament assembly, and we do not know whether hyperphosphorylation of τ is causally related to PHF assembly.

The earliest known change in the events that lead to the neurofibrillary lesions of Alzheimer's disease is the appearance of hyperphosphorylated τ protein in a pretangle stage within individual nerve cells in the transentorhinal cortex *(102)*. This probably results in the inability of τ to bind to microtubules within affected nerve cells, followed by its assembly into the PHF. This sequence of events puts hyperphosphorylation of τ before PHF assembly; however, it does not imply that hyperphosphorylation is the immediate cause of filament formation. Hyperphosphorylation may only be responsible for the inability of τ to bind to microtubules, thereby permitting it to accumulate within affected nerve cells. Other cellular components may be required for the nucleation of filament assembly. This is borne out by the relative ease with which it is possible to demonstrate the reduced ability of phosphorylated τ to bind to microtubules in vitro and by the impossibility (so far) to form bona fide PHFs from full-length hyperphosphorylated recombinant τ. Hyperphosphorylation of τ may thus be necessary, but not sufficient for PHF formation.

The majority of phosphorylated sites in normal brain τ and PHF-τ have been identified by mass spectrometry and the use of phosphorylation-dependent anti-τ antibodies. This has provided the necessary baseline for identifying protein kinases and protein phosphatases that regulate the phosphorylation state of τ. Thus, several candidate enzymes have been described that phosphorylate τ at some of the relevant sites in vitro. Similarly, apolipoprotein E3 has been shown to bind to recombinant τ, but not to phosphorylated τ in vitro, resulting in the proposal that it may modulate the rate at which τ becomes hyperphosphorylated in Alzheimer's disease brain *(103)*. However, all these studies suffer from the inherent limitation that in vitro studies are not necessarily representative of the in vivo situation.

The next step must therefore be to relate these in vitro findings to the in vivo situation. At first sight, one way to achieve this would be to compare protein kinase and protein phosphatase activities in Alzheimer's disease brain with those in control brain. Unfortunately, such an undertaking is hampered by the limited postmortem stability of protein kinase and protein phosphatase activities. An additional drawback is that, in a given piece of brain, the percentage of cells affected by the neurofibrillary pathology is only a fraction of those expressing the various enzymes, thereby rendering the interpretation of tissue homogenate measurements of enzyme activities doubtful. One way forward may be to use the information gained from in vitro studies in order to induce hyperphosphorylation of τ in intact cells and in animal brain. Studies on intact cells have already shown that overexpression of GSK3 results in hyperphosphorylation of τ *(104,105)*.

Transgenic animal technology and gene targeting are likely to play increasingly important roles in the investigation into the neurofibrillary lesions of Alzheimer's disease. One could in principle upregulate τ phosphorylation by overexpressing candidate

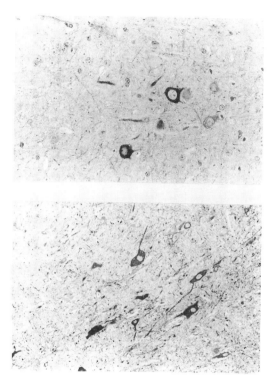

Fig. 7. Immunohistochemical staining of human τ in the brain of a mouse transgenic for the longest human brain τ isoform. The anti-τ serum 133 was used. Upper picture: section through the cerebral cortex. Lower picture: section through the brainstem. Note the strong somatodendritic staining of some nerve cells; it resembles the pretangle lesions of Alzheimer's disease.

protein kinases in nerve cells or by producing animals that lack protein phosphatases that are involved in the dephosphorylation of τ. We have taken a step in that direction by producing transgenic mice that express the longest human brain τ isoform under control of the human Thy1 promoter *(106)*. These animals show prominent axonal and somatodendritic staining of human τ in a subset of nerve cells in a number of brain regions, including cerebral cortex and hippocampal formation (Fig. 7), thereby reproducing the abnormal cellular localization of τ that is observed in Alzheimer's disease brain. Moreover, transgenic human τ is phosphorylated at some of the same sites that are hyperphosphorylated in PHF-τ. Although PHFs have not yet been detected, the transgenic human τ protein shows pretangle changes similar to those that precede the full neurofibrillary pathology of Alzheimer's disease. The hope is that these and similar approaches will result in a true animal model for the neurofibrillary lesions. It represents an essential requirement for the testing of compounds aimed at halting or preventing the intracellular pathology of Alzheimer's disease.

ACKNOWLEDGMENT

We thank D.W. Dickson for Fig. 3.

REFERENCES

1. Goedert, M. (1993) Tau protein and the neurofibrillary pathology of Alzheimer's disease, *Trends Neurosci.* **16**, 460–465.
2. Lee, V. M.-Y. (1995) Disruption of the cytoskeleton in Alzheimer's disease, *Curr. Opinion Neurobiol.* **5**, 663–668.
3. Kidd, M. (1963) Paired helical filaments in electron microscopy of Alzheimer's disease, *Nature* **197**, 192,193.
4. Braak, H. and Braak, E. (1991) Neuropathological stageing of Alzheimer-related changes, *Acta Neuropathol.* **82**, 239–259.
5. Arriagada, P. V., Growdon, J. H., Hedley-White, E. T., and Hyman, B. T. (1992) Neurofibrillary tangles but not senile plaques parallel duration and severity of Alzheimer's disease, *Neurology* **42**, 631–639.
6. Dickson, D. W., Crystal, H. A., Mattiace, L. A., Masur, D. M., Blau, A. D., Davies, P., Yen, S.-H., and Aronson, M. K. (1991) Identification of normal and pathological aging in prospectively studied non-demented elderly humans, *Neurobiol. Aging* **13**, 179–189.
7. Kowall, N. W., Beal, M. F., Busciglio, J., Duffy, L. K., and Yankner, B. A. (1991) An in vivo model for the neurodegenerative effects of β-amyloid and protection by substance P, *Proc. Natl. Acad. Sci. USA* **88**, 7247–7251.
8. Crowther, R. A. and Wischik, C. M. (1985) Image reconstruction of the Alzheimer paired helical filament, *EMBO J.* **4**, 3661–3665.
9. Wischik, C. M., Novak, M., Thogersen, H. C., Edwards, P. C., Runswick, M. J., Jakes, R., Walker, J. E., Milstein, C., Roth, M., and Klug, A. (1988) Isolation of a fragment of tau derived from the core of the paired helical filament of Alzheimer disease, *Proc. Natl. Acad. Sci. USA* **85**, 4506–4510.
10. Kondo, J., Honda, T., Mori, H., Hamada, Y., Miura, R., Ogawara, H., and Ihara, Y. (1988) The carboxyl third of tau is tightly bound to paired helical filaments, *Neuron* **1**, 827–834.
11. Greenberg, S. G. and Davies, P. (1990) A preparation of Alzheimer paired helical filaments that displays distinct tau proteins by polyacrylamide gel electrophoresis, *Proc. Natl. Acad. Sci. USA* **87**, 5827–5831.
12. Lee, V. M.-Y., Balin, B. J., Otvos, L., and Trojanowski, J. Q. (1991) A68—a major subunit of paired helical filaments and derivatized forms of normal tau, *Science* **251**, 675–678.
13. Goedert, M., Spillantini, M. G., Cairns, N. J., and Crowther, R. A. (1992) Tau proteins of Alzheimer paired helical filaments: Abnormal phosphorylation of all six brain isoforms, *Neuron* **8**, 159–168.
14. Crowther, R. A. (1991) Straight and paired helical filaments in Alzheimer disease have a common structural unit, *Proc. Natl. Acad. Sci. USA* **88**, 2288–2292.
15. Goedert, M., Jakes, R., Spillantini, M. G., and Crowther, R. A. (1994) Tau protein and Alzheimer's disease, in Microtubules (Hyams, J. S. and Lloyd, C. W., eds.), Wiley-Liss, New York, pp. 183–200.
16. Binder, L. I., Frankfurter, A., and Rebhun, L. I. (1985) The distribution of tau in the mammalian central nervous system, *J. Cell Biol.* **101**, 1371–1378.
17. Lee, G., Cowan, N., and Kirschner, M. (1988) The primary structure and heterogeneity of tau protein from mouse brain, *Science* **239**, 285–288.
18. Goedert, M., Wischik, C. M., Crowther, R. A., Walker, J. E., and Klug, A. (1988) Cloning and sequencing of the cDNA encoding a core protein of the paired helical filament of Alzheimer disease, *Proc. Natl. Acad. Sci. USA* **85**, 4051–4055.
19. Goedert, M., Spillantini, M. G., Jakes, R., Rutherford, D., and Crowther, R. A. (1989) Multiple isoforms of human microtubule-associated protein tau. Sequences and localization in neurofibrillary tangles of Alzheimer's disease, *Neuron* **3**, 519–526.
20. Goedert, M. and Jakes, R. (1990) Expression of separate isoforms of human tau protein: Correlation with the tau pattern in brain and effects on tubulin polymerization, *EMBO J.* **9**, 4225–4230.

21. Goedert, M., Spillantini, M. G., Potier, M. C., Ulrich, J., and Crowther, R. A. (1989) Cloning and sequencing of the cDNA encoding an isoform of microtubule-associated protein tau containing four tandem repeats: Differential expression of tau protein mRNAs in human brain, *EMBO J.* **8**, 393–399.

22. Butner, K. A. and Kirschner, M. W. (1991) Tau protein binds to microtubules through a flexible array of distributed weak sites, *J. Cell Biol.* **115**, 717–730.

23. Goode, B. L. and Feinstein, S. C. (1994) Identification of a novel microtubule binding and assembly domain in the developmentally regulated inter-repeat region of tau, *J. Cell Biol.* **124**, 769–782.

24. Hirokawa, N., Shiomura, Y., and Ogabe, S. (1988) Tau proteins: The molecular structure and mode of binding on microtubules, *J. Cell Biol.* **107**, 1449–1459.

25. Goedert, M., Spillantini, M. G., and Crowther, R. A. (1992) Cloning of a big tau microtubule-associated protein characteristic of the peripheral nervous system, *Proc. Natl. Acad. Sci. USA* **89**, 4378–4381.

26. Couchie, D., Mavilia, C., Georgieff, I. S., Liem, R. K. H., Shelanski, M. L., and Nunez, J. (1992) Primary structure of high molecular weight tau present in the peripheral nervous system, *Proc. Natl. Acad. Sci. USA* **89**, 4378–4381.

27. Butler, M. and Shelanski, M. L. (1986) Microheterogeneity of microtubule-associated tau protein is due to differences in phosphorylation, *J. Neurochem.* **47**, 1517–1522.

28. Burack, M. A. and Halpain, S. (1996) Site-specific regulation of Alzheimer-like tau phosphorylation in living neurons, *Neuroscience* **72**, 167–184.

29. Poulter, L., Barratt, D., Scott, C. W., and Caputo, C. B. (1993) Locations and immunoreactivities of phosphorylation sites on bovine and porcine tau proteins and a PHF-tau fragment, *J. Biol. Chem.* **268**, 9636–9644.

30. Watanabe, A., Hasegawa, M., Suzuki, M., Takio, K., Morishima-Kawashima, M., Titani, K., Arai, T., Kosik, K. S., and Ihara, Y. (1993) In vivo phosphorylation sites in fetal and adult rat tau, *J. Biol. Chem.* **268**, 25,712–25,717.

31. Kanemura, K., Takio, K., Miura, R., Titani, K., and Ihara, Y. (1992) Fetal-type phosphorylation of the tau in paired helical filaments, *J. Neurochem.* **58**, 1667–1675.

32. Bramblett, G. T., Goedert, M., Jakes, R., Merrick, S. E., Trojanowski, J. Q., and Lee, V. M.-Y. (1993) Abnormal tau phosphorylation at Ser^{396} in Alzheimer's disease recapitulates development and contributes to reduced microtubule binding, *Neuron* **10**, 1089–1099.

33. Kenessey, A. and Yen, S.-H. C. (1993) The extent of phosphorylation of fetal tau is comparable to that of PHF-tau from Alzheimer paired helical filaments, *Brain Res.* **629**, 40–46.

34. Brion, J. P., Smith, C., Couck, A. M., Gallo, J. M., and Anderton, B. H. (1993) Developmental changes in tau phosphorylation: fetal tau is transiently phosphorylated in a manner similar to paired helical filament tau characteristic of Alzheimer's disease, *J. Neurochem.* **61**, 2071–2080.

35. Hasegawa, M., Watanabe, A., Takio, K., Suzuki, M., Arai, T., Titani, K., and Ihara, Y. (1993) Characterization of two distinct monoclonal antibodies to paired helical filaments: further evidence for fetal-type phosphorylation of the tau in paired helical filaments, *J. Neurochem.* **60**, 2068–2077.

36. Goedert, M., Jakes, R., Crowther, R. A., Cohen, P., Vanmechelen, E., Vandermeeren, M., and Cras, P. (1994) Epitope mapping of monoclonal antibodies to the paired helical filaments of Alzheimer's disease: identification of phosphorylation sites in tau protein, *Biochem. J.* **301**, 871–877.

37. Matsuo, E. S., Shin, R.-W., Bilingsley, M. L., Van de Voorde, A., O'Connor, M., Trojanowski, J. Q., and Lee, V. M.-Y. (1994) Biopsy-derived adult human brain tau is phosphorylated at many of the same sites as Alzheimer's disease paired helical filament tau, *Neuron* **13**, 989–1002.

37a. Otvos, L., Feiner, L., Lang, E., Szendrei, G. I., Goedert, M., and Lee, V. M.-Y. (1994) Monoclonal antibody PHF-1 recognizes tau protein phosphorylated at serine residues 396 and 404, *J. Neurosci. Res.* **39**, 669–673.

38. Seubert, P., Mawal-Dewan, M., Barbour, R., Jakes, R., Goedert, M., Johnson, G. V. W., Litersky, J. M., Schenk, D., Lieberburg, I., Trojanowski, J. Q., and Lee, V. M.-Y. (1995) Detection of phosphorylated Ser^{262} in fetal tau, adult tau and paired helical filament tau, *J. Biol. Chem.* **270,** 18,917–18,922.

38a. Goedert, M., Jakes, R., and Vanmechelen, E. (1995) Monoclonal antibody AT8 recognises tau protein phosphorylated at both serine 202 and threonine 205, *Neurosci. Lett.* **189,** 167–170.

39. Ishiguro, K., Sato, K., Takamatsu, M., Park, J., Uchida, T., and Imahori, K. (1995) Analysis of phosphorylation of tau with antibodies specific for phosphorylation sites, *Neurosci. Lett.* **202,** 81–84.

40. Hasegawa, M., Jakes, R., Crowther, R. A., Lee, V. M.-Y., Ihara, Y., and Goedert, M. (1996) Characterization of mAb AP422, a novel phosphorylation-dependent monoclonal antibody against tau protein, *FEBS Lett.* **384,** 25–30.

41. Drewes, G., Trinczek, B., Illenberger, S., Biernat, J., Schmitt-Ulms, G., Meyer, H. E., Mandelkow, E. M., and Mandelkow, E. (1995) Microtubule-associated protein/microtubule affinity-regulating kinase (p110^{mark}), *J. Biol. Chem.* **270,** 7679–7688.

42. Ledesma, M. D., Correas, I., Avila, J., and Diaz-Nido, J. (1992) Implication of brain cdc2 and MAP2 kinases in the phosphorylation of tau in Alzheimer's disease, *FEBS Lett.* **308,** 218–224.

43. Hanger, D. P., Hughes, K., Woodgett, J. R., Brion, J. P., and Anderton, B. H. (1992) Glycogen synthase kinase-3 induces Alzheimer's disease-like phosphorylation of tau: Generation of paired helical filament epitopes and neuronal localization of the kinase, *Neurosci. Lett.* **147,** 58–62.

44. Mandelkow, E. M., Drewes, G., Biernat, J., Gustke, N., Van Lint, J., Vandenheede, J. R., and Mandelkow, E. (1992) Glycogen synthase kinase-3 and the Alzheimer-like state of microtubule-associated protein tau, *FEBS Lett.* **314,** 315–321.

45. Ishiguro, K., Shiratsuchi, A., Sato, S., Omori, A., Arioka, M., Kobayashi, S., Uchida, T., and Imahori, K. (1993) Glycogen synthase kinase-3β is identical to tau protein kinase I generating several epitopes of paired helical filaments, *FEBS Lett.* **325,** 167–172.

46. Paudel, H. K., Lew, J., Zenobia, A., and Wang, J. H. (1993) Brain proline-directed kinase phosphorylates tau on sites that are abnormally phosphorylated in tau associated with Alzheimer's paired helical filaments, *J. Biol. Chem.* **268,** 23,512–23,518.

47. Kobayashi, S., Ishiguro, K., Omori, A., Takamatsu, M., Arioka, M., Imahori, K., and Uchida, T. (1993) A cdc2-related kinase PSSALRE/cdk5 is homologous with the 30 kDa subunit of tau protein kinase II, a proline-directed protein kinase associated with microtubules, *FEBS Lett.* **335,** 171–175.

48. Baumann, K., Mandelkow, E. M., Biernat, J., Piwnica-Worms, H., and Mandelkow, E. (1993) Abnormal Alzheimer's-like phosphorylation of tau protein by cyclin-dependent kinases cdk2 and cdk5, *FEBS Lett.* **336,** 417–424.

49. Yang, S.-D., Yu, J.-S., Shiah, S.-G., and Huang, J.-J. (1994) Protein kinase F$_A$/glycogen synthase kinase-3 alpha after heparin potentiation phosphorylates tau on sites abnormally phosphorylated in Alzheimer's disease brain, *J. Neurochem.* **63,** 1416–1425.

50. Moreno, F. J., Medina, M., Pérez, M., Montejo de Garcini, E., and Avila, J. (1995) Glycogen synthase kinase-3 phosphorylates recombinant human tau protein at serine-262 in the presence of heparin (or tubulin), *FEBS Lett.* **372,** 65–68.

51. Litersky, J. M., Johnson, G. V. W., Jakes, R., Goedert, M., Lee, M., and Seubert, P. (1996) Tau protein is phosphorylated by cAMP-dependent protein kinase and calcium/calmodulin-dependent protein kinase II within its microtubule-binding domains at Ser^{262} and Ser^{356}, *Biochem. J.* **316,** 655–660.

52. Goedert, M., Cohen, E. S., Jakes, R., and Cohen, P. (1992) p42 MAP kinase phosphorylation sites in microtubule-associated protein tau are dephosphorylated by protein phosphatase 2A$_1$. Implications for Alzheimer's disease, *FEBS Lett.* **312,** 95–99.

53. Goedert, M., Jakes, R., Qi, Z., Wang, J. H., and Cohen, P. (1995) Protein phosphatase 2A is the major enzyme in brain that dephosphorylates tau protein phosphorylated by proline-directed protein kinases or cAMP-dependent protein kinase, *J. Neurochem.* **65**, 2804–2807.

54. Szücs, K., Ledesma, M. D., Dombradi, V., Gergely, P., Avila, J., and Friedrich, P. (1994) Dephosphorylation of tau protein from Alzheimer's disease patients, *Neurosci. Lett.* **165**, 175–178.

55. Fleming, L. M. and Johnson, G. V. W. (1995) Modulation of the phosphorylation state of tau in situ: the roles of calcium and cyclic AMP, *Biochem. J.* **309**, 41–47.

56. Saito, T., Ishiguro, K., Uchida, T., Miyamoto, E., Kishimoto, T., and Hisanaga, S.-I. (1995) In situ dephosphorylation of tau by protein phosphatase 2A and 2B in fetal rat primary cultured neurons, *FEBS Lett.* **376**, 238–242.

57. Dupont-Wallois, L., Sautiere, P. E., Cocquerelle, C., Bailleul, B., Delacourte, A., and Caillet-Boudin, M. L. (1995) Shift from fetal-type to Alzheimer-type phosphorylated tau proteins in SKNSH-SY5Y cells treated with okadaic acid, *FEBS Lett.* **357**, 197–201.

58. Merrick, S. E., Demoise, D. C., and Lee, V. M.-Y. (1996) Site-specific dephosphorylation of tau protein at Ser/Thr 202/205 in response to microtubule depolymerization in cultured human neurons involves protein phosphatase 2A, *J. Biol. Chem.* **271**, 5589–5594.

59. Davis, D. A., Brion, J. P., Couck, A. M., Gallo, J. M., Hanger, D. P., Ladhani, K., Lewis, C., Miller, C. C. J., Rupniak, T., Smith, C., and Anderton, B. H. (1995) The phosphorylation state of the microtubule-associated protein tau as affected by glutamate, colchicine and β-amyloid in primary rat cortical neuronal cultures, *Biochem. J.* **309**, 941–949.

59a. Arendt, T., Holzer, M., Fruth, R., Brückner, M. K., and Gärtner, U. (1995) Paired helical filament-like phosphorylation of tau, deposition of β/A4-amyloid and memory impairment in rat induced by chronic inhibition of phosphatase 1 and 2A, *Neuroscience* **69**, 691–698.

60. Sontag, E., Nunbhadki-Craig, V., Bloom, G. S., and Mumby, M. C. (1995) A novel pool of protein phosphatase 2A is associated with microtubules and is regulated during the cell cycle, *J. Cell Biol.* **128**, 1131–1144.

60a. Weingarten, M. D., Lockwood, A. H., Hwo, S.-H., and Kirschner, M. W. (1975) A protein factor essential for microtubule assembly, *Proc. Natl. Acad. Sci. USA* **72**, 1858–1862.

61. Drechsel, D. N., Hyman, A. A., Cobb, M. H., and Kirschner, M. W. (1992) Modulation of the dynamic instability of tubulin assembly by the microtubule-associated protein tau, *Mol. Cell. Biol.* **3**, 1141–1154.

62. Drubin, D. G. and Kirschner, M. W. (1986) Tau protein function in living cells, *J. Cell Biol.* **103**, 2739–2746.

63. Kanai, Y., Takemura, R., Oshima, T., Mori, H., Ihara, Y., Yanagisawa, M., Masaki, T., and Hirokawa, N. (1989) Expression of multiple tau isoforms and microtubule bundle formation in fibroblasts transfected with a single tau cDNA, *J. Cell Biol.* **109**, 1173–1184.

64. Knops, J., Kosik, K. S., Lee, G., Pardee, J. D., Cohen-Gould, L., and McColongue, L. (1991) Overexpression of tau in a nonneuronal cell induces long cellular processes, *J. Cell Biol.* **114**, 725–733.

65. Lee, G. and Rook, S. L. (1992) Expression of tau protein in non-neuronal cells: Microtubule binding and stabilization, *J. Cell Sci.* **102**, 227–237.

66. Gallo, J. M., Hanger, D. P., Twist, E. C., Kosik, K. S., and Anderton, B. H. (1992) Expression and phosphorylation of a three-repeat isoform of tau in transfected non-neuronal cells, *Biochem. J.* **286**, 399–404.

67. Kanai, Y., Chen, J., and Hirokawa, N. (1992) Microtubule bundling by tau proteins in vivo: Analysis of functional domains, *EMBO J.* **11**, 3953–3961.

68. Lo, M. M. S., Fieles, A. W., Norris, T. E., Dargis, D. G., Caputo, C. B., Scott, C. W., Lee, V. M.-Y., and Goedert, M. (1993) Human tau isoforms confer distinct morphological and functional properties to stably transfected fibroblasts, *Mol. Brain Res.* **20**, 209–220.

69. Edson, K., Weisshaar, B., and Matus, A. (1993) Actin depolymerisation induces process formation in MAP2-transfected neuronal cells, *Development* **117,** 689–700.
70. Caceres, A. and Kosik, K. S. (1990) Inhibition of neurite polarity by tau antisense oligonucleotides in primary cerebellar neurons, *Nature* **343,** 461–463.
71. Hanemaaijer, R. and Ginzburg, I. (1991) Involvement of mature tau isoforms in the stabilization of neurites in PC12 cells, *J. Neurosci. Res.* **30,** 163–171.
72. Harada, A., Oguchi, K., Okabe, S., Kuno, J., Tereda, S., Ohshima, T., Sato-Yoshitake, R., Takei, Y., Noda, T., and Hirokawa, N. (1994) Altered microtubule organization in small-calibre axons of mice lacking tau protein, *Nature* **369,** 488–491.
73. Brion, J. P., Passareiro, H., Nunez, J., and Flament-Durand, J. (1985) Mise en évidence immunologique de la protéine tau au niveau des lésions de dégénérescence neurofibrillaire de la maladie d'Alzheimer, *Arch. Biol. (Bruxelles)* **95,** 229–235.
74. Jakes, R., Novak, M., Davison, M., and Wischik, C. M. (1991) Identification of 3- and 4-repeat tau isoforms within the PHF in Alzheimer's disease, *EMBO J.* **10,** 2725–2729.
75. Bondareff, W., Wischik, C. M., Novak, M., Amos, W. B., Klug, A., and Roth, M. (1990) Molecular analysis of neurofibrillary degeneration in Alzheimer's disease: an immunohistochemical study, *Am. J. Pathol.* **37,** 711–723.
76. Wille, H., Drewes, G., Biernat, J., Mandelkow, E. M., and Mandelkow, E. (1992) Alzheimer-like paired helical filaments and antiparallel dimers formed from microtubule-associated protein tau in vitro, *J. Cell Biol.* **118,** 573–584.
77. Crowther, R. A., Olesen, O. F., Jakes, R., and Goedert, M. (1992) The microtubule-binding repeats of tau protein assemble into filaments like those found in Alzheimer's disease, *FEBS Lett.* **309,** 199–202.
78. Ksiezak-Reding, H. and Yen, S.-H. (1991) Structural stability of paired helical filaments requires microtubule-binding domains of tau: A model for self-association, *Neuron* **6,** 717–728.
79. Brion, J. P., Hanger, D. P., Bruce, M. T., Couck, A. M., Flament-Durand, J., and Anderton, B. H. (1991) Tau in Alzheimer neurofibrillary tangles: N- and C-terminal regions are differentially associated with paired helical filaments and the location of a putative abnormal phosphorylation site, *Biochem. J.* **273,** 127–133.
80. Mori, H., Kondo, J., and Ihara, Y. (1987) Ubiquitin is a component of paired helical filaments in Alzheimer's disease, *Science* **315,** 1641–1644.
81. Perry, G., Friedman, R., Shaw, G., and Chau, V. (1987) Ubiquitin is detected in neurofibrillary tangles and senile plaque neurites of Alzheimer disease brains, *Proc. Natl. Acad. Sci. USA* **84,** 3033–3036.
82. Morishima-Kawashima, M., Hasegawa, M., Takio, K., Suzuki, M., Titani, K., and Ihara, Y. (1993) Ubiquitin is conjugated with amino-terminally processed tau in paired helical filaments, *Neuron* **10,** 1151–1160.
83. Flament, S., Delacourte, A., Hémon, B., and Défossez, A. (1989) Characterization of two pathological tau protein variants in Alzheimer's disease, *J. Neurol. Sci.* **92,** 133–141.
84. Greenberg, S. G., Davies, P., Schein, J. D., and Binder, L. I. (1992) Hydrofluoric acid-treated tau PHF proteins display the same biochemical properties as normal tau, *J. Biol. Chem.* **267,** 564–569.
85. Liu, W.-K., Dickson, D. W., and Yen, S.-H. (1993) Heterogeneity of tau proteins in Alzheimer's disease, *Am. J. Pathol.* **142,** 387–394.
86. Yoshida, H. and Ihara, Y. (1993) Tau in paired helical filament is functionally distinct from fetal tau: assembly incompetence of paired helical filament tau, *J. Neurochem.* **61,** 1183–1186.
87. Hasegawa, M., Morishima-Kawashima, M., Takio, K., Suzuki, M., Titani, K., and Ihara, Y. (1992) Protein sequence and mass spectrometric analyses of tau in the Alzheimer's disease brain, *J. Biol. Chem.* **267,** 17,047–17,054.
88. Goedert, M., Jakes, R., Crowther, R. A., Six, J., Lübke, U., Vandermeeren, M., Cras, P., Trojanowski, J. Q., and Lee, V. M.-Y. (1993) The abnormal phosphorylation of tau protein

at serine 202 in Alzheimer disease recapitulates phosphorylation during development, *Proc. Natl. Acad. Sci. USA* **90**, 5066–5070.

89. Morishima-Kawashima, M., Hasegawa, M., Takio, K., Suzuki, M., Yoshida, H., Titani, K., and Ihara, Y. (1995) Proline-directed and non-proline-directed phosphorylation of PHF-tau, *J. Biol. Chem.* **270**, 823–829.

90. Drewes G., Lichtenberg-Kraag, B., Döring, F., Mandelkow, E. M., Biernat, J., Dorée, M., and Mandelkow, E. (1992) Mitogen-activated protein (MAP) kinase transforms tau protein into an Alzheimer-like state, *EMBO J.* **11**, 2131–2138.

91. Yang, S.-D., Song, J.-S., Yu, J. S., and Shiah, S.-G. (1993) Protein kinase Fa/GSK-3 phosphorylates τ on Sen^{235}-Pro and Sen^{424}-Pro that are abnormally phosphorylated in Alzheimer's disease brain, *J. Neurochem.* **61**, 1742–1747.

92. Scott, C. W., Spreen, R. C., Herman, J. L., Chow, F. P., Davison, M. D., Young, J., and Caputo, C. B. (1993) Phosphorylation of recombinant tau by cAMP-dependent protein kinase, *J. Biol. Chem.* **268**, 1166–1173.

93. Steiner, B., Mandelkow, E. M., Biernat, J., Gustke, N., Meyer, H. E., Schmidt, B., Mieskes, G., Söling, H. D., Drechsel, D., Kirschner, M. W., Goedert, M., and Mandelkow, E. (1990) Phosphorylation of microtubule-associated protein tau: Identification of the site for Ca^{2+}/calmodulin-dependent kinase and relationship with tau phosphorylation in Alzheimer tangles, *EMBO J.* **9**, 3539–3544.

94. Mawal-Dewan, M., Henley, J., Van de Voorde, A., Trojanowski, J. Q., and Lee, V. M.-Y. (1994) The phosphorylation state of tau in the developing brain is regulated by phosphoprotein phosphatases, *J. Biol. Chem.* **269**, 30,981–30,987.

95. Trojanowski, J. Q. and Lee, V. M.-Y. (1995) Phosphorylation of paired helical filament tau in Alzheimer's disease neurofibrillary lesions: focusing on phosphatases, *FASEB J.* **9**, 1570–1576.

96. Vandermeeren, M., Mercken, M., Vanmechelen, E., Six, J., Van de Voorde, A., Martin, J. J., and Cras, P. (1993) Detection of tau proteins in normal and Alzheimer's disease cerebrospinal fluid with a sensitive sandwich enzyme-linked immunosorbent assay, *J. Neurochem.* **61**, 1828–1834.

97. Hock, C., Golombowski, S., Naser, W., and Mueller-Spahn, F. (1995) Increased levels of tau in cerebrospinal fluid of patients with Alzheimer's disease—correlation with degree of cognitive impairment, *Ann. Neurol.* **183**, 43–45.

98. Jensen, M., Basum, H., and Lannfelt, L. (1995) Increased cerebrospinal fluid tau in patients with Alzheimer's disease, *Neurosci. Lett.* **186**, 189–191.

99. Mori, H., Hosoda, K., Matsubara, E., Nakamoto, T., Furiya, Y., Endoh, R., Usami, M., Shoji, M., and Maruyama, S. (1995) Tau in cerebrospinal fluid: establishment of the sandwich ELISA with antibody specific to the repeat sequence in tau, *Neurosci. Lett.* **186**, 181–183.

100. Vigo-Pelfrey, C., Seubert, P., Barbour, R., Blomquist, C., Lee, M., Lee, D., Coria, F., Chang, L., Miller, B., Lieberburg, I., and Schenk, D. (1995) Elevation of microtubule-associated protein tau in the cerebrospinal fluid of patients with Alzheimer's disease, *Neurology* **45**, 788–793.

101. Arai, H., Terajima, M., Miura, M., Higuchi, S., Muramatsu, T., Machida, N., Seki, H., Takase, S., Clark, C. M., Lee, V. M.-Y., Trojanowski, J. Q., and Sasaki, H. (1995) Tau in cerebrospinal fluid: a potential diagnostic marker in Alzheimer's disease, *Ann. Neurol.* **38**, 649–652.

102. Braak, E., Braak, H., and Mandelkow, E. M. (1994) A sequence of cytoskeleton changes related to the formation of neurofibrillary tangles and neuropil threads, *Acta Neuropathol.* **87**, 554–567.

103. Strittmatter, W. J., Saunders, A. M., Goedert, M., Weisgraber, K. H., Dong, L.-M., Jakes, R., Huang, D. Y., Pericak-Vance, M., Schmechel, D., and Roses, A. D. (1994) Isoform-specific interactions of apolipoprotein E with microtubule-associated protein tau: Implications for Alzheimer disease, *Proc. Natl. Acad. Sci.* **91**, 11,183–11,186.

104. Lovestone, S., Reynolds, C. H., Latimer, D., Davis, D. R., Anderton, B. H., Gallo, J. M., Hanger, D., Mulot, S., Marquardt, B., Stabel, S., Woodgett, J. R., and Miller, C. C. J. (1994)

Alzheimer's disease-like phosphorylation of the microtubule-associated protein tau by glycogen synthase kinase-3 in transfected mammalian cells, *Curr. Biol.* **4,** 1077–1086.

105. Sperber, B. R., Leight, S., Goedert, M., and Lee, V. M.-Y. (1995) Glycogen synthase kinase-3β phosphorylates tau protein at multiple sites in intact cells, *Neurosci. Lett.* **197,** 149–153.

106. Götz, J., Probst, A., Spillantini, M. G., Schäfer, T., Jakes, R., Bürki, K., and Goedert, M. (1995) Somatodendritic localization and hyperphosphorylation of tau protein in transgenic mice expressing the longest human brain tau isoform, *EMBO J.* **14,** 1304–1313.

13

Anatomy of Pathological Alterations in Alzheimer's Disease

Bradley T. Hyman

Even by inspection of the gross brain, it is evident that Alzheimer's disease (AD) neuropathological changes do not occur randomly or uniformly, but instead target the medial temporal lobe and association cortices of the temporal and parietal areas *(1–3)*. It might be expected, given the complex topography of brain architecture, that on finer examination, this distribution would show a pattern of vulnerability definable at the level of neural systems, cytoarchitectural fields, and even specific lamina within cytoarchitectural fields. Our anatomical studies of AD neuropathology have shown that this is indeed the case. Neurofibrillary tangles (NFT), senile plaques (SP), and neuronal loss affect individual cytoarchitectural areas and laminae in an extraordinarily specific and selective manner. Based on application of neuroanatomical principles and extrapolation of connectional data from the nonhuman primate experimental system, we have suggested that these lesions destroy major feed-forward and feedback projections, leading to disruption of neural systems related to memory and cognition *(4)*. In this chapter, I will briefly review the major themes of the anatomical alterations in AD from the perspective of the studies we have carried out over the last decade.

We have extensively mapped the distribution of NFT and SP in the cerebral cortex in AD using standard histologic and immunohistochemical techniques. We have now surveyed the entire cerebral cortex in AD *(2)* and performed detailed analyses of many regions (e.g., hippocampus, entorhinal cortex, amygdala, thalamic reticular formation, temporal pole, temporal association cortices, especially STS, and primary visual and auditory sensory and association cortices) *(4–16)*. We found that the pathological changes of AD target in a dramatic fashion certain specific lamina in consistent cytoarchitectural fields. These neurons tend to be large projection neurons; the terminal zones of these neurons are frequently affected by deposition of amyloid, and the combination of destruction of projection neurons, amyloid deposition, and synapse loss in terminal zones supports a view of specific neural system disruption. These anatomically based approaches have also led to studies of clinical–pathological correlations, highlighting the specific but widespread nature of the pathology in limbic and association cortices. Our recent studies implicate NFT and neuronal loss, rather than amyloid deposition, as the proximate cause of AD dementia *(2,7,8,12,17–19)*.

From: Molecular Mechanisms of Dementia *Edited by: W. Wasco and R. E. Tanzi Humana Press Inc., Totowa, NJ*

This anatomical approach has been powerful in terms of demonstrating the hierarchical vulnerability of different cytoarchitectural fields and even lamina for NFT and SP, and for generating hypotheses regarding the specific vulnerability of neuronal subpopulations. For example, we and others have defined both anatomically and by some biochemical criteria populations of vulnerable and spared neurons; e.g., SMI-32 positive presumed projection neurons in high-order association cortices are severely affected *(20,21)*, whereas nitric oxide synthase-containing cells are spared even within markedly affected cytoarchitectural areas *(22)*. These anatomical analyses contributed to the appreciation that there is a "preNFT" state of neurons that are immunoreactive for Alz-50 or other phospho-τ antibodies *(22,23)*.

Moreover, there appears to be a neuropathological basis for a "preclinical" state of AD in which cases with the earliest clinically recognizable symptoms seem to have already accumulated substantial Alzheimer changes in the hippocampal formation and entorhinal cortex *(3,7,24–27)*. We have recently applied stereological approaches to count the number of neurons in the entorhinal cortex in individuals who had participated in a longitudinal assessment of memory and aging at Washington University. Twenty individuals were studied, 10 of whom were believed to be cognitively normal at death and 10 of whom had AD of various severity, including 4 with a clinical dementia rating scale score of 0.5, or "very mild dementia." We found that entorhinal cortex as a whole was severely affected in AD, but that the two major projection layers, layers II and IV, were by far the most severely affected. Layer II gives rise to the perforant pathway, which is the major source of cortical and limbic input to the hippocampal formation, whereas layer IV receives a feedback projection from the hippocampal formation and, in turn, projects widely to limbic and association areas as well as the cholinergic basal forebrain. These projections are critically important for the functional integrity of neural systems related to memory, and they are markedly affected in AD. At end-stage disease (clinical dementia rating scale score of 3), there was about a 90% loss of layer II neurons. Even more strikingly, at the earliest clinically detectable point in the disease, there was a 60% loss in layer II and a 40% loss in layer IV! These data point to early, preclinical impairments that compromise the perforant pathway and related projections, and speak toward a functional reserve in these anatomical systems that is ultimately depleted by progression of the illness *(27a)*.

The fact that layer II of entorhinal cortex is severely affected suggests that the perforant pathway is essentially disconnected by the development of NFT in the cells of origin, the loss of the cells of origin, and the development of senile plaques in the terminal zone. Perforant pathway lesion has been a well-established experimental model for studies of neural plasticity, so it was natural to ask whether there was evidence of neural plasticity, i.e., of reinnervation of the deafferented perforant pathway terminal zone, in AD. Indeed, studies looking at glutamate receptors, acetylcholine histochemistry, diaphorase histochemistry, and substance P immunohistochemistry are consistent with the idea of hippocampal deafferentation and neural attempts at reinnervation *(14,15,28–32)*. This deafferentation leads to diminished metabolic activity, even in structurally intact fields *(33)*. In addition, loss of perforant pathway afferents leads to loss of glutamate and synaptophysin in the perforant path terminal zone *(34–36)*. The framework of the disconnection hypothesis, which is dramatically illustrated in the hippocampal formation, can be applied more generally, leading to the idea that there is a widespread alteration of feed-forward and feedback connections among limbic and association areas; this widespread disconnection is part of the groundwork that underlies the ideas set forth recently by Terry and colleagues and DeKosky and Scheff regarding the importance of synaptic loss in AD *(37,38)*.

In summary, what has emerged from analyzing the anatomic alterations in AD from the perspective of neuroanatomical connections is a view of AD dissecting neural systems, especially memory-related neural systems, by specifically and selectively affecting individual cytoarchitectural fields and laminae. These specific lesions tend to disrupt crucial cortico-cortical projections of the limbic system, as well as feed-forward and feedback projections in the association cortices. We believe that these lesions lead to a loss of structural and functional integrity of neural systems that underlies much of the cognitive disturbance of AD. Additional work has refined the phenotype of the neurons that are selectively affected, and has established a pattern of hierarchical vulnerability of brain regions and even individual lamina. Alterations in this brain landscape occur in AD in a systematic and consistent fashion. The challenge remains to understand why specific neurons are targeted, to understand how (and whether!) NFT and SP deposition are related to neuronal loss, and if so, to understand the pathophysiological mechanisms linking these one to another.

REFERENCES

1. Brun, A. and Gustafson, L. (1976) Distribution of cerebral degeneration in Alzheimer's disease, *Arch. Psychiatr. Nervenk* **223,** 15–33.
2. Arnold, S. E., Hyman, B. T., Flory, J., Damasio, A. R., and Van Hoesen, G. W. (1991) The topographical and neuroanatomical distribution of neurofibrillary tangles and neuritic plaques in cerebral cortex of patients with Alzheimer's disease, *Cerebral Cortex* **1,** 103–116.
3. Braak, H. and Braak, E. (1991) Neuropathological stageing of Alzheimer related changes, *Acta Neuropathol.* **82,** 239–259.
4. Hyman, B. T., Van Hoesen, G. W., and Damasio, A. R. (1990) Memory-related neural systems in Alzheimer's disease: An anatomical study, *Neurology* **40,** 1721–1730.
5. Arnold, S. E., Hyman, B. T., and Van Hoesen, G. W. (1994) Neuropathological changes of the temporal pole in Alzheimer's disease and Pick's disease, *Arch. Neurol.* in press.
6. Arriagada, P. V., Louis, D. N., Hedley-Whyte, E. T., and Hyman, B. T. (1991) Neurofibrillary tangles and olfactory dysgenesis: a test of the olfactory hypothesis of neurofibrillary tangle formation, *Lancet* **337,** 559.
7. Arriagada, P. V., Marzloff, K., and Hyman, B. T. (1992) Distribution of Alzheimer-type pathological changes in nondemented elderly matches the pattern in Alzheimer's disease, *Neurology* **42,** 1681–1688.
8. Arriagada, P. V., Growdon, J. H., Hedley-Whyte, E. T., and Hyman, B. T. (1992) Neurofibrillary tangles but not senile plaques parallel duration and severity of Alzheimer disease, *Neurology* **42,** 631–639.
9. Hyman, B. T. and Van Hoesen, G. W. (1989) Hippocampal and entorhinal cortex cellular pathology in Alzheimer's disease, in *The Hippocampus, New Vistas* (Chan-Palay, V. and Köhler, C., eds.), Liss, New York, pp. 499–512.
10. Hyman, B. T., Arriagada, P. V., and Van Hoesen, G. W. (1991) Pathological changes in the olfactory system in aging and Alzheimer's disease, in *Aging and Alzheimer's Disease* (Wurtman, R., Corkin, S., and Growdon, J. H., eds.), New York Academy of Science, New York, pp. 14–19.
11. Hyman, B. T. (1992) Down syndrome and Alzheimer's disease. Down Syndrome and Alzheimer Disease, in *Prog. Clin. Biol. Res.,* vol. 379 (Nadel, L. and Epstein, C. W., eds.), Wiley-Liss, New York, pp. 123–142.

12. Hyman, B. T., Arriagada, P. V., Van Hoesen, G. W., and Damasio, A. R. (1993) Memory impairment in Alzheimer's disease: An anatomical perspective, in *Neuropsychology of Alzheimer's Disease and other Dementias* (Parks, R. W., Zec, R. F., and Wilson, R. S., eds.), Oxford, New York, pp. 135–150.

13. Kromer-Vogt, L. J., Hyman, B. T., Van Hoesen, G. W., and Damasio, A. R. (1990) Pathological alterations in the amygdala in Alzheimer's disease, *Neuroscience* **37,** 377–385.

14. Rebeck, G. W. and Hyman, B. T. (1993) Neuroanatomical connections and specific regional vulnerability in Alzheimer's disease, *Neurobiol. Aging* **14,** 45–47.

15. Simonian, N. A., Rebeck, G. W., and Hyman, B. T. (1994) Functional integrity of neural systems related to memory in Alzheimer disease, in *Progress in Brain Research* (Bloom, F., ed.), Elsevier, Amsterdam, pp. 245–254.

16. Van Hoesen, G. W., Hyman, B. T., and Damasio, A. R. (1991) Entorhinal cortex pathology in Alzheimer's disease, *Hippocampus* **1,** 1–8.

17. Hyman, B. T., Arriagada, P. V., McKee, A., Ghika, J., Corkin, S., and Growdon, J. H. (1991) The earliest symptoms of Alzheimer disease: Anatomic correlates, *Soc. Neurosci.* **371,**

18. Hyman, B. T., Marzloff, K., and Arriagada, P. V. (1993) The lack of accumulation of senile plaques or amyloid burden in Alzheimer's disease suggests a dynamic balance between amyloid deposition and resolution, *J. Neuropathol. Exp. Neurol.* **52,** 594–600.

19. Hyman, B. T. and Tanzi, R. E. (1992) Amyloid, dementia and Alzheimer's disease, *Curr. Opinion Neurol. Neurosurg.* **5,** 88–93.

20. Hof, P. R., Cox, K., and Morrison, J. H. (1990) Quantitative analysis of a vulnerable subset of pyramidal neurons in Alzheimer's disease: I. Superior frontal and inferior temporal cortex, *J. Comp. Neurol.* **301,** 44–54.

21. Hof, P. R., Cox, K., and Morrison, J. H. (1988) Quantitative analysis of non-phosphorylated neurofilament protein (NPNFP)-immunoreactive neurons in normal and Alzheimer's disease brain, *Soc. Neurosci.* **14,** 1086.

22. Hyman, B. T., Marzloff, K. M., Wenniger, J. J., Dawson, T. M., Bredt, D. S., and Snyder, S. H. (1992) Relative sparing of nitric oxide synthase containing neurons in the hippocampal formation in Alzheimer's disease, *Ann. Neurol.* **32,** 818–821.

23. Vickers, J. C., Delacourte, A., and Morrison, J. H. (1993) Progressive transformation of the cytoskeleton associated with normal aging and Alzheimer's disease, *Brain Res.* **594,** 273–278.

24. Hyman, B. T., Van Hoesen, G. W., Kromer, L. J., and Damasio, A. R. (1986) Perforant pathway changes and the memory impairment of Alzheimer's disease, *Ann. Neurol.* **20,** 473–482.

25. Hyman, B. T. and Mann, D. M. A. (1991) Alzheimer type pathological changes in Down's syndrome individuals of various ages, in *Alzheimer's Disease: Basic Mechanisms, Diagnosis, and Therapeutic Strategies* (Iqbal, K., Mortimer, J., Winbld, B., and Wisniewski, H., eds.), Wiley, New York. pp. 105–113.

26. Bouras, C., Hof, P. R., and Morrison, J. H. (1993) Neurofibrillary tangle densities in the hippocampal formation in a nondemented population define subgroups of patients with differential early pathological changes, *Neurosci. Lett.* **153,** 131–135.

27. Price, D. L., Davis, P. B., Morris, J. C., and White, D. L. (1991) The distribution of tangles, plaques and related immunohistochemical markers in healthy aging and Alzheimer's disease, *Neurobiol. Aging* **12,** 295–312.

27a. Gomez-Igla, T., Price, J. L., McKeel, D. W., Morris, J. C., Growdon, J. J., and Hyman, B. T. (1996) Profound loss of layer II of entorhinal cortex neurons occurs in very mild Alzheimer's disease, *J. Neurosci.* **16,** 4491–4500.

28. Hyman, B. T., Kromer, L. J., and Van Hoesen, G. W. (1987) Reinnervation of the hippocampal perforant pathway zone in Alzheimer's disease, *Ann. Neurol.* **21,** 259–267.

29. Gertz, H. J., Cervos-Navarro, J., and Ewald, V. (1987) The septo-hippocampal pathway in patients suffering from senile dementia of Alzheimer's type. Evidence for neuronal plasticity? *Neurosci. Lett.* **76,** 228–232.

30. Geddes, J. W., Monaghan, D. T., Cotman, C. W., Lott, I. T., Kim, R. C., and Chui, H. C. (1985) Plasticity of hippocampal circuitry in Alzheimer's disease, *Science* **230,** 1179–1181.
31. Jaarsma, D., Sebens, J. B., and Korf, J. (1991) Reduction of adenosine A1-receptors in the perforant pathway terminal zone in Alzheimer hippocampus, *Neurosci. Lett.* **121,** 111–114.
32. Rebeck, G. W., Marzloff, K. M., and Hyman, B. T. (1993) The pattern of NADPH-diaphorase staining, a marker of nitric oxide synthase activity, is altered in the perforant pathway terminal zone in Alzheimer's disease, *Neurosci. Lett.* **152,** 165–168.
33. Harr, S., Simonian, N., and Hyman, B. T. (1995) Functional alterations in Alzheimer's disease: Decreased glucose transporter 3 immunoreactivity in the perforant pathway terminal zone, *J. Neuropath. Exp. Neurol.* **54,** 38–41.
34. Hyman, B. T., Van Hoesen, G. W., and Damasio, A. R. (1987) Alzheimer's disease: Glutamate depletion in perforant pathway terminals, *Ann. Neurol.* **22,** 37–40.
35. Cabalka, L. M., Hyman, B. T., Goodlett, C. R., Ritchie, T. C., and Van Hoesen, G. W. (1992) Alteration in the pattern of nerve terminal protein immunoreactivity in the perforant pathway in Alzheimer's disease and in rats after entorhinal lesions, *Neurobiol. Aging* **13,** 283–291.
36. Masliah, E., Terry, R. D., Alford, M., DeTeresa, R., and Hansen, L. A. (1991) Cortical and subcortical patterns of synaptophysinlike immunoreactivity in Alzheimer's disease, *Am. J. Pathol.* **138,** 235–246.
37. Terry, R. D., Masliah, E., and Salmon, D. P. (1991) Physical basis of cognitive alterations in Alzheimer's disease: Synapse loss is the major correlate of cognitive impairment, *Ann. Neurol.* **41,** 572–580.
38. De Kosky, S. T. and Scheff, S. W. (1990) Synapse loss in frontal cortex biopsies in Alzheimer's disease: correlation with cognitive severity, *Ann. Neurol.* **27,** 457–464.

14

Cerebral Zinc Metabolism in Alzheimer's Disease

Craig S. Atwood, Robert D. Moir, Xudong Huang, Rudolph E. Tanzi, and Ashley I. Bush

Most cases of Alzheimer's disease (AD) are sporadic, and overall estimates of life-time risk of developing AD in first-degree relatives of probands with AD suggest that only ≈50% of AD cases are influenced by hereditary risk factors *(1)*. Meanwhile, a relatively low concordance rate of 40% in monozygotic twins *(2)* implicates nongenetic factors in the expression of the disease. Therefore, environmental factors could have a major impact on the pathogenesis of AD. Several environmental factors have been proposed to influence the onset of AD. However, the study of the influence of a candidate stressor on the generation of hallmark pathology of AD has been a classic approach that initially implicated aluminum exposure in the generation of neurofibrillary tangles *(3,4)*. We have similarly explored candidate environmental or dietary factors that may impact on the deposition of Aβ as amyloid in the cerebral cortex—the other hallmark of AD neuropathology. Our approaches have been by studies of human amyloid protein precursor (APP) physiology, animal models, and in vitro models of Aβ aggregation. To date, although we have provocative data from in vivo studies, the in vitro studies of Aβ aggregation are most evolved. We have found that the solubility of the Aβ peptide is sensitively destabilized by the presence of zinc. This finding targets zinc as an important candidate environmental factor that could modulate Aβ solubility, since the brain is a unique compartment that sequesters zinc to high concentrations, whereas the blood–brain barrier in health serves to prevent undue exposure of the brain to this highly neurotoxic element.

1. ZINC AND APP

The APPs constitute a complex family of membrane-bound and soluble glycoproteins that are derived by alternate splicing of a gene on chromosome 21, yielding more than 10 isoforms, some of which contain a Kunitz-type protease inhibitory insert (KPI-APP). The description of two other highly homologous genes coding for amyloid precursor-like protein 1 (APLP1) *(5)*, which maps to human chromosome 19 *(6)*, and amyloid precursor-like protein 2 (APLP2) *(7)*, indicates that APP, APLP1, and APLP2 are members of a homologous superfamily whose products all carry a significantly negative charge at neutral pH (pI of 4.5, 5.5, and 4.5, respectively).

From: Molecular Mechanisms of Dementia *Edited by: W. Wasco and R. E. Tanzi Humana Press Inc., Totowa, NJ*

The function of the APP superfamily is unknown, but because all members of the superfamily share strong homology of major domains (cysteine-rich amino-terminus, zinc-binding site, negatively charged midregion, span the lipid bilayer once, short intra-cytoplasmic carboxyl-terminus), they are likely to be functionally related. APLP1 and APLP2 lack the Aβ domain and, hence, could not be amyloidogenic.

Zinc interaction is implicated in the function of the APP superfamily *(8,9)*. A novel zinc binding site has been described in the ectodomain of the protein within exon five, at the end of the cysteine-rich region. This domain is found in all known members of the APP superfamily as well as the drosophila homolog, APP-L *(10)*, and the *Caenorhabditis elegans* homolog, APL *(11)*. The affinity constant for binding is 750 nM, and binding to this site promotes the affinity of APP for heparin with an effect that saturates at 75 μM. A separate report demonstrated that zinc promoted the inhibition of coagulation factor XIa activity by KPI-APP with an effect that also saturated at 75 μM *(12)*.

Prominent among the proposed functions for APP are its possible roles in cell adhesiveness *(13)* and neurite outgrowth *(14)*. Indeed, the observation that APP is most greatly enriched in platelets and brain tissue *(15)* suggests that APP participates in tissue remodeling. It is intriguing that zinc, too, is most highly concentrated in the body in these two tissues *(16,17)*. APP is highly concentrated in vesicles in both these tissues *(15,18–22)*. Although the colocalization of APP with zinc in these vesicles has yet to be demonstrated, zinc is known to be stored in vesicles in tissues, like pancreatic β-cells, salivary secretory cells, and pituitary gland, where its function is thought to be the stabilization of intravesicular proteins and endocrine peptides, such as nerve growth factor (NGF) and insulin *(23)*. The effect of extracellular zinc on platelet function is to increase platelet adhesiveness and aggregation *(24)*. The effect of zinc on APP in increasing its affinity for heparin is reminiscent of this general effect. It will be important to determine whether extracellular zinc concentrations can also modulate neurite outgrowth and neuronal or glial adhesiveness by modifying the affinity of APP or APLP for extracellular matrix elements. Because extracellular brain zinc levels may modulate the function of APP, an understanding of the homeostatic mechanisms governing the physiology of zinc may yield insights that may be relevant to the pathophysiology of AD.

Recently, the possibility that dietary zinc exposure can impact on the metabolism of systemic and brain APP has been confirmed. Exposure of rats to dietary (Whyte, et al., manuscript submitted) or systemic zinc *(25)* specifically causes changes in brain APP metabolism, inducing the production of more full-length APP. The effect of this environmental stressor on Aβ generation is being determined.

No other dietary factor has yet been shown to modulate brain APP metabolism. These results are also unusual, since very little ingested zinc makes it into the brain, which is protected by stringent homeostatic mechanisms, including a specific metallothionein system as well as the blood–brain barrier.

2. CEREBRAL Aβ DEPOSITION IN AD

The discovery of Aβ as a normal secretion product of neuronal cell cultures and a soluble component of cerebrospinal fluid (CSF) at concentrations in the low ng/mL range *(26–28)* has propelled the inquiry into the molecular mechanisms that drive the generation of Aβ from APP. Aβ is generated from its large, transmembrane parent molecule, APP, by the combined action of proteases whose identities are still unknown (reviewed in ref. *29*), but whose activities create a variety of soluble fragments that are found in biological fluids. Of the Aβ fragments that are generated, the most abundant in the cerebrospinal fluid is the 40-residue species Aβ1–40 *(26,27,30)* which is enriched in cerebrovascular amyloid *(31,32)*. The effects of FAD-linked mutations of the presenilins and APP (reviewed in Chapters 1 and 8) seem to increase the quantity of total Aβ or the less soluble 42-residue species (Aβ1–42).

In vitro, synthetic Aβ1–42 is less soluble in neutral aqueous solutions *(33)*, than Aβ1–39 *(34)* or Aβ1–40 *(35)*, which are both soluble at millimolar concentrations. Kinetically soluble Aβ1–39/40 can be destabilized by seeding with Aβ1–42 fibrils *(36)*. This has led to a hypothesis that Aβ1–42, which is enriched in senile plaque amyloid, is a "pathogenic" species whose production is a feature of AD. There is increasing evidence that increased Aβ total concentration or an increase in Aβ1–42 induces accelerated amyloid deposition. The FAD-linked APP670/671 mutation has been shown to increase the secretion of Aβ species several-fold, whereas although the APP717 mutation (Val to Ile, downstream from the carboxyl-terminus of Aβ) does not increase the total quantity of Aβ production *(37,38)*, the mutation increases the proportion of Aβ1–42 *(39)*. Increased soluble Aβ1–42 has been found in the brains of individuals affected by Down's syndrome (DS), a condition complicated by premature AD, but was undetectable in the brains of age-matched controls *(40)*. Recently, Younkin and colleagues *(41a)* have reported increased levels of Aβ1–42 from fibroblasts and plasma of individuals affected with FAD-linked PS-1 and PS-2 mutations.

However, there are several lines of observation that indicate that overproduction of Aβ or an Aβ species alone is unlikely to account for the initiation of cerebral amyloid in sporadic AD cases. Aβ levels in the CSF are not elevated in AD *(28,42–44)*. In fact, there is evidence that Aβ1–42 levels are decreased in the CSF of AD subjects *(45)*. Elevated concentrations of Aβ alone are insufficient to induce cortical Aβ precipitation, since although one transgenic mouse model has developed amyloid pathology related to overexpression of APP and Aβ species *(46)*, similar degrees of overexpression have failed to induce amyloid deposition in other attempts to induce cortical amyloid pathology in an APP-transgenic mouse model *(47)*. To attribute amyloid initiation to the presence of Aβ1–42 alone is problematic, since this peptide is a normal component of healthy CSF. Furthermore, the focal nature of Aβ deposition close to synaptic junctions suggests that microanatomical environments might expose the soluble peptide to a focal stress originating from the synaptic region. From these sets of observations, it seems highly likely that pathogenic mechanisms apart from overproduction initiate Aβ amyloid deposition in sporadic AD.

For these reasons, we have systematically appraised the interaction of soluble synthetic Aβ with candidate neurochemical factors as a means of determining whether the peptide's vulnerabilities will yield telltale clues concerning the upstream lesions in the AD-affected brain that induce the soluble peptide to precipitate. To this end, we have found that of all the potential neurochemical environments that we have tested, the solubility of the peptide is most sensitively destabilized by the presence of low micromolar concentrations of Zn(II) *(48)* and by mildly acidic pH (5.0–7.4) *(34,49;* Atwood et al., manuscript in preparation). These in vitro data are significant because micromolar concentrations of zinc and mild acidosis are predicted to be features of the synaptic cleft affected by AD.

3. ABNORMAL CEREBRAL ZINC METABOLISM: A PRELUDE FOR Aβ AMYLOID DEPOSITION

Aβ specifically and saturably binds zinc, manifesting high-affinity binding ($K_d =$ 107 nM) with a 1:1 (zinc:Aβ) stoichiometry, and low-affinity binding ($K_d = 5.2$ μM) with a 2:1 stoichiometry *(9)*. Occupation of the zinc-binding site (between residues 6 and 28) inhibits constitutive α-secretase-type cleavage, and so may influence the production of Aβ from APP and may increase the biological half-life of the peptide *(9)*. Concentrations of zinc ≥1 μM rapidly destabilize human Aβ1–40 solutions, inducing a heterogenous product of amorphous precipitate and amyloid *(9)*. Zinc-induced Aβ amyloid formation, confirmed by a variety of techniques, is highly specific for zinc, although both copper and iron(II) can induce partial aggregation, but not amyloid formation *(50)*. Meanwhile, rat Aβ1–40 (with substitutions of Arg → Gly, Tyr → Phe, and His → Arg at positions 5, 10, and 13, respectively) binds zinc less avidly ($K_a = 3.8$ μM, with 1:1 stoichiometry) and is unaffected by zinc at these concentrations, perhaps explaining the scarcity with which these animals form cerebral Aβ amyloid *(13,51)*. We have used tritiated Aβ as well as immunodetection techniques to determine that zinc-induced Aβ precipitation is also achieved with physiological concentrations of peptide, as well as with both Aβ1–40 and Aβ1–42. The reaction also is inhibited by cerebrospinal fluid elements.

Recently, another laboratory has contended that they could not precipitate soluble Aβ with zinc at concentrations below 100 μM *(52)*. We have explored the reasons for this variance, and found that the most important variable in achieving the results we observed is the freshness of the peptide solution. When the peptide is freshly solubilized in water or neutral buffer, it is principally in the native, α-helical conformation. We have now shown that the α-helical conformation is essential for the initial interaction with zinc. In contrast to our procedure, Esler and colleagues *(52)* kept a concentrated (1 mM) stock of Aβ for months while performing experiments. We find that the ability of the synthetic peptide to be precipitated by zinc is readily lost when the radiolabeled peptide is aged. This may be owing to radiolytic damage. Additionally, we find that aged nonlabeled Aβ peptide solutions, even when centrifuged or filtered to remove aggregates, behave differently to freshly prepared peptide solutions. Aging the peptide is known to induce a decrease in α-helical conformers and an increase in random coil and β-sheet conformers. More importantly, concentrations of zinc below 10 μM have been shown by other laboratories to induce rapid precipitation of soluble Aβ1–40, corroborating our original observations (Glabe, personal communication; Zagorski, personal communication). These workers use freshly solubilized peptide.

Esler and colleagues believe that our data may have been subject to artifact owing to "inappropriate reliance on optical density to measure Aβ concentrations." These authors have not taken into account our corroborative observations of the Aβ-precipitating effects of zinc at concentrations in the low micromolar range in varied experimental systems that do not rely on optical density measurements. These observations include: zinc-modified proteolytic digestion of Aβ *(9)*, zinc-specific precipitation of Aβ into sedimentable amyloid particles assayed by Congo red staining *(48)* and corroborated by Western blot *(50)*, and zinc-specific precipitation of Aβ into filterable particles assayed by Western blot *(50)*. We have recently achieved further corroboration using three other systems to monitor Aβ concentrations: by protein assay, by using tritiated

Aβ as a marker (a means of labeling the peptide that does not disturb its interaction with zinc), and by turbidometry (Atwood et al., manuscript in preparation; Huang et al., manuscript in preparation).

Our data are at variance with those of Mantyh et al. *(53)*, who used iodinated Aβ in their studies. We found that iodinated Aβ has attenuated interaction with zinc, probably because of the presence of a relatively large iodine atom on the sole tyrosine residue at position 10. This residue is within the obligatory zinc-binding domain of Aβ, and is substituted with phenylalanine in the rat form of Aβ, which has diminished zinc-binding properties. Hence, it is not surprising that much higher concentrations of zinc are required to precipitate Aβ that is protected by iodine from coordinating with zinc *(48)*. Iodination of Aβ occurs in a region that is critical for the stability of the conformation of the molecule *(53a)*, and we have also found that iodinated Aβ does not comigrate with the unmodified peptide on native gel electrophoresis (unpublished results) bringing to doubt the validity of this reagent in in vitro systems. Mantyh and coworkers *(53)* found that Zn(II), Fe(III), and Al(III), at 200–1000 μ*M*, were capable of precipitating nanomolar concentrations of iodinated Aβ peptide in vitro. Whereas their aim of studying the behavior of the peptide at physiological concentrations is laudible, their results are difficult to interpret, since the brain environment is unlikely to generate these metal ions in such high concentrations, with the exception of zinc. Our data, using unmodified Aβ1–40 at concentrations as low as 0.8 μ*M (48)* and 6 n*M* (Atwood et al., manuscript in preparation), indicate that concentrations of zinc nearly two orders of magnitude lower induce the immediate aggregation of Aβ. Since the cortex has an abundant turnover of zinc, it is not difficult to envisage a situation where a small fraction of this metal ion could be incorrectly diverted towards an amyloidogenic pathway.

Since the APP secretase site at Lys-16 *(54,55)* in Aβ is within the obligatory zinc-binding region, the ability of Zn(II) to protect Aβ from secretase-type cleavage was tested. Amino-terminal sequence on Aβ tryptic digestion products (trypsin activity is not affected by zinc concentrations within the range employed) transferred to PVDF membrane following sodium dodecyl sulfate polyacrylamide gel electrophoresis (SDS-PAGE) indicated two detectable fragments corresponding to residues 6–40 and 17–40, and digestion was inhibited by increasing concentrations of Zn(II) *(56)*. The effects of Zn(II) on the resistance of Aβ to tryptic digestion were quantified more sensitively in that study by assaying proteolytic products for residual ability to bind ^{65}Zn. As little as 3 μ*M* Zn(II) were capable of protecting Aβ from tryptic lysis of the zinc-binding region, preserving 44% of ^{65}Zn binding to residual digestion products. These data indicate that occupation of the Zn(II)-binding site on Aβ inhibits cleavage at Lys-16, and can thus modulate the resistance of Aβ to secretase activity.

The importance of the in vitro observations of the effects of zinc ions on Aβ amyloidogenesis lies in the physiological plausibility of this metal ion encountering soluble Aβ in the brain environment. The effects of zinc on Aβ aggregation are highly specific, but we found that other neurochemical metal ions, mostly Cu(II) and Fe(II), were capable of inducing a degree of aggregation at physiologically plausible concentrations. However, Zn(II), when either compared at concentrations that reflect physiological concentration ranges or compared mole-for-mole to other metal ions, is by far the most potent means of precipitating Aβ at physiological pH *(48,50,56)*. Furthermore, Zn(II) was the only metal ion that we observed that could induce the synthetic peptide to produce congophilic amyloid. The concentrations of metal ion at which Aβ is aggregated is critical in determining the credibility of the results in a pathophysiological model. It is unlikely that Cu(II) or Fe(II), both of which are usually transported by proteins, would be available at significant concentrations to exchange with Aβ in the extracellular environment in order to induce interstitial amyloid formation. In contrast, an abundance of zinc is released into the synaptic cleft of many neurons during synaptic transmission. Although much of this zinc must be buffered in the extracellular environment, only ≈1% of the total zinc released following neurotransmission need exchange with Aβ to induce aggregation. Therefore, the mechanisms that exist to keep zinc and Aβ from reacting inappropriately must be close to 100% efficient in health, and might be a site of a potential lesion in AD.

There are two potential sources of high zinc concentrations that may inappropriately interact with soluble Aβ causing it to precipitate: the intrinsic zinc concentrated within the brain (especially at glutamatergic synaptic boutons), and the extrinsic zinc in the plasma that is customarily excluded from the brain interstitium by the filtration function of the blood–brain barrier.

4. CEREBRAL ZINC METABOLISM IN AD

The regulation of brain zinc compartmentalization and transport is governed by very strict homeostatic mechanisms. Although zinc is essential for brain development and function, the mechanisms underlying brain zinc nutriture and metabolism are poorly understood. Zinc stores are preserved in the brain, so that zinc malnutrition can be life-threatening without significantly depleting cerebral zinc stores (57–59). The consequences of clinical zinc deficiency include impaired mentation and memory functions. Conversely, zinc is neurotoxic in cell cultures in concentrations as low as 75 μM (60), and higher concentrations may be irreversibly toxic during exposures as brief as 15 min (61). AMPA receptor activation potentiates zinc-induced neurotoxicity even following brief (5 min) exposure in neuronal cell cultures (62). The peak extracellular concentration of zinc in the hippocampus rises to 300 μM during neurotransmission (63,64). Even higher concentrations might be expected at the synaptic cleft. However, because zinc can be rapidly neurotoxic at such high concentrations, active transport is likely to occur to remove the zinc from the interstitial space and to maintain homeostasis. The basis of this predicted homeostatic mechanism is still unknown.

The uptake of zinc into the brain is accomplished by an unidentified active transport mechanism. Plasma zinc, which is mainly bound to albumin, does not easily passively transfer into the central nervous system. The maximal accumulation of zinc into rat brain was shown to be only 0.5% of an ip dose and then subjected to a protracted intracerebral biological half-life in contrast to peripheral tissues (57). The blood–brain barrier and the choroid plexus appear to possess stringent means of protecting the brain from the passive zinc transfer, which would be driven by the large gradient generated by the relative concentrations of zinc in plasma (20 μM) (65) and in CSF (0.15 μM) (17).

Zinc is abundant in the brain cortex, where it is actively taken up (66,67) and stored in synaptic vesicles in nerve terminals throughout the telencephalon (68–70). The hippocampus, a critical region for memory function, contains the highest concentrations of zinc in the body, and is exposed to extreme fluctuations of extracellular zinc levels (0.15–300 μM) (17,68a), e.g., during synaptic transmission (63,64). The physiological purpose of such high zinc concentrations in the hippocampus is unclear, but Choi and coworkers *(71)* have proposed that this large transsynaptic movement of zinc may have a normal signaling function and be involved in long-term potentiation *(71)*. Sustained high levels of zinc are, however, neurotoxic *(61)*, so that an active transport system has been postulated for the reuptake of zinc following synaptic transmission *(18)*. The hippocampus is also the region of the brain that is most severely and consistently affected by the pathological lesions of AD *(72)*. Interestingly, a prominent neurochemical deficit in AD is cholinergic deafferentation of the hippocampus, which raises the concentration of zinc in this region *(73)*. Glutamatergic excitotoxicity, also thought to play a role in the pathophysiology of AD, may further raise the concentration of extracellular zinc in the cerebral cortex as a homeostatic mechanism attempting to antagonize the response of the NMDA receptor *(74)*.

Several observations indicate that zinc metabolism is altered in AD. These observations include decreased temporal lobe zinc levels *(75–78)*, increased hepatic zinc with reduced zinc bound to metallothionein *(79)*, an increase in extracellular zinc-metalloproteinase activity in AD hippocampus *(80)*, and decreased levels of the zinc-chelating protein metallothionein III *(81)*. Recently, we have observed abnormal systemic zinc homeostasis in subjects affected by presenilin-linked familial AD. Collectively, these reports indicate that there may be an abnormality in the uptake or distribution of zinc in the AD brain causing high extracellular and low intracellular concentrations in the brain.

5. SYNAPTIC ZINC HOMEOSTASIS— A THERAPEUTIC TARGET FOR AD

It has been suggested that AD is biologically inevitable, and that inheritance of the apolipoprotein E4 allele increases the risk for AD by lowering the age of onset of pathology, and that the E2 allele delays the inevitable onset of Alzheimer-type pathology *(82,83)*. In a similar vein, even the deterministic FAD-linked mutations induce amyloid deposition and dementia in an age-related manner. Children and young adults do not develop AD, but conversely, if one lives long enough, even the inheritance of the most favorable of risk factors cannot prevent the inevitable onset of AD brain pathology. These observations indicate that the biochemical lesions caused by genetic lesions and risk factors probably must combine with another age-related slowly-progressive pathological condition to yield amyloid deposition.

In one heuristic model that we contemplate (Fig. 1), mitochondrial dysfunction contributes to the generation of free radicals that may accelerate neurodegeneration *(84)* and induce amyloid crosslinking *(85)*. The energy depletion caused by mitochondrial dysfunction may, in turn, also cause abnormal zinc homeostasis by decreasing the activity of the highly energy-dependent neuronal zinc uptake mechanism *(67)*. This will cause zinc to accumulate extracellularly, thereby accelerating Aβ amyloid deposition *(48)*. The resultant intraneuronal zinc depletion that would be anticipated by this model has already been observed by several laboratories *(75–78)*. We are currently exploring this heuristic model.

Importantly, mildly acidic conditions potentiate the effect of copper (30 μ*M*) on the precipitation of Aβ (Atwood et al., manuscript in preparation). These data are important because of the likelihood that the brain is mildly acidotic in AD. Cerebral acidosis

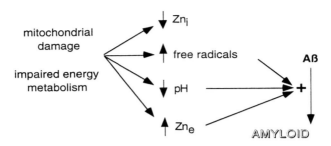

Fig. 1. Mitochondrial dysfunction: a heuristic model for the initiation of Aβ amyloid. Mitochondrial damage causes an energy debt to the neuron affecting three systems that could each lead to amyloid formation: (1) free radical formation that can crosslink soluble Aβ, (2) acidosis that can precipitate soluble Aβ, (3) impairment of the heavily energy-dependent zinc reuptake system that will lead to intracellular zinc (Zn_i) deficiency, and to an accumulation near synapses (Zn_e) where, in concert with free radicals and acidosis, soluble Aβ will be induced to precipitate.

is a consequence of cerebrovascular disease, but also can be brought about by decreased aerobic metabolism, a well-characterized complication of AD. One report has found a decrease in AD-affected cortical tissue of ≈0.5 pH u *(86)*. Taken together, our data indicate that whereas either environment could strongly promote Aβ aggregation, circumstances where both metal ion and pH homeostasis are disrupted could have profound consequences on Aβ solubility.

Several other candidate environmental factors are likely to impact on amyloid deposition in AD. Those being studied in the current literature include a history of head injury, diabetes (abnormal glycation), and exposure to free-radical-generating stressors. Genetic risk factors, such as the inheritance of an apolipoprotein E allotype, may influence amyloid deposition *(87)* by modulating the transduction of environmental stressors into the brain environment. Much work lies ahead in elaborating the biochemical pathways of each of these factors in modulating the AD amyloid phenotype.

ACKNOWLEDGMENT

Supported by grants from the NIA/NIH (R2912626), Alzheimer's Association, ILSI, and AFAR/Alliance for Aging Research (Paul Becson Award to AIB).

REFERENCES

1. Breitner, J., Siverman, J. S., Mohs, R. C., and Davis, K. L. (1988) Familial aggregation in Alzheimer's disease:comparison of risk among relatives of early- and late onset cases, and among male and female relatives in successive generations, *Neurology* **38,** 207–212.
2. Rapoport, S. I., Pettigrew, K. D., and Schapiro, M. B. (1991) Discordance and concordance of dementia of the Alzheimer type (DAT) in monozygotic twins indicate heritable and sporadic forms of Alzheimer's disease, *Neurology* **41,** 1549–1553.
3. Klatzo, I., Wisniewski, H., and Streicher, E. (1965) Experimental production of neurofibrillary degeneration. 1. Light microscopic observations, *J. Neuropathol. Exp. Neurol.* **24,** 187–199.
4. Terry, R. D. and Peña, C. (1965) Experimental production of neurofibrillary degeneration. 2. Electron microscopy, phosphatase histochemistry and electron probe analysis, *J. Neuropathol. Exp. Neurol.* **24,** 200–210.

5. Wasco, W., Bupp, K., Magendantz, M., Gusella, J. F., Tanzi, R. E., and Solomon, F. (1992) Identification of a mouse brain cDNA that encodes a protein related to the Alzheimer disease-associated β precursor protein, *Proc. Natl. Acad. Sci. USA* **89**, 10,758–10,762.

6. Wasco, W., Brook, J. D., and Tanzi, R. E. (1993) The amyloid precursor-like protein (APLP) gene maps to the long arm of human chromosome 19, *Genomics* **15**, 238,239.

7. Wasco, W., Gurubhagavatula, S., Paradis, Md, Romano, D., Sisodia, S. S., Hyman, B. T., Neve, R. L., and Tanzi, R. E. (1993) Isolation and characterization of the human APLP2 gene encoding a homologue of the Alzheimer's associated amyloid β protein precursor, *Nature Genet.* **5**, 95–100.

8. Bush, A. I., Multhaup, G., Moir, R. D., Williamson, T. G., Small, D. H., Rumble, B., Pollwein, P., Beyreuther, K., and Masters, C. L. (1993) A novel zinc(II) binding site modulates the function of the bA4 amyloid protein precursor of Alzheimer's disease, *J. Biol. Chem.* **268**, 16,109–16,112.

9. Bush, A. I., Pettingell, W. H., Paradis M., Tanzi, R. E., and Wasco, W. (1994) The amyloid β-protein precursor and its mammalian homologues: evidence for a zinc-modulated heparin-binding superfamily, *J. Biol. Chem.* **269**, 26,618–26,621.

10. Rosen, D. R., Martin-Morris, L., Luo, L., and White, K. (1989) A drosophila gene encoding a protein resembling the human β-amyloid protein precursor, *Proc. Natl. Acad. Sci. USA* **86**, 2478–2482.

11. Daigle, I. and Li, C. (1993) Apl-1, a *Caenorhabditis elegans* gene encoding a protein related to the human β-amyloid protein precursor, *Proc. Natl. Acad. Sci. USA* **90**, 12,045–12,049.

12. Komiyama, Y., Murakami, T., Egawa, H., Okubo, S., Yasunaga, K., and Murata, K. (1992) Purification of factor XIa inhibitor from human platelets, *Thromb. Res.* **66**, 397–408.

13. Shivers, B. D., Hilbich, C., Multhaup, G., Salbaum, M., Beyreuther, K., and Seeburg, P. H. (1988) Alzheimer's disease amyloidogenic glycoprotein: expression pattern in rat brain suggests role in cell contact, *EMBO J.* **7**, 1365–1370.

14. Milward, E. A., Papadopoulos, R., Fuller, S. J., Moir, R. D., Small, D., Beyreuther, K., and Masters, C. L. (1992) The amyloid protein precursor of Alzheimer's disease is a mediator of the effects of nerve growth factor on neurite outgrowth, *Neuron* **9**, 129–137.

15. Bush, A. I., Martins, R. N., Rumble, B., Moir, R., Fuller, S., Milward, E., Currie, J., Ames, D., Weidemann, A., Fischer, P., Multhaup, G., Beyreuther, K., and Masters, C. L. (1990) The amyloid precursor protein of Alzheimer's disease is released by human platelets, *J. Biol. Chem.* **265**, 15,977–15,983.

16. Baker, R. J., McNeil, J. J., and Lander, H. (1978) Platelet metal levels in normal subjects determined by atomic absorption spectrophotometry, *Thromb. Haemostasis* **39**, 360–365.

17. Frederickson, C. J. (1989) Neurobiology of zinc and zinc-containing neurons, *Int. Rev. Neurobiol.* **31**, 145–328.

18. Cole, G. M., Galasko, D., Shapiro, I. P., and Saitoh T. (1990) Stimulated platelets release amyloid β-protein precursor, *Biochem. Biophys. Res. Commun.* **170**, 288–295.

19. Smith, R. P., Higuchi, D. A., and Broze, G. J. Jr. (1990) Platelet coagulation factor XIa-inhibitor, a form of Alzheimer amyloid precursor protein, *Science* **248**, 1126–1128.

20. Van Nostrand, W. E., Schmaier, A. H., Farrow, J. S., and Cunningham, D. D. (1990) Protease nexin-II (amyloid β-protein precursor): a platelet α-granule protein, *Science* **248**, 745–748.

21. Schlossmacher, M. G., Ostaszewski, B. L., Hecker, L. I., Celi, A., Haass, C., Chin, D., Lieberburg, I., Furie, B. C., Furie, B., and Selkoe, D. J. (1992) Detection of distinct isoform patterns of the β-amyloid precursor protein in human platelets and lymphocytes, *Neurobiol. Aging* **13**, 421–434.

22. Suenaga, T., Hirano, A., Llena, J. F., Ksiezak-Reding, H., Yen, S. H., and Dickson, D. W. (1990) Modified Bielschowsky and immunocytochemical studies on cerebellar plaques in Alzheimer's disease, *J. Neuropathol. Exp. Neurol.* **49**, 31–40.

23. Frederickson, C. J., Perez-Clausell, J., and Danscher, G. (1987) Zinc-containing 7S-NGF complex. Evidence from zinc histochemistry for localization in salivary secretory granules, *J. Histochem. Cytochem.* **35**, 579–583.

24. Heyns, A. du P., Eldor, A., Yarom, R., and Marx, G. (1985) Zinc-induced platelet aggregation is mediated by the fibrinogen receptor and is not accompanied by release or by thromboxane synthesis, *Blood* **66**, 213–219.

25. Bush, A. I. (1992) Aspects of the pathophysiology and pathogenesis of Alzheimer's disease. University of Melbourne.

26. Haass, C., Schlossmacher, M. G., Hung, A. Y., Vigo-Pelfrey, C., Mellon, A., Ostaszewski, B. L., Lieberburg, I., Koo, E. H., Schenk, D., Teplow, D. B., and Selkoe, D. S. (1992) Amyloid β-peptide is produced by cultured cells during normal metabolism, *Nature* **359**, 322–325.

27. Seubert, P., Vigo-Pelfrey, C., Esch, F., Lee, M., Dovey, H., Davis, D., Sinha, S., Schlossmacher, M., Whaley, J., Swindlehurst, C., McCormack, R., Wolfert, R., Selkoe, D., Lieberberg, I., and Schenk, D. (1992) Isolation and quantification of soluble Alzheimer's β-peptide from biological fluids, *Nature* **359**, 325–327.

28. Shoji, M., Golde, T.-E., Ghiso, J., Cheung, T. T., Estus, S., Shaffer, L. M., Cai, X.-D., McKay, D. M., Tintner, R., Frangione, B., and Younkin, S. G. (1992) Production of the Alzheimer amyloid β protein by normal proteolytic processing, *Science* **258**, 126–129.

29. Evin, G., Beyreuther, K., and Masters, C. L. (1994) Alzheimer's disease amyloid precursor protein (AβPP): proteolytic processing, secretases and βA4 production, *Amyloid: Int. J. Exp. Clin. Invest.* **1**, 263–280.

30. Busciglio, J., Gabuzda, D. H., Matsudaira, P., and Yankner, B. A. (1993) Generation of β-amyloid in the secretory pathway in neuronal and nonneuronal cells, *Proc. Natl. Acad. Sci. USA* **90**, 2092–2096.

31. Prelli, F., Castaño, E., Glenner, G. G., and Frangione, B. (1988) Differences between vascular and plaque core amyloid in Alzheimer's disease, *J. Neurochem.* **51**, 648–651.

32. Miller, D. L., Papayannopoulos, I. A., Styles, J., Bobin, S. A., Lin, Y. Y., Biemann, K., and Iqbal, K. (1993) Peptide compositions of the cerebrovascular and senile plaque core amyloid deposits of Alzheimer's disease, *Arch. Biochem. Biophys.* **301**, 41–52.

33. Hilbich, C., Kisters-Woike, B., Reed, J., Masters, C. L., and Beyreuther, K. (1991) Aggregation and secondary structure of synthetic amyloid βA4 peptides of Alzheimer's disease, *J. Mol. Biol.* **218**, 149–163.

34. Burdick, D., Soreghan, B., Kwon, M., Kosmoski, J., Knauer, M., Henschen, A., Yates, J., Cotman, C., and Glabe, C. (1992) Assembly and aggregation properties of synthetic Alzheimer's A4/β amyloid peptide analogs, *J. Biol. Chem.* **267**, 546–554.

35. Tomski, S. and Murphy, R. M. (1992) Kinetics of aggregation of synthetic b-amyloid peptide, *Arch. Biochem. Biophys.* **294**, 630–638.

36. Jarrett, J. T., Berger, E. P., and Lansbury, P. T. (1993) The carboxy terminus of the b amyloid protein is critical for the seeding of amyloid formation: implications for the pathogenesis of Alzheimer's disease, *Biochemistry* **32**, 4693–4697.

37. Citron, M., Oltersdorf, T., Haass, C., McConlogue, L., Hung, A. Y., Seubert, P., Vigo-Pelfrey, C., Lieberburg, I., and Selkoe, D. J. (1992) Mutation of the β-amyloid precursor protein in familial Alzheimer's disease increases β-protein production, *Nature* **360**, 672–674.

38. Cai, X.-D., Golde, T.-E., and Younkin, S. G. (1993) Release of excess amyloid β protein from a mutant amyloid β protein precursor, *Science* **259**, 514–516.

39. Suzuki, N., Cheung, T. T., Cai, X.-D., Odaka, A., Otvos, L., Eckman, C., Golde, T.-E., and Younkin, S. G. (1994) An increased percentage of long amyloid β protein secreted by familial amyloid β protein precursor (bAPP$_{717}$) mutants, *Science* **264**, 1336–1340.

40. Teller, J. K., Russo, C., DeBusk, L. M., Angelini, G., Zaccheo, D., Dagna-Bricarelli, F., Scartezzini, P., Bertolini, S., Mann, D. M., Tabaton, M., and Gambetti, P. (1996) Presence of soluble amyloid beta-peptide precedes amyloid plaque formation in Down's syndroms, *Nat. Med.* **2**, 93–95.

41. Younkin, S., Scheuner, D., Song, X., Eckman, C., Citron, M., Suzuki, N., Bird, T., Hardy, J., Hutton, M., Lannfelt, L., Levy-Lahad, F., Peskind, E., Poorkaj, P., Schellenberg, G., Tanzi, R., Viitanen, M., Wasco, W., and Selkoe, D. (1996) The presenilin 1 and 2 mutations linked

to familial Alzheimer's disease increase the extracellular concentration of amyloid β protein (Aβ) ending at Aβ42(43), *Neurobiology of Aging* **17(4S)**, 149.
42. Nakamura, T., Shoji, M., Harigaya Y., Watanabe, M., Hosoda, K., Cheung, T. T., Shaffer, L. M., Golde, T.-E., Younkin, L. H., Younkin, S. G., and Hirai, S. (1994) Amyloid β protein levels in cerebrospinal fluid are elevated in early-onset Alzheimer's disease, *Ann. Neurol.* **36**, 903–911.
43. Nitsch, R. M., Rebeck, G. W., Deng, M., Richardson, U. I., Tennis, M., Schenk, D. B., Vigo-Pelfrey, C., Lieberburg, I., Wurtman, R. J., Hyman, B. T., et al. (1995) Cerebrospinal fluid levels of amyloid beta-protein in Alzheimer's disease: inverse correlation with severity of dementia and effect of apolipoprotein E genotype, *Ann. Neurol.* **37**, 512–518.
44. Southwick, P. C., Yamagata, S. K., Echol, C. L., Jr., Higson, G. J., Neynaber, S. A., Parson, R. E., and Munroe, W. A. (1996) Assessment of amyloid beta protein in cerebrospinal fluid as an aid in the diagnosis of Alzheimer's disease. *J. Neurochem.* **66**, 259–265.
45. Motter, R., Vigo-Pelfrey, C., Kholodenko, D., Barbour, R., Johnson-Wood, K., Galasko, D., Chang, L., Miller, B., Clark, C., Green, R., Olson, D., Southwick, P., Wolfert, R., Munroe, B., Lieberburg, I., Seubert, P., and Schenk, D. (1995) Reduction of β-amyloid peptide42 in the cerebrospinal fluid of patients with Alzheimer's Disease, *Ann Neurol.* **38**, 643–648.
46. Games, D., Adams, D., Alessandrini, R., Barbour, R., Berthelette, P., Blackwell, C., Carr, T., Clemens, J., Donaldson, T., Gillespie, F., Guido, T., Hagopian, S., Johnson-Wood, K., Khan, K., Lee, M., Leibowitz, P., Lieberburg, I., Little, S., Masliah, E., McConlogue, L., Montoya-Zavala, M., Mucke, L., Paganini, L., Penniman, E., Power, M., Schenk, D., Seubert, P., Snyder, B., Soriano, F., Tan, H., Vitale, J., Wadsworth, S., Wolozin, B., and Zhao, J. (1995) Alzheimer-type neuropathology in transgenic mice overexpressing V717F β-amyloid precursor protein, *Nature* **373**, 523–527.
47. Hsiao, K. K., Borchelt, D. R., Olson, K., Johannsdottir, R., Kitt, C., Yunis, W., Xu, S., Eckman, C., Younkin, S., Price, D., Iadecola, C., Clark, H. B., and Carlson, G. (1995) Age-related CNS disorder and early death in transgenic FVB/N mice overexpressing Alzheimer amyloid precursor proteins, *Neuron* **15**, 1203–1218.
48. Bush, A. I., Pettingell, W. H., Multhaup, G., Paradis M., Vonsattel, J.-P., Gusella, J. F., Beyreuther, K., Masters, C. L., and Tanzi, R. E. (1994) Rapid induction of Alzheimer Aβ amyloid formation by zinc, *Science* **265**, 1464–1467.
49. Barrow, C. J. and Zagorski, M. G. (1991) Solution structures of β peptide and its constituent fragments: relation to amyloid deposits, *Science* **253**, 179–182.
50. Bush, A. I., Moir, R. D., Rosenkranz, K. M., and Tanzi, R. E. (1995) Zinc and Alzheimer's disease, *Science* **268**, 1921–1923.
51. Johnstone, E. M., Chaney, M. O., Norris, F. H., Pascual, R., and Little, S. P. (1991) Conservation of the sequence of the Alzheimer's disease amyloid peptide in dog, polar bear and five other mammals by cross-species polymerase chain reaction analysis, *Mol. Brain Res.* **10**, 299–305.
52. Esler, W. P., Stimson, E. R., Jennings, J. M., Ghilardi, J. R., Mantyh, P., and Maggio, J. E. (1996) Zinc-induced aggregation of human and rat β-amyloid peptides in vitro, *J. Neurochem.* **66**, 723–732.
53. Mantyh, P. W., Ghilardi, J. R., Rogers, S., DeMaster, E., Allen, C. J., Stimson, E. R., and Maggio, J. E. (1993) Aluminum, iron, and zinc ions promote aggregation of physiological concentrations of β-amyloid peptide, *J. Neurochem.* **61**, 1171–1174.
53a. Halverson, K., Fraser, P. E., Kirschner, D. A., and Lansbury, P. T., Jr. (1990) Molecular determinants of amyloid deposition in Alzheimer's disease: conformational studies of synthetic β-protein fragments, *Biochemistry* **29**, 2639–2644.
54. Esch, F. S., Keim, P. S., Beattie, E. C., Blacher, R. W., Culwell, A. R., Oltersdorf, T., McClure, D., and Ward, P. J. (1990) Cleavage of amyloid β peptide during constitutive processing of its precursor, *Science* **248**, 1122–1124.
55. Sisodia, S. S., Koo, E. H., Beyreuther, K., Unterbeck, A., and Price, D. L. (1990) Evidence that β-amyloid protein in Alzheimer's disease is not derived by normal processing, *Science* **248**, 492–495.

56. Bush, A. I., Pettingell, W. H., Jr., Paradis, M., and Tanzi, R. E. (1994) Modulation of Aβ adhesiveness and secretase site cleavage by zinc, *J. Biol. Chem.* **269,** 12,152–12,158.
57. Kasarkis, E. J. (1984) Zinc metabolism in normal and zinc-deficient rat brain, *Exp. Neurol.* **85,** 114–127.
58. O'Neal, R. M., Pla, G. W., Fox, M. R. S., Gibson, F. S., and Fry, B. E. (1970) Effect of zinc deficiency and restricted feeding on protein and ribonucleic acid metabolism of rat brain, *J. Nutr.* **100,** 491–497.
59. Wallwork, J. C., Milne, D. B., Sims, R. L., and Sandstead, H. H. (1983) Severe zinc deficiency: effects on the distribution of nine elements (potassium, phosphorus, sodium, magnesium, calcium, iron, zinc, copper, and manganese) in regions of the rat brain, *J. Nutrition* **113,** 1895–1905.
60. Duncan, M. W., Marini, A. M., Watters, R., Kopin, I. J., and Markey, S. P. (1992) Zinc, a neurotoxin to cultured neurons, contaminates cycad flour prepared by traditional Guamanian methods, *J. Neurosci.* **12,** 1523–1537.
61. Choi, D. W., Yokoyama, M., and Koh, J. (1988) Zinc neurotoxicity in cortical cell culture, *Neuroscience* **24,** 67–79.
62. Weiss, J. H., Hartley, D. M., Koh, J., and Choi, D. W. (1993) AM, PA receptor activation potentiates zinc neurotoxicity, *Neuron* **10,** 43–49.
63. Assaf, S. Y. and Chung, S.-H. (1984) Release of endogenous Zn^{2+} from brain tissue during activity, *Nature* **308,** 734–736.
64. Howell, G. A., Welch, M. G., and Frederickson, C. J. (1984) Stimulation-induced uptake and release of zinc in hippocampal slices, *Nature* **308,** 736–738.
65. Davies, I. J.T, Musa, M., and Dormandy, T. L. (1968) Measurements of plasma zinc, *J. Clin. Pathol.* **21,** 359–365.
66. Wolf, G., Scutte, M., and Römhild, W. (1984) Uptake and subcellular distribution of [65]zinc in brain structures during the postnatal development of the rat, *Neurosci. Lett.* **51,** 277–280.
67. Wensink, J., Molenaar, A. J., Woroniecka, U. D., and Van Den Hamer, C. J. (1988) Zinc uptake into synaptosomes, *J. Neurochem.* **50,** 783–789.
68. Ibata, Y. and Otsuka, N. (1969) Electron microscope demonstration of zinc in the hippocampal formation using Timm's sulfide-silver technique, *J. Histochem. Cytochem.* **17,** 171–175.
68a. Frederickson, C. J., Klitenick, M. A., Manton, W. I., and Kirkpatrick, J. B. (1983) Cytoarchitectonic distribution of zinc in the hippocampus of man and the rat, *Brain Res.* **273,** 335–339.
69. Perez-Clausell, J. and Danscher, G. (1985) Intravesicular localization of zinc in rat telencephalic boutons, a histochemical study. *Brain Res.* **337,** 91–98.
70. Friedman, B. and Price, J. L. (1984) Fiber systems in the olfactory bulb and cortex: a study in adult and developing rats, using the Timm method with the light and electron microscope, *J. Comp. Neurol.* **223,** 88–109.
71. Weiss, J. H., Koh, J., Christine, C. W., and Choi, D. W. (1989) Zinc and LTP, *Nature* **338,** 212.
72. Hyman, B. T., Van Hoesen, G. W., Kroner, L. J., and Damasio, A. R. (1986) Perforant pathway changes and the memory impairment of Alzheimer's disease, *Ann. Neurol.* **20,** 472–481.
73. Stewart, G. R., Frederickson, C. J., Howell, G. A., and Gage, F. H. (1984) Cholinergic denervation-induced increase of chelatable zinc in mossy-fiber region of the hippocampal formation, *Brain Res.* **290,** 43–51.
74. Choi, D. W. (1990) Possible mechanisms limiting *N*-Methyl-D-Aspartate receptor overactivation and the therapeutic efficacy of *N*-Methyl-D-Aspartate antagonists, *Stroke* **21(Suppl. III),** 20–22.
75. Wenstrup, D., Ehmann, W. D., and Markesbery, W. R. (1990) Trace element imbalances in isolated subcellular fractions of Alzheimer's disease brains, *Brain Res.* **533,** 125–131.
76. Constantinidis, J. (1990) Maladie d'Alzheimer et la théorie du zinc, *L'Encephale* **16,** 231–239.
77. Corrigan, F. M., Reynolds, G. P., and Ward, N. I. (1993) Hippocampal tin, aluminum and zinc in Alzheimer's disease, *Biometals* **6,** 149–154.

78. Deng, Q. S., Turk, G. C., Brady, D. R., and Smith, Q. R. (1994) Evaluation of brain element composition in Alzheimer's disease using inductively-coupled plasma mass spectrometry, *Neurobiol. Aging* **15(Suppl. 1)**, S113 (Abstract).
79. Lui, E., Fisman, M., Wong, C., and Diaz, F. (1990) Metals and the liver in Alzheimer's disease: an investigation of hepatic zinc, copper, cadmium, and metallothionein, *J. Am. Geriatr. Soc.* **38**, 633–639.
80. Backstrom, J. R., Miller, C. A., and Tökés, Z. A. (1992) Characterization of neutral proteinases from Alzheimer-affected and control brain specimens: identification of calcium-dependent metalloproteinases from the hippocampus, *J. Neurochem.* **58**, 983–992.
81. Uchida, Y., Takio, K., Titani, K., Ihara, Y., and Tomonaga, M. (1991) The growth-inhibitory factor that is deficient in the Alzheimer's disease brain is a 68-amino acid metallothionein-like protein, *Neuron* **7**, 337–347.
82. Corder, E. H., Saunders, A. M., Risch, N. J., Strittmatter, W. J., Schmechel, D. E., Gaskell, P. C., Rimmler, J. B., Locke, P. A., Conneally, P. M., Schmader, K. E., et al. (1994) Protective effect of apolipoprotein E type 2 allele for late onset Alzheimer's disease, *Nature Genet.* **7**, 180–184.
83. Corder, E. H., Saunders, A. M., Strittmatter, W. J., Schmechel, D. E., Gaskell, P. C., Small, G. W., Roses, A. D., Haines, J. L., and Pericak-Vance, M. A. (1993) Gene dose of apolipoprotein E type 4 allele and the risk of Alzheimer's disease in late onset families, *Science* **261**, 921–923.
84. Busciglio, J. and Yankner, B. A. (1995) Apoptosis and increased generation of reactive oxygen species in Down's syndrome neurons in vitro, *Nature* **378**, 776–779.
85. Dyrks, T., Dyrks, E., Hartmann, T., Masters, C., and Beyreuther, K. (1992) Amyloidogenicity of βA4 and βA4-containing amyloid protein precursor fragments by metal-catalyzed oxidation, *J. Biol. Chem.* **267**, 18,210–18,217.
86. Yates, C. M., Butterworth, J., Tennant, M. C., and Gordon, A. (1990) Enzyme activities in relation to pH and lactate in postmortem brain in Alzheimer-type and other dementias. *J. Neurochem.* **55**, 1624–1630.
87. Rebeck, G. W., Reiter, J. S., Strickland, D. K., and Hyman, B. T. (1993) Apolipoprotein E in sporadic Alzheimer's disease: allelic variation and receptor interactions, *Neuron* **11**, 575–580.

15

Potassium Channels and Calcium Release

Pathophysiological and Diagnostic Implications
for Alzheimer's Disease

René Etcheberrigaray and Daniel L. Alkon

1. INTRODUCTION

The number of diverse factors implicated in the etiology of Alzheimer's disease (AD) suggests that it can arise through distinct cascades of pathophysiologic and molecular events. These include specific genetic defects involving amyloid precursor protein (APP) and its metabolism, aging itself, prior history of head trauma, and ApoE. Of these, only aging impacts on a majority of all AD cases *(1–5)*. Considering the multifactorial nature of AD etiology as well as the number of afflicted individuals (approx 4,000,000 in the US alone), it is noteworthy that the almost universal symptom for all AD patients is early memory loss *(6,7)*. Characteristically, other dementias are revealed by constellations of symptoms, such as motor deficits with Parkinson's disease, Huntington's Chorea, and Wernicke-Korsakoff's syndrome; sensory deficits of vitamin B12 deficiency; and mood alterations of depressive disorders *(8)*.

The specificity of early memory loss suggests the possibility that lesions occur first in brain structure(s) critical for memory storage, such as the hippocampus, related regions of the amygdala, and/or the nucleus basalis. However, despite initial suggestions, pathologic changes in these regions (much more than others) have not clearly correlated with early AD. For that matter, the pathologic hallmarks of AD, β-amyloid plaques and neurofibrillary tangles, although present in AD brains, are in most cases only loosely correlated in number, size, and distribution with the severity of the disease *(9,10)*.

Why else, then, would AD in its initial stages, despite the diversity of its etiologic cascades, produce memory loss and not typically other neurologic deficits of sensation, coordination, arousal state, and motor strength? We hypothesized that human memory depends on molecular and biophysical events that, even before plaques and tangles, are uniquely susceptible to early Alzheimer's pathophysiology—independent of which contributing factor predominates.

From: Molecular Mechanisms of Dementia *Edited by: W. Wasco and R. E. Tanzi Humana Press Inc., Totowa, NJ*

This chapter will review:

1. The molecular cascades implicated in memory acquisition and storage;
2. Evidence for AD-specific dysfunction of critical steps within these cascades; and
3. The potential for future investigative directions suggested by this convergence of molecular memory methods and AD pathophysiology.

The study of molecular mechanisms of associative memory and learning in animal models, both vertebrates and invertebrates, has revealed a discrete number of molecular components and cellular events that are critical for the acquisition and storage of associative learning *(11,12)*. These steps, identified in both invertebrate and mammalian species, begin with temporally specific training stimuli in such paradigms as Pavlovian conditioning, spacial water maze learning, and olfactory discrimination learning. Initial observations showed that cell excitability of the Hermissenda's B photoreceptor was enhanced after the animal acquired a conditioned response, which was later discovered to be the result of a long-lasting reduction of specific potassium currents *(13,14)*. It was also discovered that activation and/or injection of protein kinase C (PKC) caused a reduction of the same currents, mimicking the effects of conditioning *(15)*. Single-channel studies confirmed that classical conditioning and PKC activation have similar effects on specific K^+ channels *(16)*. K^+ channels and PKC were also found to play a fundamental role in associative learning in mammals. The afterhyperpolarization (AHP) and the potassium current subserving the AHP were reduced in CA1 hippocampal cells of conditioned rabbits *(17,18)*. PKC studies revealed that the membrane-associated form of this enzyme was enriched in the CA1 region of trained rabbits *(19,20)*. In addition, the phosphorylated form of ≈ 20 kDa GTP-binding protein was found increased in nerve cells of Hermissenda *(21)*. This protein, later identified as a member of the ARF class proteins, was found to be a potent regulator of K^+ channels (in a conditioning-like manner) *(22,23)*, to induce conditioning-like changes of synaptic terminal branches *(24)*, to regulate axonal transport *(25)*, and to regulate mRNA turnover *(26)*. This protein has been identified in vertebrates, including humans *(27,28)*.

Because this sequence of events uny%rlying memory storage is apparently conserved in highly diverse species, it may also have relevance for human memory, which is characteristically associative *(29)*. Hypothesizing that AD has systemic expression *(30–32)*, we proposed that cellular changes in peripheral cells (such as skin fibroblasts, olfactory neuroblasts, lymphocytes, and so forth) might be analyzed with less interference by secondary pathologic consequences of the disease, such as occurs with widespread plaque deposits in the brain. Skin fibroblasts have been successfully used to study other neurological disorders *(33,34)* and provide an adequate cellular system to study molecular changes *(30–32)* without interference of a more generalized pathological process, such as that which occurs in the brains of AD patients.

2. POTASSIUM CHANNEL ALTERATIONS IN FIBROBLASTS FROM AD PATIENTS

Potassium channel function was studied using conventional patch-clamp techniques *(35,36)*. We found that a ≈ 113-pS, tetraethylammonium (TEA)-sensitive channel was consistently missing in fibroblasts from AD patients, although it was present in approx 60% of patches from young and age-matched controls. A second K^+ channel of ≈ 166

was present with about the same frequency (30–40% of patches) and with similar kinetics (percentage of open time ≈10%) (Fig. 1). A lack of TEA sensitivity was a common feature of this 166-pS channel in patches from AD and control fibroblasts *(37)*. These results indicate that the effects on the 113-pS K^+ channel are specific and not the reflection of a pathological process that has generalized effects on membrane proteins, such as ion channels.

In addition to the patch-clamp methodology, we also used measurement of intracellular calcium increases ($[Ca^{2+}]_i$) in response to depolarization induced by blockade of K^+ channels as an independent method of studying these channels. Since the 113-pS K^+ channel was sensitive to TEA, calcium elevation after bath application of TEA should reflect the blockade of this channel. As expected from the patch-clamp analyses, TEA-induced $[Ca^{2+}]_i$ elevation was observed only in fibroblasts from control individuals, whose functional 113-pS K^+ channels were susceptible to TEA blockade. No TEA-induced $[Ca^{2+}]_i$ elevations were observed in cell lines from AD patients *(37)*. Elimination of external Ca^{2+} abolished the responses in fibroblasts from all groups, indicating that the $[Ca^{2+}]_i$ elevation was the result of Ca^{2+} influx from the extracellular medium. Depolarization induced with elevated external KCl (50 mM) caused comparable $[Ca^{2+}]_i$ elevations in cells from control and AD patients, suggesting that voltage-activated calcium channels are functional in fibroblasts from AD patients and are not the primary site of defect.

3. INTRACELLULAR CALCIUM RELEASE IN AD FIBROBLASTS

Intracellular calcium handling in AD has been the subject of numerous studies, and although there was evidence suggesting differences between AD and controls, there was no general agreement on the exact nature and/or direction of the change *(38–43)*. In our studies, we explored the calcium release mediated by IP_3 generation because of its relevance for memory storage *(44)*. Intracellular calcium changes were measured after stimulation with the peptide bombesin (a peptide with multiple actions in various organs *[45]*, known to induce G-protein/phospholipase C-mediated IP_3 generation *[45–50]*) in AD and control fibroblasts. Calcium elevations were consistently larger in AD fibroblasts, compared to all control cell lines *(51)*. These differences were more significant in the relaxation phase following the peak response. The responses and differences were still present in the absence of external calcium, indicating that calcium release from IP_3-sensitive stores accounts for the calcium elevation, including the enhanced response in AD observed after bombesin stimulation. Biochemical analyses demonstrated that bombesin receptor numbers and/or affinity *(51)* cannot account for the observed differences in bombesin responses. More recently, we have reported that application of low concentrations (0.1 nM) of bradykinin, which also induces IP_3 generation, induces calcium responses almost exclusively in AD cell lines, whereas controls exhibited virtually no calcium elevations *(52)* (Fig. 2). In agreement with this finding, other reports have shown that IP_3 generation is indeed enhanced in AD fibroblasts *(53)*. Thapsigargin-induced Ca^{2+} release (IP_3-independent *[54–56]*) was similar in AD and control cells, indicating that $[Ca^{2+}]_i$ pools and buffering systems are also preserved in AD fibroblasts. Therefore, increased IP_3 generation and/or enhanced IP_3 receptor sensitivity is a likely candidate to explain the observed differences in the bombesin responses in AD fibroblasts.

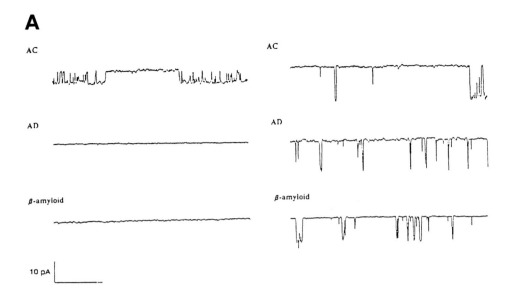

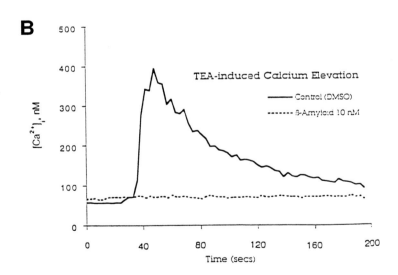

Fig. 1. Potassium channels in human fibroblasts. **(A)** Sample traces of the 113-pS K^+ channel present control fibroblasts (top left). The unitary current size (cell-attached, 0-mV pipet potential) was ≈ 4.5 pA. The channel remains largely in the open state (60% open time), with frequent but relatively short closures (upward deflections). This channel was functionally absent in AD fibroblasts and in control fibroblasts treated with 10 nM β-amyloid (bottom left). A 166-pS K^+ channel (right traces) was observed with about the same frequency in control and AD fibroblasts. In addition, this channel was not affected by β-amyloid treatment. **(B)** The TEA-induced response observed in control cell lines was missing in AD cell lines, and was also eliminated in control cells treated with β-amyloid (adapted with permission from ref. *62*).

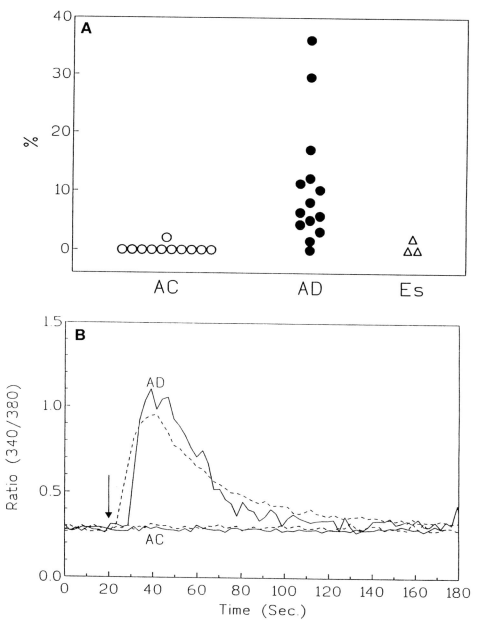

Fig. 2. Bradykinin-induced responses. Calcium elevations in response to 100 p*M* bradykinin were almost exclusively observed in AD cell lines. The graph represents each cell line tested (**A**). The degree of responsiveness is expressed as % of cells responding to the challenge (no differences in the peak or integrated area were observed among responding cells). All but one of the AD cell lines responded, and the vast majority had higher % of responding cells than the one control that exhibited a response. Cell lines from Es have responses comparable to the control group. A representative trace of the response is depicted in **B**. Solid lines are cell from the Coriell Cell Repositories. Broken lines are cells of Italian origin. The arrow indicates drug application (adapted with permission from ref. *52*).

4. Cp20 DEFICIT IN AD FIBROBLASTS

As previously stated, the small GTP-binding protein Cp20 is another critical molecule implicated in storage of associative memory. Immunoblotting techniques *(57)* were used to assess Cp20 content in fibroblasts from AD and age-matched control donors. The analyses revealed a significant reduction in Cp20 content in fibroblasts from AD patients compared to the age-matched control-group. A third group of cells from asymptomatic individuals (escapees, Es), members of a well-characterized AD Canadian family *(58,59)*, and with first-degree relatives affected, also showed a marked decrease in Cp20 content. These results suggest that Cp20 not only identifies symptomatic patients, but may also be a marker for members of this and perhaps other families with the familial form of the disease. Analyses of total protein profiles and detailed quantitative analysis of proteins with molecular weights of 200, 66–33, and 20 kDa ruled out a nonspecific, generalized protein decrease in AD fibroblasts.

5. SOLUBLE β-AMYLOID EFFECTS ON MARKERS

β-amyloid is the main component of neuritic plaques and is widely believe to play a critical role in the pathophysiology of AD. Nevertheless, no complete or satisfactory explanation exists for the mechanisms by which β-amyloid causes cell derangement and clinical symptoms *(2–4,60,61)*.

Since the potassium channel dysfunction was a clear and specific marker for AD in fibroblasts, we decided to explore the potential effects of β-amyloid on this AD marker. Fibroblasts from control individuals, known to have functional 113-pS channels and normal TEA-induced $[Ca^{2+}]_i$ elevations, were treated for 48 h with low concentrations (10 nM) of soluble β-amyloid. This concentration of β-amyloid does not cause increases in basal Ca^{2+} levels. The electrophysiological analysis revealed, however, that the 113-pS channel was missing in patches from β-amyloid-treated cells. The 166-pS channel, not affected in AD fibroblasts, was also not affected by the treatment. Thus, the β-amyloid-treated fibroblasts presented an AD-like phenotype for potassium channel function. Moreover, only the 113-pS channel was affected, indicating specificity and not a generalized toxic effect of soluble β-amyloid *(62)*. Accordingly, TEA responses were also abolished or greatly reduced in β-amyloid-treated cells, confirming that the treatment induces a K^+ channel dysfunction similar to that naturally observed in AD fibroblasts (*see* Fig. 1).

Since Cp20 was also a specific marker for AD fibroblasts, similar β-amyloid treatment was conducted prior to Cp20 measurements. Treatment of control cells with 10 nM β-amyloid for 48 h induced a significant reduction in Cp20 content, comparable to the levels observed in AD patients *(28)*. Quantitative total protein analyses indicated that, as was the case for K^+ channels, the effect of soluble β-amyloid was specific for Cp20 and not a generalized effect on protein content.

Treatment with 10 nM β-amyloid, contrary to the observed marked effects on K^+ channel function and Cp20 content, had no effect on the bombesin-induced responses *(62)*. This lack of effect of β-amyloid treatment suggests that the enhanced IP_3-induced calcium elevation in AD fibroblasts might be independent of the β-amyloid mediated pathological effects.

6. POTASSIUM CHANNELS AS TARGETS OF β-AMYLOID

In addition to the aforementioned studies on K^+ channels, a few other studies have addressed ion channel and membrane conductance changes in the general context of AD and/or in particular related to β-amyloid effects. A brief discussion of reported total membrane conductance changes will precede a more detailed discussion of reports that have specifically studied K^+ channels.

6.1. Membrane Conductances

A report *(63)* showed that sympathetic bullfrog neurons treated with relatively high concentrations of β-amyloid 25–35 (10–100 μ*M*) exhibited a nonspecific membrane conductance increase 3–4 min after drug application. This increase in membrane conductance partially reverted toward basal levels on removal of the peptide. The authors also reported a disruption of the time-dependent Ca^{2+} and K^+ currents normally present in these cells. Nevertheless, no specific channel was identified as the main current carrier. Galdizcki et al. initially reported a dose-dependent (4.6–46 μ*M*) passive membrane conductance increase in pc12 cell treated for 12 h with β-amyloid 1–40 *(64)*. In a later and expanded communication *(65)*, the authors reported that there is a choline conductance increase in pc12 cells after β-amyloid treatment.

6.2. Artificial Lipid Bilayer Studies

Using this technique, it has been shown that β-amyloid itself can form large conductance, cationic selective, multilevel ion channels with high calcium permeability. These ion channel-forming properties would arise from the formation of a complex of peptides *(61)*. The authors of the original studies have also proposed that the calcium-carrying capacity of these channels might constitute a significant pathophysiological event in AD. An independent study using the 25–35 β-amyloid fragment also showed ion channel-forming capabilities for β-amyloid with some differences in terms of the biophysical properties of the channels compared to the original studies *(66)*. These studies provided novel and intriguing pathophysiological alternatives. Nevertheless, it remains to be demonstrated that similar ion channels are indeed formed in cellular systems. A related study showing attenuation of β-amyloid toxicity by Ca^{2+} blockers also indirectly suggests that ion channels (calcium) and intracellular calcium may be part of the β-amyloid-induced alterations *(67)*.

6.3. Potassium Channels

In addition to our studies discussed above *(62)*, a few other reports have directly demonstrated effects of β-amyloid/APP on K^+ channels. Good et al. *(68)* reported that acute application (delivered close to the cell) of β-amyloid 1–40 (also 1–28 and 1–39) caused a marked decrease in rat hippocampal K^+ currents, particularly the fast-inactivating (I_A) K^+ component. Noticeable changes were observed at an estimated concentration of 10 μ*M* for the I_A. The observed effects were reversible on removal of the peptide. Other ion channels (Na^+, Ca^{2+}) were unaffected. A related study *(69)* explored the effects of secreted amyloid precursor proteins (APPs) on K^+. In concordance with other studies, the effect was the opposite. The K^+ currents were enhanced after bath application of APPs in the n*M* range in a dose-dependent manner. Single K^+ channel measurements confirmed the effect by showing a dramatic increase in the open probability of the channel after APP application. The effects of APP 695 and APP 751 were similar. The use of pharmacological tools suggested that cGMP and protein dephosphorylation mediate the APPs' effects on K^+ channels. One report using freshly isolated lymphocytes *(70)* did not find significant differences in K^+ currents after bath treatment with β-amyloid 25–35. Five days' exposure to the 1–40 peptide also was without effect on maximal K^+ conductance. Methodological differences and cell type could explain these apparently discordant results. In addition, it should be emphasized that the previously reported effects are not generalized for **all** K^+ channels and/or currents. For instance, we *(62)* reported a selective effect on the 113 pS channel, whereas a 166-pS channel was unaffected. Similarly, in the report by Good et al., only the I_A current was clearly and most significantly affected *(69)* by the treatment. Therefore, the lack of effect on the K_v current in lymphocytes might be equivalent to the lack of effect on the 166-pS channels or on other K^+ currents (different than I_A) in hippocampal rat neurons.

6.4. Potassium Channels as Therapeutic Targets?

Agents acting on K^+ channels have been in use in clinical practice, such as in diabetes (blockers) and cardiovascular diseases (mainly openers). A few studies have used blockers in AD mainly as a way to induce depolarization that would result in more neurotransmitter release. The results are mixed and not very promising (for reviews, *see* refs. *71* and *72*). Nevertheless, we could speculate—in part based on the above-discussed result on K^+ involvement in AD and their clear relationship to β-amyloid/APP—that a more direct approach using K^+ channel openers may prove useful. Consistent with such a possibility, an interesting article on ischemic injury *(73)* showed the usefulness of K^+ openers in preventing the postinjury expression or early genes, heat-shock protein, and APP. This last finding is particularly relevant in light of the relationships between head injury and/or trauma and AD, and in particular the subsequent β-amyloid deposition.

7. A DIAGNOSTIC MOLECULAR PROFILE FOR AD

Each individual molecular alteration described in AD fibroblasts *(37,51,52)* has a high degree of specificity and sensitivity, i.e., "correctly" identifies and separates AD cases from controls in the vast majority of the cases. Nevertheless, for potential diagnostic purposes, it would be desirable to maximize specificity and sensitivity. Therefore, we devised a combined scoring system taking into account all observable altered and normal responses in fibroblasts from AD and control cells, respectively. The scoring system also takes, into account the degree of "responsiveness" and/or "unresponsiveness" of each particular cell line *(52)*. The combined score generates a numerical index whose negative values indicate the pathological response for each challenge. Positive values indicate the opposite. A combined index value <0 indicates AD, and values ≥0.5 would identify normal or non-AD conditions. Control cell lines have positive scores, whereas AD cells have negative scores. Only one of the control lines had a score of 0, which is still greater than all AD cell lines. Statistical analyses of the index revealed a highly significant difference between AD and controls, $p < 0.0001$ (Mann-Whitney). Figure 3 depicts the distribution of the scores of controls and AD cell lines.

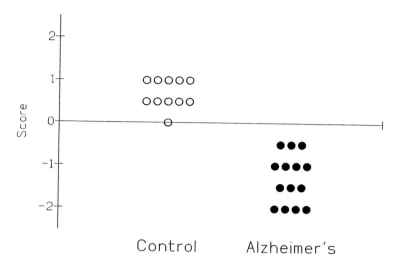

Fig. 3. Index for AD. Dots represent the combined score value for each particular cell line. As can be clearly observed from the figure, controls (open symbols) have significantly higher values than AD cell lines (solid symbols), $p < 0.001$. The two groups also segregate without overlap (adapted with permission from ref. *52*).

8. DISCUSSION

The data show that elements important in memory storage, such as K^+ channels, Cp20, and intracellular calcium release, are affected by AD. In addition, it has been shown that PKC, also implicated in memory storage and closely related to the above-mentioned components, is altered in AD fibroblasts *(74,75)*. We have also shown that fibroblasts from Alzheimer's patients exhibit a unique profile of molecular alterations. Such a profile might have significance for diagnostics and for better understanding of the pathophysiology of the disease. The results clearly indicated that taking into account the overall profile of responses does enhance the diagnostic value of these cellular alterations. Even though some AD fibroblasts do not express all AD "molecular phenotypes," in combination, they express sufficient alterations to be correctly identified by the index system. Thus, this method of considering all three responses adds significant diagnostic specificity and sensitivity. In addition, explaining why some cell lines do not express the full AD phenotype could help elucidate part of AD pathophysiology. For example, it is possible that some alterations are related to β-amyloid metabolism, whereas others are part of a more generalized pathological process. Also the changes could occur at different stages of the disease process, making some evident earlier than others. The study of familial cases and escapees has provided some indications that indeed some molecular alterations are present even before clinical symptoms are evident *(28,52)*.

Of particular pathophysiological importance is the fact that soluble β-amyloid induces AD-like alterations for K^+ channels and Cp20 in otherwise normal fibroblasts. Overall, these results suggest that the changes observed in fibroblasts might indeed occur in the brains of AD patients and may constitute molecular substrates contributing to AD symptoms, in particular early memory loss.

In addition to alterations in K^+ channels, altered regulation of IP_3-mediated calcium release occurs in AD fibroblasts. Bombesin and bradykinin induce an enhanced IP_3-mediated Ca^{2+} release in AD fibroblasts. The bombesin and bradykinin results are consistent since both agents induce IP_3 generation. More importantly, the bradykinin results are in agreement with independent studies *(53)* using a different methodology and experimental approach showing an enhanced IP_3 generation in AD fibroblasts, which consequently should produce a higher calcium signal. Responses induced by 100 p*M* bradykinin turned out to have an even higher degree of specificity for identifying AD cells than TEA or bombesin-induced responses. Higher bradykinin concentrations (1 and 10 n*M*) caused calcium elevations that were not significantly different in AD and control cell lines. These results are in agreement with a previous report showing no differences between AD and controls, using 25 n*M* bradykinin *(41)*. Another report *(42)* showed a small difference (application of 10 and 100 n*M* bradykinin) in the opposite direction, but with significant overlap. Overall, these results clearly indicate that the enhanced bradykinin sensitivity can only be observed at the subnanomolar range, and differences are obscured at higher doses. It has been suggested that the upregulation of the bradykinin-mediated response might be related to a constitutive reduction of PKC in AD fibroblasts *(53)*. It is worth noting that some of the Italian cell lines used in our study were the same in which defective PKC activity and immunoreactivity were demonstrated *(52,74,75)*. Interestingly, in these AD fibroblasts, the reduced PKC activity has been correlated with a reduced ability to secrete soluble APP *(76)*. Therefore, the AD-specific defect of Cp20 *(28)*, a highly specific substrate for the α-isozyme of PKC, may be related to these PKC differences *(74,75)*.

In summary, we provide additional evidence in peripheral tissues of AD patients that molecular changes do occur. These changes, when analyzed together, generate a unique "AD-molecular signature" that could be used as a highly specific and sensitive diagnostic tool. This is particularly relevant, since at most, genetically defined AD is only about 10% of the cases. Therefore, the vast majority of the AD cases are not amenable to detection with genetic tools. Furthermore, multiple genes are now being linked to AD, making the genetic screening even more difficult. A disease, such as cystic fibrosis (CF), which presents several different mutations, constitutes a clear example of the need to have more than the genetic criteria as a diagnostic tool. In CF, in spite of the detailed genetic knowledge, measuring sweat electrolytes remains the principal diagnostic tool *(77)*. Finally, these molecular alterations might also be of use for future research on the etiology and pathophysiology of AD.

REFERENCES

1. Katzman, R. and Kawas, C. H. (1994) The epidemiology of dementia and Alzheimer disease, in *Alzheimer Disease* (Terry, R. D., Katzman, R., and Bick, K. L., eds.), Raven, New York, pp. 105–122.
2. Selkoe, D. J. (1994) Normal and abnormal biology of the β-amyloid precursor protein, *Ann. Rev. Neurosci.* **17,** 489–517.
3. Cotman, C. W. and Pike, C. J. (1994) β-amyloid and its contributions to neurodegeneration in Alzheimer disease, in *Alzheimer Disease* (Terry, R. D., Katzman, R., and Bick, K. L., eds.), Raven, New York, pp. 305–315.
4. Ashall, F. and Goate, A. M. (1994) Role of β-amyloid precursor protein in Alzheimer's disease, *TIPS* **19,** 42–46.

5. Hardy, J. (1995) Apolipoprotein E in the genetics and epidemiology of Alzheimer's disease, *Am. J. Med. Genet.* **60**, 456–460.
6. Petersen R. C., Smith, G. E., Ivnick, R. J., Kokmen, E., and Tangalos, E. G. (1994) Memory function in very early Alzheimer's disease, *Neurology* **44**, 867-872.
7. Bondi, W. B., Salmom, D. P., and Butters, N. (1994) Neuropsychological features of memory disorders in Alzheimer disease, in *Alzheimer Disease* (Terry, R. D., Katzman, R., and Bick, K. L., eds.), Raven, New York, pp. 41–63.
8. Adams, R. D. and Victor, M. (1993) Dementia and the amnesic (Korsakoff) syndrome, in *Principles of Neurology* (Adams, R. D. and Victor, M., eds.), McGraw-Hill, pp. 364–377.
9. Terry, R. D., Masliah, E., and Hansen, L. A. (1994) Structural basis of the cognitive alterations in Alzheimer disease, in *Alzheimer Disease* (Terry, R. D., Katzman, R., and Bick, K. L., eds.), Raven, New York, pp. 179–196.
10. Nagy, S. Joshi, K. A., Esiri, M. M., Morris, J. H., King, E. M.-F., MacDonald, B., Litchield, S., Barnetson, L., and Smith (1996) Hippocampal pathology reflects memory deficits and brain imaging measurements in Alzheimer's disease: clinicopathologic correlations using three sets of pathologic diagnostic criteria, *Dementia* **7**, 76–81.
11. Alkon, D. L. (1987) *Memory Traces in the Brain*, Cambridge University Press, New York.
12. Alkon, D. L. (1989) Memory storage and neural systems, *Sci. Am.* **260**, 42–50.
13. Alkon, D. L. (1984) Calcium-mediated reduction of ionic currents: a biophysical memory trace, *Science* **226**, 1037–1045.
14. Collin, C., Ikeno, H., Harrigan, J. F., Ledelhendler, I., and Alkon, D. L. (1988) Sequential modification of membrane currents with classical conditioning, *Biophys. J.* **55**, 955–960.
15. Alkon, D. L., Naito, S., Kubota, M., Chen, C., Bank, B., Smallwood, J., Gallant, P., and Rasmussen, H. (1988) Regulation of Hermissenda K^+ channels by cytoplasmic and membrane-associated C-kinase, *J. Neurochem.* **51**, 903–917.
16. Etcheberrigaray, R., Matzel, D. L., Lederhendler, I. I., and Alkon, D. L. (1992) Classical conditioning and protein kinase C activation regulate the same single potassium channel in Hermissenda, *Proc. Natl. Acad. Sci. USA* **89**, 7184–7188.
17. Coulter, D. A., Lo Turco, J. J., Kubota, M., Disterhoft, J. F., Moore, J. W., and Alkon, D. L. (1989) Classical conditioning reduces amplitude and duration of calcium-dependent afterhyperpolarization in rabbit hippocampal pyramidal cells, *J. Neurophysiol.* **61**, 971–981.
18. Sánchez-Andrés, J. V. and Alkon, D. L. (1991) Voltage-clamp analysis of the effects of classical conditioning on the hippocampus, *J. Neurophysiol.* **65**, 796–807.
19. Bank, B., DeWeer, A., Kuzirian, A. M., Rasmussen, H., and Alkon, D. L. (1988) Classical conditioning induces long-term translocation of protein kinase C in rabbit hippocampal CA1 cells, *Proc. Natl. Acad. Sci. USA* **85**, 1988–1992.
20. Olds, J. L., Anderson, M. L., McPhie, D. L., Stanten, L. D., and Alkon, D. L. (1989) Imaging of memory-specific changes in the distribution of protein kinase C in the hippocampus, *Science* **245**, 866–869.
21. Neary, T. J., Crow, T., and Alkon, D. L. (1981) Change in a specific phosphoprotein band following associative learning in Hermissenda, *Nature* **293**, 658–660.
22. Nelson, T. J., Yoshioka, T., Toyoshima, S., Han, Y. F., and Alkon, D. L. (1994) Characterization of a GTP-binding protein implicated in both memory storage and interorganelle vesicle transport, *Proc. Natl. Acad. Sci. USA* **91**, 9287–9291.
23. Nelson, T. J., Collin, C., and Alkon, D. L. (1990) Isolation of a G protein that is modified by learning and reduces potassium currents in Hermissenda, *Science* **247**, 1479–1483.
24. Alkon, D. L., Ikeno, H., Dworkin, J., McPhie, D. L., Olds, J. L., Lederhendler, I., Matzel, L. D., Schreurs, B. G., Kuzirian, A., Collin, C., and Yamoah, E. (1990) Contraction of neuronal branching volume: an anatomical correlate of Pavlovian conditioning, *Proc. Natl. Acad. Sci. USA* **87**, 1611–1614.
25. Moshiach, S., Nelson, T., Sánchez-Andrés, J. V., Sakakibara, M., and Alkon, D. L. (1993) G-protein effects on retrograde axonal transport, *Brain Res.* **605**, 298–304.

26. Nelson, T. J., Olds, J. L., Kim, H., and Alkon, D. L. (1994) Activation of DNA transcription in neuronal cells by ARF-like GTP-binding protein, submitted.
27. Nelson, T. J., Sánchez-Andrés, J. V., Schreurs, B. G., and Alkon, D. L. (1991) Classical conditioning-induces changes in low-molecular-weight GTP-binding proteins in rabbit hippocampus, *J. Neurochem.* **57**, 2065–2069.
28. Kim, C. S., Han, Y.-F., Etcheberrigaray, R., Nelson, T. J., Olds, J. L., Toshioka, T., and Alkon, D. L. (1995) A memory-associated GTP-binding protein (Cp20) deficit in Alzheimer's and β-amyloid treated fibroblasts, *Proc. Natl. Acad. Sci. USA* **92**, 3060–3064.
29. Alkon, D. L. (1992) *Memory's Voice*, HarperCollins, New York.
30. Baker, A. C., Ko, L.-W., and Blass, J. P. (1988) Systemic manifestations of Alzheimer's disease, *Age* **11**, 60–65.
31. Scott, R. B. (1993) Extraneuronal manifestations of Alzheimer's disease, *JAGS* **41**, 268–276.
32. Hsueh-Meei, H., Martins, R., Gandy, S., et al. (1994) Use of cultured fibroblasts in elucidating the pathophysiology and diagnosis of Alzheimer's disease, *Proc. N. Y. Acad. Sci.* **747**, 225–244.
33. Seegmiller, J. E., Rosenbloom, F. M., and Kelley, N. W. (1967) An enzyme defect associated with a sex-linked human neurological disorder and an excessive purine synthesis, *Science* **155**, 1682–1686.
34. Okada, S. and O'Brien, J. S. (1969) Tay-Sachs disease: generalized absence of a beta-d-N-acetylhexosaminidase component, *Science* **165**, 698–701.
35. French, A. S. and Stockbridge, L. L. (1988) Potassium channels in human and avian fibroblasts, *Proc. R. Soc. Lond.* **232**, 395–412.
36. Sakmann, B. and Neher, E. (1995) *Single-Channel Recordings*. Plenum, New York.
37. Etcheberrigaray, R., Ito, E., Oka, K., Tofel-Grehl, B., Gibson, G. E., and Alkon, D. L. (1993) Potassium channel dysfunction in fibroblasts, *Proc. Natl. Acad. Sci. USA* **90**, 8209–8213.
38. Peterson, C., Ratan, R. R., Shelanski, M. L., and Goldman, J. E. (1986) Cytosolic free calcium and cell spreading decreases during aging and Alzheimer's disease, *Proc. Natl. Acad. Sci. USA* **83**, 7999–8001.
39. Gibson, G. E., Nielsen, P., Sherman, K. A., and Blass, J. P. (1987) Diminished mitogen-induced calcium uptake by lymphocytes from Alzheimer patients, *Biol. Psychiatry* **22**, 1079–1086.
40. Peterson, C., Ratan, R. R., Shelanski, M. L., and Goldman, J. E. (1988) Altered response of fibroblasts from aged and Alzheimer donors to drugs that elevate cytosolic free calcium, *Neurobiol. Aging* **9**, 261–266.
41. Borden, L. A., Maxfield, F. R., Goldman, J. E., and Shelanski, M. L. (1992) Resting $[Ca^{2+}]_i$ and $[Ca^{2+}]_i$ transients are similar in fibroblasts from normal and Alzheimer's donors, *Neurobiol. Aging* **13**, 33–38.
42. McCoy, K. R., Mullins, R. D., Newcornb, T. G., Ng, G. M., Pavlinkova, G., Polinsky, R. J., Nee, L. E., and Sisken, J. E. (1993) Serum- and bradykinin-induced calcium transients in familial Alzheimer's fibroblasts, *Neurobiol. Aging* **14**, 447–455.
43. Le Quang Sang, K. H., Mignot, E., Gilbert, J. C., et al. (1993) Platelet cytosolic free-calcium concentration is increased in aging and Alzheimer's disease, *Biol. Psychiatry* **3**, 391–393.
44. Sakakibara, M., Alkon, D. L., Neary, J. T., Heldman, E., and Gould, R. (1986) Inositol trisphosphate regulation of receptor membrane currents, *Biophys. J.* **50**, 797–803.
45. Spindel, E. R., Giladi, E., Segerson, T. P., and Nagalla, S. (1993) *Recent Prog. Hormone Res.* **48**, 365–391.
46. Lloyd, A. C., Davies, S. A., Crossley, I., Whitaker, M., Houslay, M. D., Hall, A., Marshall, C. J. and Wakelam, M. J. O. (1989) Bombesin stimulation of inositol 1,4,5-trisphosphate generation and the intracellular release is amplified in a cell line overexpressing the N-ras proto-oncogene, *Biochem. J.* **260**, 813–819.
47. Matozaki, T., Zhu, W.-Y., Tsunoda, Y., Göke, B., and Williams, J. A. (1991) Intracellular mediators actions on rat acinar cells, *Am. J. Physiol.* **260**, G858–G864.

48. Murphy, A. C. and Rozengurt, E. (1992) Pasteurella multocida toxin selectively facilitates phosphatidylinositol 4-5-bisphosphate hydrolysis by bombesin, vasopresin, and endothelin. Requirement for a functional G protein, *J. Biol. Chem.* **267,** 25,296–25,303.

49. Streb, H., Irvine, R. F., Berridge, M. J., and Schultz, I. (1983) Release of Ca^{2+} from nonmitochondrial intracellular stores in pancreatic acinar cells by inositol-1,4,5-trisphosphate, *Nature* **306,** 67–69.

50. Berridge, M. J. (1993) Inositol trisphosphate and calcium signalling, *Nature* **361,** 315–325.

51. Ito, E., Oka, K., Etcheberrigaray, R., et al. (1994) Internal Ca^{2+} mobilization is altered in fibroblasts from patients with Alzheimer disease, *Proc. Natl. Acad. Sci. USA* **91,** 534–538.

52. Hirashima, N., Etcheberrigaray, R., Bergamaschi, S., Racchi, M., Battaini, F., Binetti, G., Govoni, S., and Alkon, D. L. (1996) Calcium responses in human fibroblasts: a diagnostic molecular profile for Alzheimer's disease, *Neurobiol. Aging,* **17,** 549–555.

53. Huang, H.-M., Lin, T.-A., Sun, G. Y., and Gibson, G. E. (1995) Increased inositol 1,4,5-triphosphate accumulation correlates with an up-regulation of bradykinin receptors in Alzheimer's disease. *J. Neurochem.* **64,** 761–766.

54. Thastrup, O., Linnebjerg, H., Bjerrum, P. J., Knudsen, J. B., and Christensen, S. B. (1987) *Biochim. Biophys. Acta* **927,** 65–73.

55. Takemura, H., Hughes, A. R., Thastrup, O., and Putney, J. W., Jr. (1989) Activation of calcium entry by the tumor promoter thapsigargin in parotid acinar cells, *J. Biol. Chem.* **264,** 12,266–12,271.

56. Thastrup, O., Cullen, P. J., Drøbak, B. J., Hanley, M. R., and Dawson, A. P. (1990) Thapsigargin, a tumor promoter, discharges intracellular Ca^{2+} stores by specific inhibition on endoplasmic reticulum Ca^{2+}-ATPase, *Proc. Natl. Acad. Sci. USA* **87,** 2466–2470.

57. Dunbar, B. S. (1994) *Protein Blotting: A Practical Approach.* Oxford University Press, New York.

58. Nee, L. E., Polinsky, R. J., Roswell, E., Weingartner, H., Smallberg, S., and Ebert, M. (1983) A family with histologically confirmed Alzheimer's disease, *Arch. Neurol.* **40,** 203–208.

59. National Institute of Aging (1991) *Catalog of Cell Lines.*

60. Mattson, M. P., Cheng, B., Davis, D., Bryant, K., Lieberburg, I., and Rydel, R. E. (1992) β-amyloid peptides destabilize calcium homeostasis and render human cortical neurons vulnerable to excitotoxicity, *J. Neurosci.* **12,** 376–389.

61. Arispe, N., Pollard, H. B., and Rojas, E. (1993) Giant multilevel cation channels formed by Alzheimer's disease amyloid, β-protein [AβP-(1-40)] in bilayer membranes, *Proc. Natl. Acad. Sci. USA* **90,** 10,573–10,577.

62. Etcheberrigaray, R., Ito, E., Kim, C. S., and Alkon, D. L. (1994) Soluble β-amyloid induction of Alzheimer's phenotype for human fibroblasts K^+ channels, *Science* **264,** 276–279.

63. Simmons, M. A. and Schneider, C. R. (1993) Amyloid β peptides act directly on single neurons, *Neurosci. Lett.* **150,** 133–136.

64. Galdzicki, Z., Furuyama, R., Waldhwani, K. C., Ehrenstein, G., and Rapoport, S. I. (1993) Alzheimer disease β-amyloid polypeptide increases permeability of PC12 cells membrane, *Soc. Neurosci. Abs.* **19,** 397a.

65. Galdzicki, Z., Furuyama, R., Waldhwani, K. C., Rapoport, S. I., and Ehrenstein, G. (1994) β-Amyloid increases choline conductance of PC12 cells: possible mechanism of toxicity in Alzheimer's disease, *Brain Res.* **646,** 332–336.

66. Mirzabekov, T., Lin, M.-C., Yuan, W.-L., Marshall, P. J., Carman, M., Tomaselli, K., Liebeburg, I., and Kagan, B. L. (1994) Channel formation in planar lipid bilayers by a neurotoxic fragment of beta-amyloid peptide, *Biochem. Biophys. Res. Commun.* **202,** 1142–1148.

67. Weiss, J. H., Pike, C. J., and Cotman, C. W. (1994) Ca^{2+} channel blockers attenuate β-amyloid peptide toxicity to cortical neurons in culture, *J. Neurochem.* **62,** 372–375.

68. Good, T. A., Smith, D. O., and Murphy, R. M. (1996) β-Amyloid peptide blocks the fast-inactivating K^+ current in rat hippocampal neurons, *Biophys. J.* **70,** 296–304.

69. Furukawa, K., Barger, S. W., Blalock, E. M., and Mattson, M. P. (1996) Activation of K^+ channels and suppression of neural activity by secreted β-amyloid-precursor protein, *Nature* **379**, 74–78.
70. Cohen, C. D., Vollmayr, B., and Aldenhoff, J. B. (1996) *Neurosci. Lett.* **202**, 177–180.
71. Wiseman, E. J. and Jarvik, L. F. (1996) Potassium channel blockers: could they work in Alzheimer disease?, *Alzheimer Disease and Associated Disorders* **5**, 25–30.
72. Lavretsky, E. P. and Jarvik, L. F. J. (1992) A group of potassium-channel blockers-acetylcholine releasers: new potentials for Alzheimer disease?, *Clin. Psychopharmacol.* **12**, 110–118.
73. Heurteaux, C., Bertaina, V., Widmann, C., and Lazdunzki, M. (1993) K^+ openers prevent global ischemia-induced expression of c-fos, c-jun, heat shock protein, and amyloid β-protein precursor genes and neuronal death in rat hippocampus, *Proc. Natl. Acad. Sci. USA* **90**, 9431–9435.
74. Govoni, S., Bergamaschi, S., Racchi, M., Battaini, F., Binetti, G., Bianchetti, A., and Trabucchi, M. (1993) Cytosol protein kinase C down regulation in fibroblasts from Alzheimer's disease patients, *Neurology* **43**, 2581–2586.
75. Racchi, M., Wetsel, W. C., Trabucchi, M., Govoni, S., Battaini, F., Binetti, G., Bianchetti, A., and Bergamaschi, S. (1994) Reduced protein kinase C immunoreactivity in fibroblasts from patients with Alzheimer's disease, *Neurology* **44**, A164.
76. Bergamaschi, S., Racchi, M., Battaini, F., Trabucchi, M., Bianchetti, A., Binetti, G., and Govoni, S. (1994) Protein kinase C regulates β-amyloid precursor secretion in fibroblasts from control and Alzheimer's disease patients, *Soc. Neurosci. Abs.* **20**, 849.
77. Boucher, R. (1994) Cystic fibrosis, in *Harrison's principles of internal medicine* (Isselbacher, K. S., Brauwald, E., Wilson, J. D., Martin, J. B., Fauci, A. S., and Kasper, D. L., eds.), McGraw-Hill, New York, pp. 1194–1197.

16

Pick Disease

Jean Paul G. Vonsattel, Giuliano Binetti, and Lynne M. Kelley

INTRODUCTION

Lobar atrophy is a clinically diverse group of rare, non-Alzheimer, neurodegenerative disorders that often run in families, and includes the rarely occurring Pick disease.

Clinically, Pick disease mimics Alzheimer's disease (AD). However, distinctive symptoms, such as palilalia, echolalia, stereotypy (PES syndrome), language disturbances personality changes, bipolar mood changes, and bulimia, are much more striking in Pick disease than in AD. On gross examination of the brain, Pick disease is characterized by circumscribed atrophy, especially in the fronto-temporo-parietal region (Figs. 1–5). On microscopical examination, "typical" Pick disease is remarkable for neuronal loss, gliosis, and status spongiosus, principally involving the atrophic areas; also present are cortical, limbic, and striatal neurons with a single, round, intracytoplasmic, argyrophilic inclusion or Pick body (Fig. 6), and with ballooned neurons or Pick cells (Figs. 7 and 8). Furthermore, neurofibrillary tangles of Alzheimer and neuritic plaques are absent or rare.

As yet, there is no consensus on the diagnostic criteria of Pick disease. For some investigators, the presence of lobar atrophy, gliosis, and neuronal loss with or without Pick bodies is the prerequisite for diagnosing Pick disease *(1–8)*. Others require that Pick bodies and ballooned neurons be present in addition to the circumscribed atrophy with neuronal loss, and that neurofibrillary tangles of Alzheimer and neuritic plaques be absent or rare *(9–15)*. For these investigators, the brains from demented patients with lobar atrophy, but without Pick bodies are categorized in groups with the following designations: "'atypical' Pick disease" *(16)*, "fronto-temporal degeneration" *(17)*, "frontal lobe dementia" *(18,19)*, "frontal lobe dementia of non-Alzheimer type" *(18,20)*, "frontal lobe degeneration" *(6)*, "dementia of frontal lobe type" *(19–21)*, "primary progressive aphasia" *(22–24)*, or "dementia lacking distinctive histopathology" *(16,25,26)*.

Tissot et al. *(27,28)*, and Constantinidis *(29)* proposed a classification often referred to in publications on Pick disease; this classification embraces the three following subgroups of non-Alzheimer dementia brains with lobar atrophy:

1. Group A includes those brains with Pick bodies and ballooned neurons;
2. Group B includes those brains with ballooned neurons and no Pick bodies; and
3. Group C includes those brains with neither Pick bodies nor ballooned neurons.

From: Molecular Mechanisms of Dementia *Edited by: W. Wasco and R. E. Tanzi Humana Press Inc., Totowa, NJ*

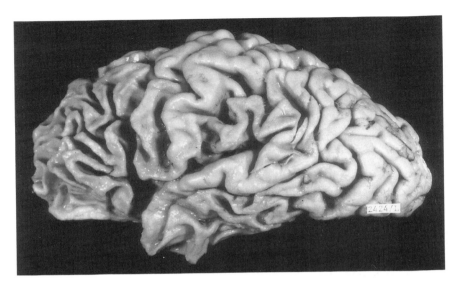

Fig. 1. Pick disease. Lateral aspect of the left cerebral hemisphere after removal of the lep-tomeninges (brain weight 860 g). Note widening of the sulci, and severe narrowing of the gyri (knife-edge appearance) involving the frontal and temporal lobes. The atrophy encroaches on both the frontal and parietal opercula; it involves the supramarginal gyrus. The caudal third of the superior temporal gyrus, and the pre- and postcentral gyri (except for the opercular area) are relatively preserved. The occipital lobe is normal.

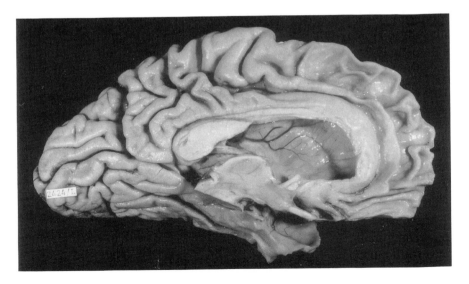

Fig. 2. Medial aspect of the left cerebral hemisphere with lateral ventricular dilatation (same brain as in Fig. 1). Knife-edge appearance of the frontal and temporal gyri, with abrupt transi-tion between atrophic and relatively preserved parts. Note the atrophy of the rostral two-thirds of the corpus callosum, and the apparently normal splenium corpori callosi.

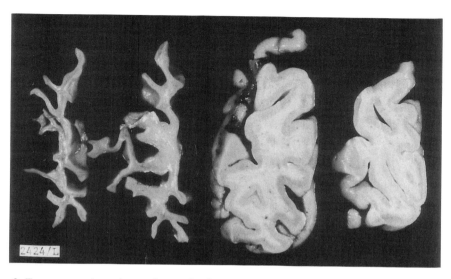

Fig. 3. Four coronal sections of same brain as in Fig. 1. The two coronal sections on the left are passing rostral to the rostrum corpori callosi, and show extreme cortical and white-matter atrophy. The two coronal sections on the right are passing caudal to the splenium corpori callosi, and show minimal atrophy, if at all.

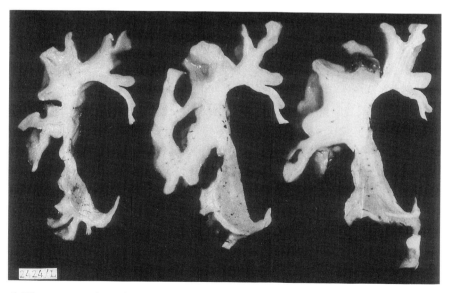

Fig. 4. Three coronal sections of same brain as Fig. 1, passing through the rostral tip of the neostriatum (left) and anterior white commissure (right). There is pan-laminar *(see text)* atrophy involving cortex, white matter, and striatum, and striking ventricular dilatation. Note that the head of the caudate nucleus is more severely atrophic than the putamen.

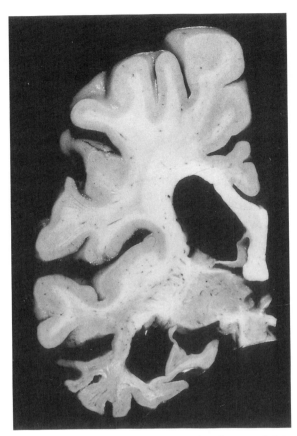

Fig. 5. Coronal section of same brain as Fig. 1, passing just caudal to the lateral geniculate body. Note the striking atrophy of the hippocampal formation and temporal lobe, except for the superior temporal gyrus. Also relatively preserved are the gyrus precentralis, and the gyrus postcentralis. There is marked atrophy of the parietal cortex and subcortical white matter (between the superior temporal gyrus, and the gyrus postcentralis).

In the International Classification of Diseases (ICD-10), there is no reference to Pick bodies in the definition of Pick disease, and the neuropathological picture is described as a selective atrophy of the frontal and temporal lobes without the occurrence of the neuritic plaques and neurofibrillary tangles in excess of what is seen in normal aging.

More recent diagnostic concepts on Pick disease are discussed by Baldwin and Förstl *(10)*, and Jellinger *(13)*. According to these new concepts, Pick disease should not or cannot be diagnosed on the basis of frontotemporal degeneration alone; truly, the pathology associated with the frontotemporal degeneration is too heterogeneous. The presence of ballooned neurons is not specific to Pick disease, since ballooned neurons are seen in many other neurodegenerative conditions *(2,30)*, including AD, corticobasal degeneration, corticonigral degeneration, primary progressive aphasia, and progressive supranuclear palsy *(22,31–38)*. However, special emphasis is now made on the presence of Pick bodies for diagnosing "typical" Pick disease, since Pick bodies are almost never identified in conditions other than those combining dementia and circumscribed

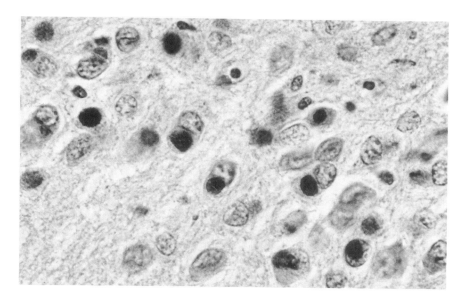

Fig. 6. Microphotograph of the dentate gyrus of the hippocampus showing approx 10 Pick bodies detected with antibodies recognizing abnormal τ (×700).

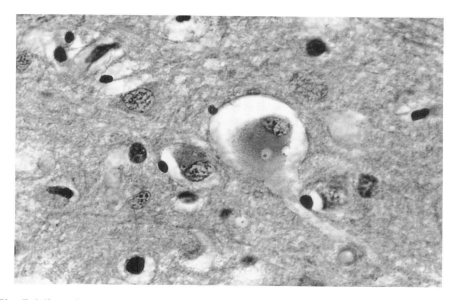

Fig. 7. Microphotograph with a ballooned neuron (Pick cell) containing two vacuoles, each with a granule. Granulovacuolar changes are also present in the smaller neuron on the left of the ballooned neuron. Superior frontal gyrus. Stained with Luxol-fast-blue and counterstained with H&E (×700).

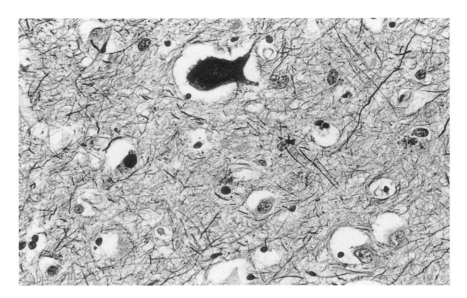

Fig. 8. Microphotograph from the transition zone between severely atrophic and relatively preserved areas. There is an argyrophilic ballooned neuron, and, located at approx 7 o'clock, a small neuron with an argyrophilic Pick body. Note numerous normal looking neurons and axons. Superior frontal gyrus. Stained with Bielschowsky silver method (×440).

cerebral atrophy. Therefore, the features that are gaining acceptance as being characteristic of "typical" Pick disease may be summarized as follows: speech impairment, emotional instability often with moriatic syndrome (hebetude, foolishness, dullness of comprehension, mental state marked by frivolity, joviality, inability to take anything seriously); cognitive deterioration and dementia, circumscribed fronto-temporo-parietal atrophy (lobar atrophy often including the hippocampal formation, amygdala, and deep gray nuclei, especially in the anterior portion of the striatum, with relative preservation of the caudal third of the superior temporal gyrus); status spongiosus, neuronal loss in the atrophic areas, and the presence of Pick bodies, usually with ballooned neurons.

2. HISTORICAL OVERVIEW

Arnold Pick claimed that, in some instances, "senile brain atrophy" was circumscribed and not diffuse, challenging the dogmatic belief, defended by Wernicke, that senile cerebral atrophy was always a diffuse process *(39)*. To support his claim, Pick presented, along with the clinical data, the macroscopical findings of the neuropathological evaluation performed by Chiari of the brain from V. J., who died at the age of 60. The clinical hallmarks relevant to the present understanding of the disease include: family burden of mental illness involving at least a sister; "amnesic" aphasia, however, with preserved ability to recite the months serially; memory loss, stereotypy, and apraxia. The neuropathological hallmarks provided are: brain weight 1105 g (right hemisphere 485 g; left hemisphere 460 g); severe atrophy involving the frontal lobes and the left inferior parietal lobule; mild atrophy involving the right inferior parietal lobule, and the bilateral temporal and occipital lobes; there was no atrophy of the precentral gyri or superior parietal lobules. No microscopical evaluation was performed. This early publication emphasized that cerebral degeneration can be circumscribed and asymmetric, and that the condition might be hereditary.

The description and association of the Pick bodies and ballooned neurons with circumscribed cerebral atrophy was done by Alzheimer, who also pointed out the absence of neuritic plaques, the lack of neurofibrillary tangles, and the relative preservation of the superior temporal gyrus as compared to the severely atrophic middle and inferior temporal gyri *(40)*. Lüers and Spatz noted that, in 1918, H. Richter described lobar atrophy in a 42-yr-old woman, indicating that the condition was not restricted to old people; they also claim that, in 1930, Grünthal observed the occurrence in siblings of what was then already referred to as Pick disease *(2)*. Recent studies have been crucial in defining Pick disease and in distinguishing it from AD *(2,3,27)*. Unfortunately, universally accepted diagnostic criteria for Pick disease are still lacking, as previously mentioned.

3. CLINICAL ASPECTS

Currently, the reliability of the diagnosis of Pick disease depends on both the clinical course and the results of the postmortem evaluation. Most clinical data available about Pick disease patients with detailed neuropathological evaluations are derived from individuals having discrete frontotemporal atrophy, either with or without parietal involvement, Pick bodies, or mild concomitant Alzheimer pathology. Therefore, this clinical review reflects data obtained from series of patients categorized as having Pick disease according to the criteria described by Tissot et al. *(27)*, or according to criteria closely resembling them, since Pick bodies or ballooned neurons are not sensitive indicators of the whole range of reported Pick disease *(2,3,41)*.

Pick disease is rare and is often confused with AD; clarification is then brought by postmortem evaluation. Pick disease is observed in areas where reliable clinical and pathological evaluations of dementias can be performed. Sporadic Pick disease is more frequent than familial. A literature search identified 16 pedigrees, including two or more affected family members, at least one of which had lobar atrophy and Pick bodies. Fourteen of the 16 pedigrees showed Pick disease in two or more generations. Additional studies of large families also suggest an inheritance pattern compatible with an autosomal-dominant gene *(41–43)*. The frequency of Pick disease is described in comparison to AD: in individuals aged 65 or older, the prevalence of Pick disease is estimated to be 5–6/1000 persons *(28)*, whereas the prevalence of AD is estimated to be between 3 and 11/100 persons in this same age group *(44,45)*. Women are more frequently involved than men at a ratio of up to 2:1 *(2,27,28,41)*. The onset of symptoms occurs most often during the sixth decade of life; however, it has also been observed during the second and ninth decades *(2,27)*. Patients with early onset of symptoms have a shorter clinical course, increased familial incidence, and more severe pathology (involvement of the deep gray nuclei) than patients with late onset *(2,9)*. Survival from onset of symptoms to death ranges from 1 to 15 yr *(3,27,42)*. The increased apolipoprotein E ε4 allele frequency is a well-recognized risk factor for AD; however, in Pick disease, it was found to be either slightly increased *(8)* or indistinguishable from the control population *(46)*.

The symptoms observed in Pick disease are determined by the pathology character-istic of the disease, i.e., predominantly circumscribed frontotemporal atrophy with rela-tive preservation of the rest of the brain. Arnold Pick himself noticed speech abnormalities in the presence of severe frontotemporal atrophy, and claimed that the atrophy of the left temporal lobe could be diagnosed *intra vitam*.

The initial symptoms are variable, and they apparently affect the personality or character of the patient rather than formal intelligence *(2)*. Behavioral disturbances, personality changes (socially inappropriate activity, sexual indiscretions, loss of per-sonal propriety, and other disinhibition), hyperorality, excessive manual exploration (hypermetamorphosis), emotional blunting, altered dietary preferences, apathy, irri-tability, depression, jocularity, euphoria, echolalia, and mutism are reported as early symptoms *(47)*. An isolated progressive aphasia, characterized by the presence of word finding difficulties, paraphasic errors, circumlocution, occasional jargon, echolalia, and verbal stereotypy, is the second most prominent presentation of the disease.

The following anomalies gradually appear and worsen with time: dysexecutive syn-drome, loss of interest in the usual activities, inability to manage intellectual capacity, euphoria, depression, disproportionate reactions, poor hygiene, and inappropriate sexual behavior (at times, including Klüver-Bucy syndrome, often early in the disease), all without the patient's awareness; other symptoms include megalomania, compul-sive–obsessive disorder, stereotypy, dysarthria, apraxia, imbalance with frequent falls, and bulimia. In contrast to AD, perception and orientation (visuospatial skills) and memory are relatively preserved; e.g., the bulimic Pick disease patient looks for food in an organized fashion *(3,47–49)*.

Pyramidal signs might occur when the circumscribed atrophy includes the precen-tral gyrus *(42)*. Extrapyramidal signs (troncular rigidity, cogwheel rigidity, stooped posture, festinating gait, tremor, choreoathetosis) are less frequently observed than would be expected, since striatopallidonigral degeneration is observed between 62 and 78% of the Pick disease brains *(see below) (4,9)*.

Three syndromes summarize the clinical findings often observed in Pick disease: Moriatic syndrome (or moria), PES syndrome, and PEMA syndrome, which includes palilalia, echolalia, mutism, and amimia *(3,18,27)*.

The association of Pick disease and amyotrophic lateral sclerosis occurs more fre-quently than just by chance, and was identified as early as 1932 *(2)*. The association of Pick disease with amyotrophic lateral sclerosis appears to take place especially when there is "total frontal atrophy" with involvement of the precentral gyrus. In such instances, the entire motor system, including the spinal motor neurons, might degenerate *(2)*.

There are reports of the association of Pick disease with corticobasal degeneration *(50,51)*, striatopallidonigral degeneration *(52)*, or progressive supranuclear palsy *(53)*. The concomitant occurrence of Pick disease (with Pick bodies) and AD does happen occasionally, and is probably coincidental *(11,54)*. Similarly, some Alzheimer changes are often (if not always) apparent, but only to a degree that is insufficient to meet the neuropathological criteria of AD *(11)*.

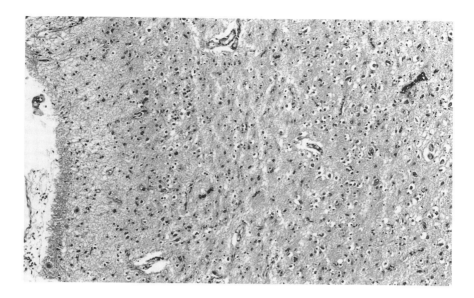

Fig. 9. Microphotograph of the cortex of the occipitotemporalis gyrus with pial surface on the left, showing neuronal loss, and loose textured neuropil (status spongiosus). Stained with Luxol-fast-blue and counterstained with H&E (×85).

4. NEUROPATHOLOGY

As previously mentioned, there is no consensus on the neuropathological diagnosis of Pick disease, the trend now being the requirement of the presence of Pick bodies assessed microscopically, which is not universally accepted.

Because of their importance in Pick disease, we will first present and define key features encountered in this disease: Pick bodies (Figs. 6 and 8), ballooned neurons (Figs. 7 and 8), and status spongiosus (Fig. 9).

As mentioned, Pick bodies were initially described by Alzheimer while evaluating brains with circumscribed atrophy from demented patients. Alzheimer's description *(40)* is as follows:

Sections prepared with Bielschowsky method show small pyramidal cells containing an argyrophilic, sometimes structureless ball near the nucleus, whose size varies from half to twice that of the nucleus. The inclusion is either above or below the nucleus, which is displaced accordingly downward or upward.

In addition to being argyrophilic, Pick bodies are weakly basophilic. Ultrastructurally, the inclusions are membraneless, composed of straight filaments, 15–18 nm in diameter, without sidearm or fuzzy material attached to them *(9,55,56)*.

In the classification of Tissot et al. *(27)*, Pick bodies are found in 31% of brains with lobar atrophy; at about the same frequency reported earlier *(2)*. However, according to the new trend of categorization, Pick bodies must be present.

The sites of predilection for Pick bodies are the hippocampal formation (subiculum, indusium griseum, and stratum granulosum of the dentate gyrus); entorhinal cortex, amygdala, septal nuclei, and the second, third, and sixth cortical layers of the frontal, cingulate, and temporal neocortices, except in the caudal third of the superior temporal gyrus *(11,12,27)*. Pick bodies, which are apparently free in the neuropil, are occasionally present in the cortical areas displaying extreme atrophy *(27)*. Pick bodies may be prominent in the anterior neostriatum (caudate nucleus, putamen, and nucleus accumbens) and hypothalamus *(9,27)*, but are rarely found in the globus pallidus (personal observation).

Pick bodies are stained with antibodies to ubiquitin, chromogranin A *(13,57)*, phosphorylated neurofilaments epitopes (Fig. 6), τ, or to A2B5, which recognizes neuronal surface ganglioside, indicating that membrane proteins may be incorporated into the inclusions *(38,58,59)*, the N-terminal, and the intermediate segments of β-amyloid precursor protein *(60)*.

Immunoblot evaluation of brain samples containing Pick bodies revealed abnormally phosphorylated 55- and 64-kDa τ protein doublets. This differs from the triplet τ profile (55, 64, and 69) of the paired helical filaments in AD *(14)*. Buée-Scherrer et al. *(61)* confirmed this particular τ profile in brains with Pick bodies, but without neurofibrillary tangles of Alzheimer; however, they also demonstrated that the τ profile of Pick disease brains containing both Pick bodies and neurofibrillary tangles of Alzheimer was similar to that of AD (τ 55, 64, and 69).

In some instances, cortical Lewy bodies are strongly argyrophilic and therefore may be difficult to differentiate from Pick bodies by usual staining methods; hence, discrimination between cortical Lewy bodies and Pick bodies may require ultrastructural evaluation *(56)*.

Ballooned neurons (Figs. 7 and 8) are swollen ganglia cells with convex contours, homogeneous glassy, pale, eosinophilic cytoplasm, and eccentric nuclei. The cytoplasm is diffusely argyrophilic with variable intensity (Fig. 8). At times, cytoplasmic vacuoles with or without a centrally located granule are present (Fig. 7) *(3,30,32,41)*. Ultrastructurally, ballooned neurons have variable features; some are filled with straight filaments similar to those found in Pick bodies, and others contain normal elements with admixed straight filaments of variable density *(9,41,55)*. Ballooned neurons can be distinguished from swollen chromatolytic neurons, suggesting different pathogenesis *(32)*.

In the classification of Tissot et al. *(27)*, ballooned neurons are found in 62% of brains with lobar atrophy. They are scattered, especially in the intermediary zones between the severely affected and the relatively preserved areas of the neocortex and entorhinal cortex. They are frequently observed in the anterior cingulate gyrus, insular cortex, and claustrum. At times, they are found in the anterior neostriatum *(27)*.

Ballooned neurons share most of the immunocytochemical characteristics with the filaments in Pick bodies *(13,32,41)*; many ballooned neurons in Pick disease are positive with antibodies to αB-crytallin *(6)*, or Alz-50 *(5)*.

Microscopically, the atrophic, severely gliotic parenchyma is often vacuolated or loose-textured; the outer layers of the cortical ribbon are especially involved (Fig. 9). Unfortunately, many terms are used to designate these changes that are best referred to as status spongiosus, which is defined as follows: "nonspecific, and characteristically is the manifestation of end-stage gliosis; it consists of irregular cavitation of the neuropil in the presence of a dense glial meshwork" *(62)*. Status spongiosus is to be distinguished from spongiform changes, which consist of the presence of small round or ovoid vacuoles within the neuropil, and which are striking features of the spongiform encephalopathies *(43,62)*. To some extent, spongiform changes are also observed in diffuse Lewy body disease, AD-Lewy body variant, and in some cases of AD *(63–66)*.

The average brain weight and volume of one lateral ventricle obtained from our series (n = 20 women and 15 men; 23 with Pick bodies) are as follows: women (known weight and ventricular volume, n = 18), 955 ± 174 g; 25.6 ± 13.2 cc (normal 7–10 cc); men (known weight, n = 14; known ventricular volume, n = 11), 1085 ± 172 g; 28.5 ± 14.6 cc. The average Pick brain weight reported is 900–1000 g for women and 1000–1220 g for men *(27,41)*.

Pick disease brains show circumscribed bilateral, symmetric, or asymmetric, pan laminar (*see below*) frontotemporal atrophy, and may be with or without parietal involvement. The atrophy is evidenced by widening of the sulci and narrowing of the gyri. It can be so severe that the gyri may resemble a knife edge (Figs. 1 and 2). When more than one lobe is involved (at times referred to as mixed atrophy), the atrophy can be harmonious or can predominate in either of them. The involvement can encompass the whole lobe or part of it; it might be more severe medially than laterally, or vice versa. About 60% of the Pick disease brains show more atrophy on one side than on the other, most frequently on the left. The transition between the atrophic and relatively preserved areas is abrupt, or when gradual, is usually confined over a narrow band (Fig. 2). Often, the caudal third of the superior temporal gyrus is relatively preserved (Fig. 5). Exceptionally, the atrophy also involves the occipital lobe *(47)*, or is mainly confined to the parietal lobe on one side *(50)*.

Pan laminar atrophy refers to the involvement of all the structures included in the circumscribed atrophic area; for example, if the lobar atrophy extends from the frontal pole to the precentral gyrus, including the temporal lobe, usually the pathological changes will be conspicuous in the cortex, white matter, anterior portion of the striatum and thalamus with mesencephalic extension, and amygdala and hippocampal formation (Fig. 4). In contrast to Huntington's disease *(67)*, the atrophy of the rostral portion of the neostriatum can be extreme, whereas the caudal portion is relatively preserved. Furthermore, the head of the caudate nucleus and nucleus accumbens are more atrophic than the nearby putamen, which shows more pathological changes along the internal capsule than along the external capsule (Fig. 4).

Neuronal loss, cortical status spongiosus, myelin and axonal loss, and astrogliosis are striking in the atrophic areas of gray or white matter. In addition, in "typical" Pick disease, scattered neurons are present with Pick bodies and ballooned neurons. The three outer cortical layers are more prone to degenerate than the inner layers (Fig. 9). Proliferation of microglial cells was found to be striking in both atrophic cortex and white matter using the microgliocytes marker KiM1P *(68)*. Scattered astrocytes and oligodendrocytes with τ-positive inclusions were observed *(38,58)*. The density of neurons, fibers, or myelin may be apparently normal in nonatrophic areas (Fig. 10). In contrast to AD, the amygdala in Pick disease is diffusely damaged, without apparent nuclear selectivity *(47)*.

Tissot et al. *(27)* found in their series (n = 32, 10 with Pick bodies) atrophy and gliosis of the caudate nucleus in 69%, of the globus pallidus in 56%, of the thalamus in 62%, and of the substantia nigra in 59% of the brains. Striatopallidonigral degeneration was found in 78% of the 41 brains (11 with Pick bodies) evaluated by Kosaka et al. *(4)*.

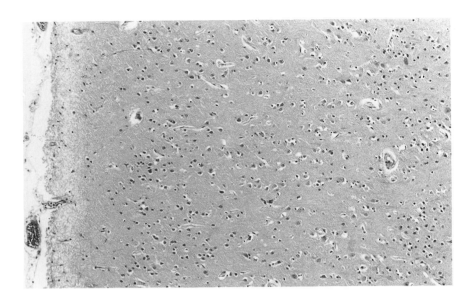

Fig. 10. Microphotograph of the relatively preserved cuneal cortex (pial surface on the left) for comparison with Fig. 9 (same magnification same staining).

In addition to the nigral damage, two features may be striking: in the brainstem, fiber loss in the crus cerebri; and severe neuronal loss and gliosis in the inferior olivary nucleus *(2,27)*.

Munoz-Garcia et al. *(9)* proposed to subcategorize Pick disease brains into two groups (classic and generalized) on the basis of the involvement of the subcortical structures and on the distribution, histochemical, immunochemical, and ultrastructural characteristics of the Pick bodies. According to this scheme, the "classic" group includes those brains with predominately cortical atrophy, and with Pick bodies that stain with antibodies to neurofilament proteins and tubilin. The "generalized" group includes those brains with subcortical and cortical atrophy, and with weakly argyrophilic Pick bodies containing RNA, which stained poorly with antibodies to neurofilaments or to microtubules. As pointed out, there are brains from patients that are clinically and pathologically indistinguishable from those categorized as "typical" Pick disease, except for the absence of Pick bodies; these could be referred to as "atypical" Pick disease, or better Pick disease without Pick bodies, Pick disease type B, or Pick disease type C according to Tissot et al. *(27)*.

It is still controversial whether Pick bodies must be present for diagnosing Pick disease or, conversely, whether the lack of Pick bodies rules out the diagnosis of Pick disease. From a practical, neuropathological point of view, the requirement of the presence of Pick bodies for the diagnosis of Pick disease is seductive, yet perhaps too rigid, especially for clinicians. Indeed, it would raise the question of whether it would be appropriate to diagnose Pick disease *intra vitam (69)*. Interestingly, the original observation by Arnold Pick was clinical, and the first clinicopathological correlation was based only on the gross examination of the brain, which is inappropriate to assess the presence or absence of Pick bodies.

We systematically evaluated 35 brains with circumscribed lobar atrophy; 23 of them had unequivocal Pick bodies (many in 12; rare in 11) evidenced with Bielschowsky silver impregnation. However, using antibodies for τ and ubiquitin, scattered cortical or limbic Pick bodies, although rare, were found in 5 of the 12 brains in which no Pick bodies could be found with the Bielschowsky method during the initial evaluation. These "Bielschowsky false-negative" brains were those with the most severe pathology. Pick bodies might fail to stain when silver impregnation is not optimal *(27)*. Furthermore, Pick bodies stain poorly with silver and with antibodies to neurofilaments or microtubules in addition to straight filaments, when they contain granular material possibly derived from ribosomes *(9)*. Perhaps there are brains in which Pick bodies are hard to find when the pathology is extreme, in the way neurofibrillary tangles can be difficult to detect in brains of patients with very severe AD *(70)*. The presence of Pick bodies (and ballooned neurons) may be a transient event and only apparent in the early stages of the disease *(31,41)*, although many Pick bodies were observed even in severely involved areas *(12)*. The reservation in categorizing brains that have all the features of Pick disease except for the presence of Pick bodies within the groups, including frontal lobe dementia, or dementia lacking distinctive histology, is justified for the following reasons:

1. The lack of methodological guidelines (silver stain, immunoperoxidase evaluation) to determine the presence or absence of Pick bodies;
2. The lack of data about the minimal number of Pick bodies and about their distribution for diagnostic inclusion or exclusion;
3. The current cloudiness surrounding the definitions of frontal lobe dementia, or dementia lacking distinctive histology is striking; and
4. The possibility of dissuading clinicians to consider using this term, at a time when Pick disease is increasingly recognized *intra vitam (16,18,19,25,26,71)*.

Brains with circumscribed atrophy from demented patients could simply be categorized as either "lobar atrophy with Pick bodies" or "lobar atrophy without Pick bodies," and then those brains without Pick bodies could be assigned to the diverse groups of frontal lobe atrophy according to their individual characteristics.

The problem of categorizing Pick disease stresses the limits of evaluations resting on morphological features, despite the availability of immunohistochemical methods. In addition, it emphasizes the need for a multidisciplinary strategy that includes molecular biology methods to unveil the mystery of this puzzling and dramatic neurodegenerative disease.

ACKNOWLEDGMENTS

This work was supported in part by NIH grants NINCDS 31862 (Brain Tissue Resource Center, J. P. V.), NS 163 67 (Huntington's Disease Center Without Walls, J. P. V.), and NIA 2P50-AGO 5134-10 (J. P. V., G. B., L. M. K.).

Special thanks are given to Yan Zhao, Wendy Hobbs, Timothy Wheelock, Stephanie Lenzi, and Larry Cherkas for advice and technical assistance. We owe an exceptional debt of gratitude to Edward P. Richardson, for his immense support, and for his special role in getting us interested in neurodegenerative diseases.

REFERENCES

1. Spatz, H. (1952) La maladie de Pick, les atrophies systématisées progressives et la sénescence cérébrale prématurée localisée, in *The Proceedings of the First International Congress of Neuropathology*, vol. 2. Rosenberg and Sellier, Torino, pp. 375–406.
2. Lüers, Th. and Spatz, H. (1957) Picksche Krankheit (Progressive umschriebene Grosshinratrophie), in *Handbuch der speziellen pathologischen Anatomie und Histologie* (XIII/1 Bandteil A) (Lubarsch, O., Henke, F., Rössle, R., and Scholz, W., eds.), Springer Verlag, Berlin, pp. 614–715.
3. Brion, S., Plas, J., and Jeanneau, A. (1991) La maladie de Pick. Point de vue anatomo-clinique, *Rev. Neurol.* **147,** 693–704.
4. Kosaka, K., Ikeda, K., Kobayashi, K., and Mehraein, P. (1991) Striatopallidonigral degeneration in Pick's disease: a clinicopathological study of 41 cases, *J. Neurol.* **238,** 151–160.
5. Wood, B. T. and McKee, A. C. (1992) Case Records of the Massachusetts General Hospital. Case 6-1992, *N. Engl. J. Med.* **326,** 397–405.
6. Cooper, P. N., Jackson, M., Lennox, G., Lowe, J., and Mann, D. M. A. (1995) τ, ubiquitin, and αB-crystallin immunohistochemistry define the principal causes of degenerative frontotemporal dementia, *Arch. Neurol.* **52,** 1011–1015.
7. Hansen, L. A. and Crain, B. (1995) Making the diagnosis of mixed and non-Alzheimer's disease, *Arch. Pathol. Lab. Med.* **119,** 1023–1031.
8. Schneider, J. A., Gearing, M., Robbins, R. S., de l'Aune, W., and Mirra, S. S. (1995) Apolipoprotein E genotype in diverse neurodegenerative disorders, *Ann. Neurol.* **38,** 131–135.
9. Munoz-Garcia, D. and Ludwin, S. K. (1984) Classic and generalized variants of Pick's disease: a clinicopathological, ultrastructural, and immunocytochemical comparative study, *Ann. Neurol.* **16,** 467–480.
10. Baldwin, B. and Förstl, H. (1993) "Pick's disease"—101 years on still there, but in need of reform, *Br. J. Psychiatry* **163,** 100–104.
11. Hof, P. R., Bouras, C., Perl, D. P., and Morrison, J. H. (1994) Quantitative neuropathologic analysis of Pick's disease cases: cortical distribution of Pick bodies and coexistence with Alzheimer disease, *Acta Neuropathol.* **87,** 115–124.
12. Jellinger, K. A. (1994) Quantitative neuropathologic analysis of Pick's disease cases, *Acta Neuropathol.* **87,** 223,224.
13. Jellinger, K. A. (1995) Neuropathological criteria for Pick's disease and frontotemporal lobe dementia, in *Neuropathological Diagnostic Criteria for Brain Banking* (Cruz-Sánchez, F. F., Ravid, R., and Cuzner, M. L., eds.), IOS Press, Amsterdam, pp. 35–54.
14. Delacourte, A., Robitaille, Y., Sergeant, N., Buée, L., Hof, P. R., Wattez, A., Laroche-Cholette, A., Mathieu, J., Chagnon, P., and Gauvreau, D. (1996) Specific pathological Tau protein variants characterize Pick's disease, *J. Neuropathol. Exp. Neurol.* **55,** 159–168.
15. Litvan, I., Hauw, J. J., Bartko, J. J., Lantos, P. L., Daniel, S. E., Horoupian, D. S., McKee, A., Dickson, D., Bancher, C., Tabaton, M., Jellinger, K., and Anderson, D. W. (1996) Validity and reliability of the preliminary NINDS neuropathologic criteria for progressive supranuclear palsy and related disorders, *J. Neuropathol. Exp. Neurol.* **55,** 97–105.
16. Giannakopoulos, P., Hof, P. R., and Bouras, C. (1995) Dementia lacking distinctive histopathology: clinicopathological evaluation of 32 cases, *Acta Neuropathol.* **89,** 346–355.
17. The Lund and Manchester Groups (1994) Clinical and neuropathological criteria for frontotemporal dementia, *J. Neurol. Neurosurg. Psychiatry* **57,** 416–418.
18. Gustafson, L., Brun, A., and Passant, U. (1992) Frontal lobe degeneration of non-Alzheimer type, in *Baillière's Clinical Neurology. International Practice and Research. Unusual Dementias* (Rossor, M. N., ed.), Baillière Tindall/W. B. Sounders, London, pp. 559–582.
19. Mann, D. M. A., South, P. W., Snowden, J. S., and Neary, D. (1993) Dementia of frontal lobe type: neuropathology and immunohistochemistry, *J. Neurol. Neurosurg. Psychiatry* **56,** 605–614.

20. Neary, D. (1990) Non Alzheimer's disease forms of cerebral atrophy, *J. Neurol. Neurosurg. Psychiatry* **53**, 929–931.
21. Wightman, G., Anderson, V. E. R., Martin, J., Swash, M., Aderton, B. H., Neary, D., Mann, D., Luthert, P., and Leigh, P. N. (1992) Hippocampal and neocortical ubiquitin-immunoreactive inclusions in amyotrophic lateral sclerosis with dementia, *Neurosci. Lett.* **139**, 269–274.
22. Lippa, C. F., Cohen, R., Smith, T. W., and Drachman, D. A. (1991) Primary progressive aphasia with focal neuronal achromasia, *Neurology* **41**, 882–886.
23. Mesulam, M. M. and Weintraub, S. (1992) Spectrum of primary progressive aphasia, in *Baillière's Clinical Neurology. International Practice and Research. Unusual Dementias* (Rossor, M. N., ed.), Baillière Tindall/W. B. Sounders, London, pp. 583–609.
24. Scheltens, P., Ravid, R., and Kamphorst, W. (1994) Pathologic findings in a case of primary progressive aphasia, *Neurology* **44**, 279–282.
25. Knopman, D. S., Mastri, A. R., Frey, W. H., Sung, J. H., and Rustan, T. (1990) Dementia lacking distinctive histologic features: a common non-Alzheimer degenerative dementia, *Neurology* **40**, 251–256.
26. Jackson, M. and Lowe, J. (1996) The new neuropathology of degenerative frontotemporal dementias, *Acta Neuropathol.* **91**, 127–134.
27. Tissot, R., Constantinidis, J., and Richard, J. (1975) La maladie de Pick. Masson, Paris.
28. Tissot, R., Constantinidis, J., and Richard, J. (1985) Pick's disease, in *Handbook of Clinical Neurology,* vol. 2 (46): *Neurobehavioural Disorders* (Frederiks, J. A. M., ed.), Elsevier Science Publishers B. V., Amsterdam, pp. 233–246.
29. Constantinidis, J. (1985) Pick Dementia: Anatomical correlations and pathophysiological considerations, *Interdiscipl. Topics Geront.* **19**, 72–97.
30. Williams, H. W. (1935) The peculiar cells of Pick's disease. Their pathogenesis and distribution in disease, *Arch. Neurol. Psychiatry* **34**, 508–519.
31. Clark, A. W., Manz, H. J., White, C. L. III, Lehmann, J., Miller, D., and Coyle, J. T. (1986) Cortical degeneration with swollen chromatolytic neurons: its relationship to Pick's disease, *J. Neuropathol. Exp. Neurol.* **45**, 268–284.
32. Dickson, D. W., Yen, S.-H., Suzuki, K. I., Davies, P., Garcia, J. H., and Hirano, A. (1986) Ballooned neurons in select neurodegenerative diseases contain phosphorylated neurofilament epitopes, *Acta Neuropathol.* **71**, 216–223.
33. Gibb, R. G., Luthert, P. J., and Marsden, C. D. (1989) Corticobasal degeneration, *Brain* **112**, 1171–1192.
34. Lippa, C. F., Smith, T. W., and Fontneau, N. (1990) Corticonigral degeneration with neuronal achromasia. A clinicopathologic study of two cases, *J. Neurol. Sci.* **98**, 301–310.
35. Feany, M. B. and Dickson, D. W. (1995) Widespread cytoskeletal pathology characterizes corticobasal degeneration, *Am. J. Pathol.* **146**, 1388–1396.
36. Mackenzie, I. R. A. and Hudson, L. P. (1995) Achromatic neurons in the cortex of progressive supranuclear palsy, *Acta Neuropathol.* **90**, 615–619.
37. Pillon, B., Blin, J., Vidailhet, M., Deweer, B., Sirigu, A., Dubois, B., and Agid, Y. (1995) The neuropsychological pattern of corticobasal degeneration: comparison with progressive supranuclear palsy and Alzheimer's disease, *Neurology* **45**, 1477–1483.
38. Feany, M. B., Mattiace, L. A., and Dickson, D. W. (1996) Neuropathologic overlap of progressive supranuclear palsy, Pick's disease and corticobasal degeneration, *J. Neuropathol. Exp. Neurol.* **55**, 53–67.
39. Pick, A. (1906) Über einen weiteren Symptomenkomplex im Rahmen der Dementia senilis, bedingt durch umschriebene stärkere Hirnatrophie (gemischte Aparxie), *Monatsschrift für Psychiatrie und Neurologie* **19**, 97–108.
40. Alzheimer, A. (1911) Über eigenartige Krankheitsfälle des späteren Alters, *Zentralblatt für die gesamte Neurologie und Psychiatrie* **4**, 356–385.
41. Brown, J. (1992) Pick's disease, in *Baillière's Clinical Neurology. International Practice and Research. Unusual Dementias* (Rossor, M. N., ed.), Baillière Tindall/W. B. Sounders, London, pp. 535–557.

42. Groen, J. J. and Endtz, L. J. (1982) Herediraty Pick's disease second re-examination of a large family and discussion of other hereditary cases, with particular reference to electroencephalography and computerized tomography, *Brain* **105**, 443–459.

43. Collinge, J., Palmer, M. S., Sidle, K. C. L., Mahal, S. P., Campbell, T., Brown, J., Hardy, J., Brun, A. E., Gustafson, L., Bakker, E., Roos, R., and Groen, J. J. (1994) Familial Pick's disease and dementia in frontal lobe degeneration of non Alzheimer type are not variants of prion disease, *J. Neurol. Neurosurg. Psychiatry* **57**, 762.

44. Corey-Bloom, J., Thal, L. J., Galasko, D., Folstein, M., Drachman, D., Raskind, M., and Lanska, D. J. (1995) Diagnosis and evaluation of dementia, *Neurology* **45**, 211–218.

45. Van Broeckhoven, C. L. (1995) Molecular genetics of Alzheimer disease: identification of genes and gene mutations, *Eur. Neurol.* **35**, 8–19.

46. Gomez-Isla, T., West, H. L., Rebeck, G. W., Harr, S. D., Growdon, J. H., Locascio, J. J., Perls, T. T., Lipsitz, L. A., and Hyman, B. T. (1996) Clinical and pathological correlates of apolipoprotein E ε4 in Alzheimer's disease, *Ann. Neurol.* **39**, 62–70.

47. Cummings, J. L. and Duchen, L. W. (1981) Kluver-Bucy syndrome in Pick disease: clinical and pathologic correlations, *Neurology* **31**, 1415–1422.

48. Holland, A. L., McBurney, D. H., Moossy, J., and Reinmuth, O. M. (1985) The dissolution of language in Pick's disease with neurofibrillary tangles: a case study, *Brain and Language* **24**, 36–58.

49. Hodges, J. R. and Gurd, J. M. (1994) Remote memory and lexical retrieval in a case of frontal Pick's disease, *Arch. Neurol.* **51**, 821–827.

50. Lang, A. E., Bergeron, C., Pollanen, M. S., and Ashby, P. (1994) Parietal Pick's disease mimicking cortico-basal ganglionid degeneration, *Neurology* **44**, 1436–1440.

51. Jendroska, K., Rossor, M. N., Mathias, C. J., and Daniel, S. E. (1995) Morphological overlap between corticobasal degeneration and Pick's disease: a clinicopathological report, *Movement Disord.* **10**, 111–114.

52. Horoupian, D. S. and Dickson, D. W. (1991) Striatonigral degeneration, olivopontocerebellar atrophy and "atypical" Pick disease, *Acta Neuropathol.* **81**, 287–295.

53. Arima, K., Murayama, S., Oyanagi, S., Akashi, T., and Inose, T. (1992) Presenile dementia with progressive supranuclear palsy tangles and Pick bodies: An unusual degenerative disorder involving the cerebral cortex, cerebral nuclei, and brain stem nuclei, *Acta Neuropathol.* **84**, 128–134.

54. Smith, D. A. and Lantos, P. L. (1983) A case of combined Pick's disease and Alzheimer's disease, *J. Neurol. Neurosurg. Psychiatry* **46**, 675–677.

55. Wisniewski, H. M., Coblentz, J. M., and Terry, R. D. (1972) Pick's disease. A clinical and ultrastructural study, *Arch. Neurol.* **26**, 97–108.

56. Tiller-Borcich, J. K. and Forno, L. S. (1988) Parkinson's disease and dementia with neuronal inclusions in the cerebral cortex: Lewy bodies or Pick bodies, *J. Neuropathol. Exp. Neurol.* **47**, 526–535.

57. Dickson, D. W., Wertkin, A., Kress, Y., Ksiezak-Reding, H., and Yen, S.-H. (1990) Ubiquitin immunoreactive structures in normal human brains. Distribution and developmental aspects, *Laboratory Investigation* **63**, 87–99.

58. Iwatsubo, T., Hasegawa, M., and Ihara, Y. (1994) Neuronal and glial tau-positive inclusions in diverse neurologic diseases share common phosphorylation characteristics, *Acta Neuropathol.* **88**, 129–136.

59. Yasuhara, O., Matsuo, A., Tooyama, I., Kimura, H., McGeer, E. G., and McGeer, P. L. (1995) Pick's disease immunohistochemistry: New alterations and Alzheimer's disease comparisons, *Acta Neuropathol.* **89**, 322–330.

60. Yasuhara, O., Aimi, Y., McGeer, E. G., and McGeer, P. L. (1994) Accumulation of amyloid precursor protein in brain lesions of patients with Pick disease, *Neurosci. Lett.* **171**, 63–66.

61. Buée-Scherrer, V., Hof, P. R., Buée, L., Leveugle, B., Vermersch, P., Perl, D. P., Olanow, C. W., and Delacourte, A. (1996) Hyperphosphorylated tau proteins differentiate corticobasal degeneration and Pick's disease, *Acta Neuropathol.* **91**, 351–359.

62. Masters, C. L. and Richardson, E. P., Jr. (1978) Subacute spongiform encephalopathy (Creutzfeldt-Jakob disease). The nature and progression of spongiform change, *Brain* **101,** 333–344.
63. Smith, T. W., Anwer, U., DeGirolami, U., and Drachman, D. A. (1987) Vacuolar change in Alzheimer's disease, *Arch. Neurol.* **44,** 1225–1228.
64. Hansen, L., Salmon, D., Galasko, D., Masliah, E., Katzman, R., DeTeresa, R., Thal, L., Pay, M. M., Hofstetter, R., Klauber, M., Rice, V., Butters, N., and Alford, M. (1990) The Lewy body variant of Alzheimer's disease: a clinical and pathologic entity, *Neurology* **40,** 1–8.
65. Lippa, C. F., Smith, T. W., and Swearer, J. M. (1994) Alzheimer's disease and Lewy body disease: a comparative clinicopathological study, *Ann. Neurol.* **35,** 81–88.
66. Kazee, A. M. and Han, L. Y. (1995) Cortical Lewy bodies in Alzheimer's disease, *Arch. Pathol. Lab. Med.* **119,** 448–453.
67. Vonsattel, J-P., Myers, R. H., Stevens, T. J., Ferrante, R. J., Bird, E. D., and Richardson, E. P., Jr. (1985) Neuropathological classification of Huntington's disease, *J. Neuropathol. Exp. Neurol.* **44,** 559–577.
68. Paulus, W., Bancher, C., and Jellinger, K. (1993) Microglial reaction in Pick's diseae, *Neurosci. Lett.* **161,** 89–92.
69. Mowadat, H. R., Kerr, E. E., and St. Clair, D. (1993) Sporadic Pick's disease in a 28-year-old woman, *Br. J. Psychiatry* **162,** 259–262.
70. Khachaturian, Z. S. (1985) Diagnosis of Alzheimer's disease, *Arch. Neurol.* **42,** 1097–1105.
71. Hulette, C. M. and Crain, B. J. (1992) Lobar atrophy without Pick bodies, *Clin. Neuropathol.* **11,** 151–156.

17

Ischemia

Raymond T. F. Cheung and Vladimir Hachinski

1. INTRODUCTION

Dementia may be defined as any acquired condition of chronic global cognitive decline severe enough to interfere with an independent social or occupational existence. Despite methodological differences, prevalence studies reveal a consistent relationship between the prevalence of dementia and age, with rates doubling every 5 yr of age *(1)*. The worldwide increasing proportions of older age groups within populations and the rising incidence of dementia among people of advancing age make dementia a great challenge to neurologists, geriatricians, psychiatrists, neuropsychologists, epidemiologists, sociologists, demographers, nurses, care-givers, the pharmaceutical industry, government, and society.

Three broad etiological groups of dementia can be recognized:

1. Primary degenerative dementia, such as Alzheimer's disease (AD) and diffuse Lewy body disease;
2. Vascular dementia; and
3. Other dementia.

Although AD and other primary degenerative dementia are the leading causes of dementia in most Western countries, vascular dementia appears to be the leading type in Orientals (Japan and China), Russians, and Swedes *(1–5)*. In addition, the vascular component of the so-called mixed (degenerative and vascular) dementia should not be underestimated, since vascular dementia or the vascular component is the only major treatable or preventable cause of dementia.

2. HISTORICAL OVERVIEW

At the turn of the century, failure of cerebral function and cognition, which affected the small proportion of elderly in the population, was attributed to "hardening of the arteries" or "cerebral arteriosclerosis" *(6)*. This old vascular concept of dementia assumed that critical narrowing of cerebral arteries owing to atherosclerosis caused a state of chronic ischemia with progressive loss of "starving" neurons with dementia being the final result. In the early 1900s, Alzheimer made the critical observation that atherosclerotic and senile processes were unrelated *(6)*, and he also described the neu-

From: Molecular Mechanisms of Dementia Edited by: W. Wasco and R. E. Tanzi Humana Press Inc., Totowa, NJ

ropathological changes of the disease that was named after him. However, the concept of atherosclerotic dementia prevailed well into 1960s when AD gained increasing recognition. Currently, the clinical, neurobehavioral, and pathological features of AD are well established, and validated clinicopathological diagnostic criteria are available. In the 1960s, Fisher suggested that blood vessel disease caused mental impairment through stroke of all sizes *(7)*. The seminal work of Tomlinson and colleagues not only distinguished clearly between the pathological features of AD and dementia owing to multiple infarcts, but also showed a relationship between the total volume of infarction and the presence of dementia *(8)*. Critical reassessment in the 1970s led to the concept of multi-infarct dementia, which emphasized the underlying vascular causes *(9)*. Unfortunately, multi-infarct dementia became equivalent to vascular dementia and was regarded as uncommon until "Binswanger's disease" was rediscovered. Binswanger described in 1894 eight patients having what he termed "encephalitis subcorticalis chronica progressiva," but he provided only the macroscopic description in one case *(10)*. The advent in neuroimaging resulted in an epidemic of clinically diagnosed "Binswanger's disease," which "is neither Binswanger's nor a disease" *(11)*. Controversies about vascular dementia have led to futile arguments over whether vascular dementia is under- or overdiagnosed *(12,13)*.

3. VASCULAR DEMENTIA—PREVENTABLE SENILITY

In the broadest sense, vascular dementia refers to all dementias in which one or more vascular mechanisms, including ischemia, hypoxia, hemorrhage, and blood–brain barrier dysfunctions, play a pathogenic role in the causation of the dementia or in the aggravation of an underlying dementing process resulting from other causes. However, the mere coexistence of a vascular mechanism (without any contribution to the dementia) and an underlying primary dementing disease may be impossible to be recognized with certainty.

Since more than one vascular mechanism may be operating in different degrees to produce lesions of different number, size, side, and location, vascular dementia does not have a uniform pattern of clinical presentation and progression or a unique set of diagnostic pathological findings; this is in contrast to AD. Despite the efforts of different research groups in attempting to establish the clinical diagnostic criteria for vascular dementia, no validated criteria exist for antemortem diagnosis of all types of vascular dementia. On the other hand, the pathological diagnosis of vascular dementia, which relies on the presence of prominent vascular damage to the brain in the absence of obvious pathological changes of primary degenerative dementia, is imperfect, because this implies a diagnosis by exclusion and because the contributions of individual vascular lesion, if any, to the dementia cannot be determined, not to mention the relative pathogenic importance of the various vascular mechanisms. In addition, the relative contributions of the vascular and degenerative components in cases with mixed pathologies are unknown. Finally, the opportunities for prevention and treatment are lost. All these factors hinder research in the area and account for the relative lack of advancement in our understanding of vascular dementia in the past few decades.

The broad definition of vascular dementia suggests that it may share many, if not all, of the risk factors for stroke, coronary artery disease, atherosclerosis, and arteriosclerosis. Since recent research work has shown promising results on the preventable and treatable aspects of stroke, coronary artery disease, and atherosclerosis, vascular dementia is potentially amenable for intervention and prevention.

4. PATHOGENIC MECHANISMS OF VASCULAR DEMENTIA

Our brain is a highly complex and integrated organ operated through highly efficient interconnected neural networks. The presence of redundancy in our brain permits proper functioning despite a limited amount of damage and partial recovery in functions after an irreversible insult *(14)*. The degree of redundancy in cerebral neural circuitry may vary among people; thus, cerebrovascular damage may be present to a similar extent by volume and location in both demented and nondemented patients. Similarly, a small volume of cerebral damage may be tolerated without cognitive impairment until the total volume of damage exceeds a certain threshold level for a particular individual. From the point of view of prevention and early intervention, all pathogenic mechanisms of cerebrovascular damage are important for early recognition, and these vascular mechanisms include small and large brain infarcts, ischemic white-matter damage, blood–brain barrier dysfunctions, impaired cerebrovascular autoregulation and hemodynamic mechanisms, and intracranial hemorrhages *(15–17)*.

4.1. Cerebral Infarction

Stroke is one of the most important causes of morbidity and mortality in the world, particularly in the elderly, and ischemic cerebral infarction is the most common subtype. Although stroke typically causes focal neurological deficits, it is generally accepted that stroke may cause disturbances in higher cerebral function, including dementia, particularly if it is extensive and/or multiple. Kotila and colleagues noted that 3 of their 37 patients, who had ischemic stroke but not dementia initially, developed new dementia (according to the *Diagnostic and Statistical Manual of Mental Disorders*, 3rd ed.) over an observation period of 4 yr *(18)*. Repeated computed tomographic examination of the head showed new infarctions in two of the three patients when the dementia was diagnosed. Tatemichi and colleagues reported the prevalence of dementia (according to the examining neurologist's best judgment) in survivors of their Stroke Data Bank cohort: 116 (16%) of 726 testable patients were "demented" when examined within 10 d of stroke onset; the prevalence was related to age, previous stroke, and previous myocardial infarction *(19)*. More interestingly, Kaplan-Meier analysis of the incidence of new dementia during a 2-yr follow-up among the 610 patients, who were not initially demented at the stroke onset, revealed the effects of age on the 1-yr risk of new-onset dementia: 5.4% for patients aged 60 yr and 10.4% for patients aged 90 yr.

Cerebral infarction of various sizes can be caused by artery-to-artery embolism (including embolism from the aorta), thrombosis of an extracranial or intracranial artery, cardiogenic embolism, lacunar infarcts and small vessel disease, ischemic destruction of the white matter, hypoperfusion of the brain (causing watershed infarcts), inflammatory and noninflammatory (amyloid angiopathy) cerebral arteriopathies, hereditary vascular diseases, and rheological (hyperviscosity) factors. Proven effective measures are available for many of these pathogenic causes. To achieve effective treatment and prevention, it is crucial to deal with the relevant pathogenic causes operating in individuals who have vascular dementia or are at risk of developing vascular dementia in the near future.

Two puzzling issues concern dementia as a result of cerebral infarction, single or multiple. Why is it that only some stroke patients become demented and others do not? Why are acute neurological deficits followed by chronic progressive mental decline, which often occurs some time after the stroke? Although there is little evidence for any proven explanation of these puzzling issues, the following factors are of theoretical importance:

1. The degree of redundancy in the neural network (threshold);
2. The total volume of infarcted brain tissue;
3. Bilaterality vs unilaterality of lesions;
4. The strategically located lesions of any size;
5. The side of the lesions in relation to the dominant hemisphere;
6. The total number of lesions;
7. The degree of coexisting white-matter lesions; and
8. The presence of a coexisting dementing process, particularly AD *(15,19–21)*.

The concept of a threshold level for mental decline after cerebrovascular insults comes from the daily clinical experience of silent stroke and infrequent occurrence of dementia in the large population of stroke patients with various degrees of permanent neurological deficits and different number of stroke. In fact, recovery of function after stroke is often observed despite persistence of the causative lesion in the brain. Recent functional mapping studies in the cerebral cortex reveal that brain functions are highly adaptive and that the cortical maps undergo plastic changes even in adult life *(14)*. Functional neuroimaging studies show reorganization in both the damaged and undamaged hemispheres in patients with functional recovery after motor stroke, and thus suggest that parallel redundant pathways or circuits may be recruited after damage to the classical central motor pathway and that the parallel pathways exist in both hemispheres.

The critical threshold separating normal cognition from dementia is also dependent on the criteria used in defining dementia. Unfortunately, the currently used diagnostic criteria of vascular dementia are modeled on AD, so the importance of memory impairment is overemphasized. The multifactorial and multifocal nature of vascular dementia demands that all higher mental functions or various cognitive domains should be assessed. In particular, emphasis should be given to the frontal subcortical networks or systems, because these systems make humans different from other animals and because our frontal lobes are relatively big and so are often affected by vascular insults.

Tomlinson and colleagues reported in 1970 the pathological features of 50 demented patients and compared the findings with 28 nondemented controls *(8)*. Although brains of the nondemented controls had total infarct volume (expressed as the volume of cerebral softening) of <50 mL, brains of demented patients often had more than 50 mL; only demented patients had more than 100 mL of cerebral softening. Although the importance of total volume of infarcts was well illustrated by this study, more recent clinicopathological studies on vascular dementia indicated that the volume of infarction was much less than 100 mL *(22)*. Thus, volume of infarction is just one parameter for the development of dementia after cerebral infarction.

The structures subserving memory function are bilateral in location. Clinicopathological studies also suggested that bilateral lesions were more significant than unilateral lesions *(19–21)*. However, bilaterality may not be an independent parameter, but is related to the total volume of lesions and/or the availability of parallel pathways (or redundancy).

Because different cerebral functions are carried out by different brain regions interconnected as networks, small, especially bilateral, lesions in critical areas may result in severe deficits in memory and/or other higher cognitive functions. The importance of location is illustrated by the concept of strategic-infarct dementia *(15,23,24)*. Angular gyrus infarction in the dominant cerebral hemisphere, paramedial thalamic (especially bilateral) infarction, or infarction of the caudate head produces multiple, significant cognitive and neuropsychological deficits consistent with dementia. In addition to direct destruction, diaschisis owing to functional disconnection may result in metabolic suppression of unaffected, but neurally connected regions, as shown in functional neuroimaging studies *(25)*.

Dementia is also associated with infarcts in the hemisphere dominant for language *(20,21)*. Although the language ability may be highly relevant to the performance in neuropsychological tests, stroke patients with severe dysphasia are often untestable and, thus, eliminated from any formal assessment of cognitive functions.

The number of infarcts is probably not an independent factor, but relates to the total volume, location, and bilaterality *(20)*. For example, two lesions at different sites of the same neural circuit or at similar sites of two parallel circuits may cause serious dysfunctions in the circuit: synergistic or multiplicative effects. In addition, multiple lacunar infarcts or lacunar state may be associated with dementia, illustrating the combined effects of location, bilaterality, and number of small deep infarcts.

The concept of chronic ischemia has recently been suggested again as a cause of vascular damage and vascular dementia *(26)*. However, there is no convincing evidence for long-standing chronic brain ischemia *(24,27)*. Elevated regional oxygen extraction fraction indicating ongoing ischemia has been shown in only a few patients with vascular dementia or stroke, and the chronicity of this ongoing ischemia is uncertain *(24,28)*.

4.2. White-Matter Lesions—Leukoaraiosis

Gross infarction of the white matter causes disconnection and functional deficits; its role in vascular dementia would resemble cerebral infarcts in the gray matter *(29)*. Nevertheless, both vascular and nonvascular factors lead to noninfarct pathological changes in the white matter. Advent in neuroimaging has caused an epidemic of "Binswanger's disease." Widespread noninfarct changes of the white matter occur in vascular dementia, AD, demyelinating disorders, and normal aging. The matter of white matter in vascular dementia is more complicated than brain infarcts: not only are the presence or absence, location, and extent of white-matter lesions important, but the pathological correlates of white-matter lesions are multiple and unpredictable among individuals.

White-matter changes on neuroimaging should not be designated "Binswanger's disease." It is unclear what disease Binswanger described in 1894 *(10)*. The clinical feature is that of transient or permanent focal symptoms with a slowly relentlessly progressive mental decline in the sixth decade. The gross pathological changes in one case were extensive white-matter atrophy in a periventricular and temporo-occipital distribution, sparing the cortical and deep gray matter. Binswanger suggested that the condition was different from neurosyphilis. In 1902, Alzheimer described the microscopic findings of "Binswanger's disease": focal degeneration and glial proliferation in the white matter with relative sparing of the cortex and the subcortical short association arcuate or U fibers *(6)*. In addition, Alzheimer noted severe atherosclerosis of the long-penetrating arteries and suggested that white-matter atrophy was caused by ischemia from arteriosclerosis. In 1962, Olszewski translated key parts of the original article by Binswanger, Alzheimer, and Nissl and presented two more cases *(30)*. Olszewski could not conclude that there was a disease: the presences of associated lacunes and cortical infarcts were emphasized and the title "subcortical arteriosclerotic encephalopathy" was suggested. Nevertheless, "Binswanger's disease" was considered rare, as Babikian and Ropper found only 46 pathologically confirmed cases reported in the literature by 1987 *(31)*.

Computed tomographic studies reported prevalence rates of 0.15–16% for "Binswanger's disease" in different series of elderly and demented individuals *(32,33)*. The reduced attentuation of the white matter in computed tomographic studies, which was erroneously attributed to "Binswanger's disease" (thus implying an ischemic cause), has been shown to represent a wide spectrum of pathological correlates, including partial loss of myelin, axons and oligodendrocytes, diffuse demyelination, reactive astrocytic gliosis, small infarcts, arteriolar sclerosis, dilatation of the ventricular system or perivascular spaces, and vascular ectasia *(17,34)*. A simple descriptive term for white-matter changes on computer tomographic studies without implying an underlying mechanism or pathology is leukoaraiosis *(35)*.

Leukoaraiosis is shown as white-matter hyperintensities on T_2-weighted magnetic resonance imaging of head. A recent study on the pathologic correlates of increased signals of the centrum ovale on magnetic resonance imaging in 15 unselected autopsies revealed two types of hyperintensities: extensive and punctate *(36)*. Extensive hyperintensities correspond to broad areas of loss of axons, myelin, and oligodendrocytes, together with spongiosis, but not infarction. Punctate hyperintensities are less well defined, with dilated perivascular spaces being the common correlates.

Studies have shown that the presence of leukoariaosis is common in both demented and nondemented subjects. The frequency of leukoaraiosis among nondemented subjects increases with increasing age, increasing intellectual decline, high systolic blood pressure, a history of stroke, the presence of gait disorder, and a tendency to fall *(17,37–40)*. The frequency of leukoaraiosis in both AD and vascular dementia appears to be higher than in age-matched controls. Leukoaraiosis appears to be more extensive in different types of vascular dementia than in AD. About 30% of patients with AD have leukoaraiosis, and these patients are older and more severely demented than those without leukoaraiosis *(41)*. In AD, age and vascular factors, like hypertension, hypotension, arteriosclerosis, cerebral amyloid angiopathy, impaired cerebral autoregulation, and leaky blood–brain barrier, have been associated with leukoaraiosis *(17)*.

Magnetic resonance studies on the white-matter changes show that the technology is more sensitive, but nonspecific, making interpretations difficult *(17)*. In general, the findings of magnetic resonance studies on the white-matter changes in normal aging, AD, and vascular dementia are reminiscent of those of computer tomographic studies with two exceptions: the prevalence rates are higher with magnetic resonance studies and the association between white-matter hyperintensities and cognitive decline is weak or absent *(42–44)*. White-matter hyperintensities in normal subjects have been linked to arterial hypertension, cardiovascular disorders, cerebrovascular disorders, Hachinski's ischemic score, and diabetes mellitus *(17)*. However, tiny hyperintensities around the frontal and occipital horns, narrow periventricular linings, and punctate hyperintensities in subcortical white matter probably do not have clinical significance *(45)*.

Controversies on leukoaraiosis or white-matter hyperintensities are owing to a combination of lack of understanding in vascular dementia, lack of validated clinico-radiological and pathological diagnostic criteria of vascular dementia, and the heterogeneous nature of white-matter changes. Patchy or diffuse white-matter changes are observed in a wide variety of neurological conditions, including multiple sclerosis, leukodystrophies with defective myelination, mitochondrial encephalomyopathies, hypertensive encephalopathy, hydrocephalus, cerebral edema, brain irradiation, intrathecal chemotherapy, cerebral amyloid angiopathy, Creutzfeldt-Jakob disease, AIDS encephalopathy, subacute sclerosing encephalopathy, progressive multifocal leukoencephalopathy, systemic lupus erythematosus, polymyalgia rheumatica, Behcet's disease, neurosarcoidosis, and others *(17)*.

The concept of incomplete infarcts refers to ischemic lesions of the white matter identifiable as loss of axons, myelin, and oligodendrocytes in the presence of few macrophages *(26)*. The latter feature is regarded as evidence against the alternative diagnosis of an infarct. As long as there is no definite evidence that ischemia is the cause of these lesions, the term should be used with caution to avoid confusion.

Vascular mechanisms for ischemic white-matter changes are similar to those for cerebral infarction, but small vessel disease, hypoperfusion of the brain (causing watershed damage), and inflammatory and noninflammatory (amyloid angiopathy) cerebral arteriopathies may be more important than others. Pathogenic mechanisms for nonischemic white-matter changes are diverse and related to the underlying pathologies. Thus, the treatment and prevention of white-matter changes may be less effective than those of cerebral infarction.

4.3. Blood–Brain Barrier Dysfunctions

Cerebrospinal fluid studies have shown a significantly higher albumin level or ratio in vascular dementia than the control group or AD, suggesting abnormal blood–brain barrier functions *(46,47)*. A correlation between the cerebrospinal fluid protein abnormalities and leukoaraiosis has been made *(48)*, and the possibility of altered blood–brain barrier functions in AD has also been raised *(49)*. In acute ischemic events, cerebral infarcts are associated with a deficient blood–brain barrier, but the deficiency appears to recover within 4 wk or less *(46)*. In vascular dementia, the blood–brain barrier appears to reflect a persistent vessel wall disturbance rather than effects of an acute stroke, since there is usually no new stroke within 3 mo prior to the time of cerebrospinal fluid studies.

Factors causing the blood–brain barrier dysfunction are largely unknown. Further studies in this area are needed to permit an effective intervention.

4.4. Impaired Cerebrovascular Autoregulation and Hemodynamic Mechanisms

Autoregulation of cerebral blood flow protects the brain from vascular injury under normal circumstances, despite the normal fluctuations of blood pressure with diurnal variation, activity, and emotional changes. The upper and lower blood pressure limits for autoregulation are known to change under conditions of persistent hypertension and perhaps hypotension. Cerebral atherosclerosis and arteriosclerosis and amyloid angiopathy may result in stiffening of cerebral arteries, and thus impaired cerebrovascular autoregulation. Effective treatment for hypertension and atherosclerosis may be able to prevent impairment in cerebrovascular autoregulation. However, the use of antihypertensives in the presence of impaired autoregulation may prevent the attainment of a very high level of blood pressure in cerebral microvasculature (with increased risk for intracerebral hemorrhage), but exacerbate the damage owing to episodes of hypoperfusion. Studies measuring the cerebrovascular reactivities to changing levels of carbon dioxide have shown impairment in vascular dementia *(50)*.

Impaired cerebrovascular autoregulation leaves the brain unprotected to hemodynamic disturbances. Systemic hypotension resulting from cardiovascular disorders, cerebral hypoperfusion owing to carotid occlusion or severe carotid stenosis, or severe hypoxia resulting from pulmonary disorders can cause ischemic or anoxic pathological changes, which resemble cerebral infarction. Nevertheless, the location of hemodynamic damage is in the vascular watershed areas: in the cerebral cortex between the territories of the major cerebral arteries, in the basal area between the head of caudate nucleus, the internal capsule and the putamen, and in the periventricular white-matter areas *(16)*. Refinement or improvement in antihypertensive therapy and appropriate medical and/or surgical treatment for cardiopulmonary disorders and severe carotid stenosis are important in preventing cerebral damage from hemodynamic mechanisms.

4.5. Intracranial Hemorrhages

Intercranial hemorrhage, including intracerebral hemorrhage, subarachnoid hemorrhage, subdural hematoma, and extradural hematoma, can cause widespread cerebral destruction and produce space-occupying effect (to cause increase in intracranial pressure and compression on nearby structures). Multiple intracerebral hemorrhage owing to hypertension, cerebral amyloid angiopathy or hereditary cause, obstructive hydrocephalus, and subdural hematoma have been described to cause dementia *(51)*. Although the high fatality rate of these hemorrhagic conditions did not result in a large number of survivors with dementia, the preventable and treatable aspects warrant their exclusion early in the course of assessment in patients with newly diagnosed dementia.

5. CLINICAL MODELS OF VASCULAR DEMENTIA

Vascular dementia is a heterogeneous condition, and coexisting primary degenerative dementia is common. There exist, however, a number of "pure" forms of vascular dementia. In practice, a combination of these "pure" forms predominates.

5.1. Multi-Infarct Dementia

Multi-infarct dementia is characterized by transient ischemic attacks or stroke episodes in relation to the development of dementia. The pathological correlates are cerebral infarcts of various sizes, number, and locations. The background is comprised of various vascular risk factors. History of cerebrovascular disease with stepwise deterioration, asymmetric focal neurological signs and multiple cortical and subcortical infarcts, lacunes, and white-matter changes on neuroimaging are hallmarks of multi-infarct dementia *(9)*.

5.2. Strategic-Infarct Dementia

The clinical syndromes resulting from small, localized ischemic damage in critical cortical and subcortical areas illustrate the importance of infarct location *(15,23,24)*. Dominant angular gyrus infarction may present acutely with fluent aphasia, alexia, agraphia, memory disturbance, spatial disorientation, and constructional disturbances. Thromboembolic occlusion of the thalamo-perforating branches of the posterior cerebral artery may cause bilateral thalamic infarcts with severe memory loss. Basal forebrain lesions or anterior cerebral artery infarcts may present with abulia, transcortical motor aphasia, memory impairment, dyspraxia, and other behavioral changes. Some patients with parietal infarcts may have impaired visuo-spatial perception as well as serious cognitive and behavioral disturbances. The diagnosis of strategic-infarct dementia is relatively straightforward and relies on the recognition of the clinical features and the use of appropriate neuropsychological assessment and neuroimaging tests.

5.3. Subcortical Dementia

Characteristic features of subcortical dementia include chronic progressive neurological decline, episodes of stroke, multifocal neurological deficits, dysarthria, a small-step gait, imbalance, incontinence, pseudobulbar palsy, extrapyramidal features, memory deficits, impaired executive function, mental slowness, psychomotor retardation, and apathy *(52)*. The main pathological correlates are lacunes and white-matter infarcts and/or demyelination. Pathogenic factors may include small vessel disease, hypertension, diabetes mellitus, hemodynamic mechanisms, impaired autoregulation, and blood–brain barrier dysfunction.

Lacunes are small, deep infarcts that are located in the putamen, caudate nucleus, thalamus, pons, internal capsule, and subcortical white-matter *(17,53)*. Lacunes range from 0.5 to 15 mm in diameter and are caused by occlusion of small penetrating arteries of 200–900 µm: atheroma blocking the origin, embolic occlusion, or lipohyalinosis. Hypertension is the main risk factor. Multiple lacunar strokes (lacunes) of the basal ganglia and frontal subcortical white matter may be associated with subcortical dementia *(54)*. Ischemic damage to the white matter with or without frank infarction may contribute to the overall neurologic and cognitive deficits through disconnection and diaschisis *(25)*.

5.4. Mixed Dementia

Pathological studies on demented patients often revealed both degenerative changes and vascular lesions of sufficient severity in causing the dementia; the diagnosis of mixed dementia is appropriate. Clinically diagnosed cases of primary degenerative dementia may turn out to be vascular dementia or mixed dementia on pathological examination, and similar errors also apply to clinically diagnosed cases of vascular dementia. To count mixed dementia as a distinct entity or to include it with primary degenerative or vascular dementias contributes to the over- and underdiagnosis of vascular dementia *(12,13)*. Since there is no effective measure of treatment or prevention for primary degenerative dementia, the vascular component of mixed dementia should be emphasized irrespective of classification. In mixed dementia, the vascular component may be large or small cerebral infarcts, lacunes, leukoaraiosis, hematoma, or a combination of these. Presumably, the presence of vascular lesions may accelerate the clinical onset and course of the primary degenerative dementia.

Studies on AD have reported that leukoaraiosis is correlated with age or more severe degree of dementia *(17,41)*. In AD, cerebral amyloid angiopathy and/or blood–brain barrier dysfunctions may lead to leukoaraiosis *(16,49)*. Recent studies have shown that apolipoprotein E ε4 allele may be a susceptibility factor and ε2 allele a protective factor for the development of AD *(55,56)*. Given the role of apolipoprotein E in lipid metabolism and the association of apolipoprotein E with coronary artery disease and atherosclerosis, and given the association of AD with leukoaraiosis, cerebral amyloid angiopathy, and blood–brain barrier dysfunctions, "pure" AD may have a treatable vascular component, making it a special form of vascular dementia *(16)*.

5.5. *Hereditary Vascular Dementia*

Hereditary vascular dementia is rare, but well documented. An autosomal-dominant familial presenile dementia with spastic paralysis has been described; the pathological findings consist of diffuse white-matter changes, cortical infarcts, medial hyaline sclerosis of small arteries, and "peculiar plaque-like structures" around small vessels *(17)*. Another dominantly inherited cerebral amyloid (containing cystatin C protein) angiopathy without hypertension, clinically manifested as increasing loss of mental function and recurring hemorrhages, has been described in Iceland *(57)*. A mutation of the amyloid precursor protein gene (chromosome 21) is responsible for the hereditary cerebral hemorrhage with amyloidosis of the Dutch type (HCHWA-D) *(57)*. In cerebral autosomal-dominant arteriopathy with subcortical infarcts and leukoencephalopathy (CADASIL), the causative gene was localized to chromosome 19q12 *(58)*. CADASIL presents clinically in the third to seventh decades with recurrent stroke and transient ischemic attacks, followed by progressive pseudobulbar palsy, cerebellar signs, and subcortical dementia *(59)*. Migraine and psychiatric complaints, particularly depression, are commonly associated. The underlying vascular lesion affects the small arteries of the white matter and basal ganglia and occasionally the small leptomeningeal arteries; the affected arteries have extensive deposition of a granular, nonfibrinoid, eosinophilic material in the media and frequent fragmentation and/or reduplication of the internal elastic lamina *(59,60)*.

In general, a strong family history, young-onset neurological episodes and dementia, and characteristic neuroimaging findings and pathological features assist in the differential diagnosis. Genetic markers are available for positive diagnosis of some types of hereditary dementia. More importantly, the pathogenesis may be illustrative in the non-hereditary types of vascular dementia.

6. ANIMAL MODELS OF "VASCULAR" DEMENTIA

In general, animal models of human disease are helpful in understanding the pathophysiology and in testing potentially effective therapeutic measures. Our understanding of dementia would be improved if there were appropriate animal models. Recently, transgenic mice overproducing amyloid precursor protein are available as potential models for AD. Although there are many animal models for stroke, good models for vascular dementia are lacking. This is because of the multifactorial and heterogeneous nature of vascular dementia and because there are only limited ways of assessing the animal's "higher mental functions" or "cognition" by behavioral tests.

Experimental approaches to vascular dementia have been largely confined to investigations of memory impairments in rodent ischemic models *(61–63)*. Unilateral middle cerebral artery occlusion, multiple small embolization, and transient four-vessel or chronic three-vessel occlusion in rats produced acute single or multiple infarctions. In these rats, significant impairment in spatial memory acquisition and retention occurs during the subacute and chronic phases *(61–63)*. Results also suggest that memory impairment owing to ischemic causes may be partially reversible if the infarctions occur only once and blood flow is adequately restored. However, chronic recurrent ischemia or chronic hypoperfusion causes permanent and sometimes progressive memory impairment. The pathological correlate of the degree of memory impairment is the extent of hippocampal necrosis and/or degree of neuronal apoptosis in the hippocampus. It has been suggested that chronic cerebrovascular insufficiency in aging rats mimics the memory deficits, behavioral effects, biochemical, and pathological changes of AD in early stage *(62,63)*.

7. CLINICAL DIAGNOSTIC CRITERIA OF VASCULAR DEMENTIA

7.1. Hachinski's Ischemic Score or Modified Ischemic Scores for Multi-Infarct Dementia

Hachinski and colleagues proposed an ischemic score in 1975 for the differentiation between multi-infarct dementia and AD *(64)*. In this original ischemic score, 13 items were scored one or two points; a sum score of four or less would indicate primary degenerative dementia and a sum score of seven or more for multi-infarct dementia. Rosen and colleagues introduced a modified ischemic score in 1980 (Table 1) *(65)*. Clinicopathological studies have confirmed the usefulness of ischemic scores in differentiation between AD from vascular dementia and mixed dementia; the scores do not differentiate between vascular and mixed dementias *(66)*.

Ischemic scores have been used in numerous clinical dementia studies. Basically, presence of the ischemic score items indicates the presence of prominent vascular risk factors and/or cerebrovascular disease, but does not establish a cause and effect relationship. A near maximal ischemic score does not imply more vascular damage than a midvalue ischemic score. In addition, information from neuroimaging is not considered. Other problems of ischemic scores include lack of objective definitions of the individual score item and a lack of temporal connection between the items and development of cognitive deficits.

7.2. The Diagnostic and Statistical Manual *(3rd ed., rev.)* Criteria for Multi-Infarct Dementia

The diagnostic criteria for multi-infarct dementia were defined in the American Psychiatric Association's *Diagnostic and Statistical Manual*, 3rd ed. (DSM-III) and subsequently in the revised third edition (DSM-III-R; Table 2) *(53)*. These criteria are based on clinical descriptions, including dementia, features of focal ischemic brain lesions, and evidence of significant cerebrovascular disease that is considered to be etiologically related to the dementia. Since the descriptions are not defined in detail and are difficult to operationalize, a low accuracy in the antemortem diagnosis compared to postmortem verification has been found *(53)*. In addition, neuroimaging findings are not included, and all subtypes of vascular dementia are considered as multi-infarct dementia.

Table 1
Hachinski's Original and Rosen's Modified Ischemic Scores
(64,65)

	Hachinski (1975)	Rosen (1980)
1 Abrupt onset	2	2
2 Stepwise deterioration	1	2
3 Fluctuating course	2	
4 Nocturnal confusion	1	
5 Preserved personality	1	
6 Depression	1	
7 Somatic complaints	1	1
8 Emotional incontinence	1	1
9 Hypertension	1	
10 History of stroke	2	2
11 Associated atherosclerosis	1	
12 Focal neurological symptoms	2	2
13 Focal neurological signs	2	2
Maximum	18	12
For Alzheimer's dementia	≤ 4	≤ 2
For multi-infarct dementia	≥ 7	≥ 4

Table 2
**Criteria for Multi-Infarct Dementia Modified from the American Psychiatric
Association: DSM-III-R** *(53)*

Presence of Dementia:
  Impaired short- and long-term memory
  Impaired higher mental function in at least one of the following: abstract thinking; judge-
    ment; aphasia, apraxia, agnosia, constructional difficulty or other cortical functions;
    and personality change
  Severe enough to interfere with social or occupational activities
  Absence of delirium
  Evidence of a specific organic causal factor(s) and/or absence of a nonorganic mental
    disorder
A course of stepwise deterioration with "patchy" distribution of deficits in the early stage
Focal neurological symptoms and signs
Significant cerebrovascular disease that is considered to be etiologically relevant to the
  dementia

7.3. The 10th Revision of the Manual of the International Statistical Classification of Diseases Criteria for Vascular Dementia and Its Subtypes

In the 9th revision of the *Manual of the International Statistical Classification of Diseases* (ICD-9), definition of arteriosclerotic dementia was outlined. Recently, the World Health Organization introduced, in Chapter V (Mental and Behavioral Disorders Including Disorders of Psychological Development) of the new 10th revision of

Table 3
Criteria for Subtypes of Vascular Dementia Modified from the ICD-10 of the World Health Organization *(67)*

Subtypes of Vascular Dementia	
Acute onset	The dementia develops rapidly within 1–3 mo after a series of strokes, or rarely after a single large infarction
Multi-infarct	The dementia develops gradually within 3–6 mo after a number of strokes and/or transient ischemic attacks
Subcortical	There is both history of hypertension and evidence (from clinical examination and investigations) of vascular disease in the deep white-matter, with preservation of the cerebral cortex
Mixed cortical and subcortical	Mixed cortical and subcortical components of the vascular dementia are suspected from the cinical features, investigations, or both
Other	No guideline is given
Unspecified	No guideline is given

the *Manual of the International Statistical Classification of Diseases* (ICD-10), operationalized diagnostic guidelines for dementia, vascular dementia, and subtypes of vascular dementia *(67)*. The dementia is objectively verifiable by history from the patient/care-giver and/or neuropsychological examination:

1. Decline in memory;
2. Decline in other cognitive abilities;
3. Preserved awareness of the environment;
4. Decline in emotional control or motivation, or a change in social behavior; and
5. At least 6 mo in duration for memory decline.

Three levels of severity are considered according to the impairment of performance in activities of daily living (mild, moderate, and severe). The ICD-10 research criteria for vascular dementia requires:

1. ICD-10 criteria for dementia;
2. Unequal distribution of deficits in higher cognitive functions;
3. Focal neurological signs; and
4. Significant cerebrovascular disease (from history, examination, and/or tests) that is considered etiologically related to the dementia.

Subtypes of vascular dementia in the ICD-10 are summarized in Table 3. Some shortcomings are obvious. The etiological link between vascular damage and dementia remains weak and is dependent on subjective judgment. The subclassification of vascular dementia is heterogeneous and lacks etiological reasoning. Finally, nonfocal neurological features and neuroimaging findings are not considered.

7.4. The State of California Alzheimer's Disease Diagnostic and Treatment Centers Criteria for Ischemic Vascular Dementia

Chui and colleagues reported the criteria for diagnosis of ischemic vascular dementia as proposed by the State of California Alzheimer's Disease Diagnostic and Treat-

Table 4
Criteria for Ischemic Vascular Dementia from the State of California ADDTC *(68)*

Dementia
    A newly stated definition is given with emphasis on objective confirmation of deterioration in intellectual functions independent of the conscious state by history and mental status testing; more detailed neuropsychological tests, which are quantifiable and reproducible, are encouraged
Probable ischemic vascular dementia
    Requires the presence of dementia, evidence of two or more ischemic strokes (from history, examination, and/or neuroimaging studies), and evidence of at least one infarct outside the cerebellum by neuroimaging studies; occurrence of a single stroke with a clear temporal relationship to the onset of dementia is also allowed
    Includes supporting, associated, and negative features
Possible ischemic vascular dementia
    Requires the presence of dementia and either evidence of a single stroke or Binswanger's disease (from symptoms, signs, vascular risk factors, and neuroimaging findings)
Definite ischemic vascular dementia
    Requires the presence of dementia and pathological confirmation of multiple infarcts
Mixed dementia
    Requires the presence of one or more other systemic or cerebral disorders that are considered to be etiologically related to the dementia
    The degree of confidence of ischemic vascular dementia should be specified as possible, probable, or definite
Research classification
    Requires the location, size, distribution, severity, and etiology of the infarcts to be specified

ment Centers (ADDTC) (Table 4) *(68)*. These criteria specifically address cognitive impairment resulting from ischemic, but not hemorrhagic or hypoxic insults. Three categories of ischemic vascular dementia (definite, probable, and possible), as well as a separate category of mixed dementia are recognized, in parallel to the diagnostic criteria for AD proposed by the National Institute of Neurological and Communicative Disorders and Stroke (NINCDS) and the AD and Related Disorders Association (ADRDA). In addition, a research classification is included with specification on the location, size, distribution, severity, and etiology of infarcts. Conceptually, these criteria are very similar to the criteria proposed by the National Institute of Neurological Disorders and Stroke and the Association Internationale pour la Recherche et l'Enseignement en Neurosciences (NINDS-AIREN).

7.5. The NINDS-AIREN Criteria for Vascular Dementia

These criteria have been proposed for epidemiological studies and are based mainly on the infarct concept, including both infarcts and ischemic white-matter changes *(23,69)*. However, hypoperfusion, hemorrhagic stroke, and unknown mechanisms are permitted as the cause for vascular damage and dementia (Table 5). The criteria emphasize on the location of the vascular lesions, and the causal and temporal link between vascular damage and cognitive impairment. The focus is on the consequence of cere-

Table 5
The NINDS-AIREN Criteria for Vascular Dementia *(23,69)*

Clinical diagnosis of probable vascular dementia requires all of the following: dementia as defined by the ICD-10; cerebrovascular disease, defined by neurological signs and/or neuroimaging studies (showing multiple large-vessel infarcts, single strategically placed infarct, multiple lacunes, or extensive white-matter change); and onset within 3 mo of stroke, abrupt onset of dementia, or fluctuating, stepwise progression of dementia

Clinical features consistent with the diagnosis of probable vascular dementia include: early onset of gait disturbance; history of unsteadiness or frequent unprovoked falls; early neurogenic urinary symptoms; pseudobulbar palsy; and personality change

Negatively associated features include: early onset memory deficit and progressive worsening of memory and other cognitive functions in the absence of corresponding focal lesions on neuroimaging studies; absence of focal neurological signs; and absence of cerebrovascular lesions on neuroimaging studies

Clinical diagnosis of possible vascular dementia may be made in the presence of dementia and focal neurological signs in the absence of neuroimaging studies, clear temporal relationship between stroke and dementia, or typical onset and/or progression of the dementia

Definite vascular dementia is diagnosed in the presence of both clinical criteria for probable vascular dementia and histopathological evidence of cerebrovascular disease, but in the absence of histopathological evidence of AD or other organic cause of dementia

Cortical vascular dementia, subcortical vascular dementia, Binswanger's disease, thalamic dementia, and other subcategories may be defined for research purposes on the basis of clinical, radiological, and neuropathological features

The term "mixed dementia" is avoided; a term of "Alzheimer's disease with cerebrovascular disease" is used for patients fulfilling the clinical criteria for possible Alzheimer's disease and who have clinical and/or radiological evidence of cerebrovascular disease

brovascular disease. Neuroimaging findings are considered, and different (definite, probable, and possible) levels of certainty are included. "AD with cerebrovascular disease" is used instead of "mixed dementia."

7.6. Overview of the Clinical Diagnostic Criteria

The ischemic scores, the DSM-III-R definitions of multi-infarct dementia, and ICD-10 definition of vascular dementia contain variable mixes of clinical and neuropsychological features without neuroimaging findings. Mixed vascular and degenerative dementia is not included in both DSM-III and ICD-10 criteria. The criteria proposed by ADDTC and NINDS-AIREN represent recent efforts in laying the groundwork for future clarification of the persisting controversy about the definition of vascular dementia, the relationship between vascular brain damage and dementia, and the ante-mortem differentiation between vascular and primary degenerative dementias *(70)*. Both ADDTC and NINDS-AIREN criteria require:

1. Presence of dementia;
2. Evidence of vascular brain lesions; and
3. Appropriate temporal and/or possible causal relationship between the two.

The importance of neuropsychological assessment has been stressed. The validity or otherwise of both sets of criteria is to be established by prospective clinicopathological studies.

8. VASCULAR COGNITIVE IMPAIRMENT

An alternative approach to vascular dementia, by applying the scientific method with emphasis on treatment and prevention, has been proposed *(71)*. The first step is to avoid the term vascular dementia: "vascular" is too generic and "dementia" too late for intervention *(72)*. The next step is to have a set of hierarchical, quantitative, standardized instruments to assess the degree of cognitive impairment from very mild to severe. The simplest should be clinical, and the assessment may be based on the individual's behavior and mental status as related to the previous level, the history obtained from the family or the care-giver, and a simple instrument like the Mini-Mental State Examination. A set of minimal, but comparable standardized tests is important for comparison across different studies in different parts of the world. Additional sophisticated neuropsychological, neuroimaging, and other laboratory tests are performed as permitted by the availability in individual centers. The latter may include a blood sample for future genetic and other analyses.

As long as there is no effective treatment or antemortem confirmatory test for AD, the instrument should be highly sensitive to recognize the presence of vascular mechanisms in individuals with any degree of cognitive impairment and in those at risk of developing cognitive impairment in the future; the vascular component of mixed dementia should be recognized. The purpose is to recognize the clincal problem of vascular cognitive impairment at three stages:

1. Brain-at-risk stage;
2. Predementia stage; and
3. Dementia stage *(71)*.

The specific vascular mechanisms operating in individuals with vascular cognitive impairment should be detected and treated with clinically proven measures. Longitudinal follow-up studies on these patients with postmortem confirmation of diagnosis would provide, retrospectively, information on the relative importance of the different vascular mechanisms. Pooling of databases for meta-analyses will provide highly testable and important hypotheses.

9. TREATMENT AND PREVENTION

Treatment and prevention should be applied early to patients at different stages of their vascular cognitive impairment *(71)*. Currently, most patients with vascular dementia come to medical attention too late for any effective intervention. In addition, prevention of vascular insults in patients destined to develop AD may retard the clinical onset and progression of the neurodegenerative process and prolong the duration of a meaningful and independent living.

9.1. Brain-at-Risk Stage

Elderly, hypertensives, smokers, diabetics, atrial fibrillators, cardiac patients, and patients with asymptomatic extracranial stenosis may be at risk of developing cognitive impairment owing to vascular causes in the future. Therapeutic measures depend on the conditions: smoking cessation (for smokers), exercise (for general health, coronary artery diseases, and diabetes mellitus), diet (for diabetes mellitus, obesity, hyperlipidemias, and hypertension), potassium supplementation (for its vascular protective effect), estrogen replacement for postmenopausal women (for atherosclerosis and coronary heart disease), antihypertensives (angiotensin-converting enzyme inhibitors and calcium channel blockers may be preferred), lipid-lowering agents (for hyperlipidemias), anticoagulants (for atrial fibrillators and patients at risk of cardiac source of embolism), and aspirin (for selected high-risk patients).

9.2. Predementia Stage

This stage is characterized by transient ischemic attacks, stroke, subtle cognitive impairment, silent cerebral infarctions, leukoaraiosis, or other causes of stroke. Therapeutic measures may include: carotid endarterectomy (for severe and symptomatic carotid artery stenosis), anticoagulants (for cardiac source of embolism), aspirin or ticlopidine (for prophylaxis of stroke), antiamyloid agents (for cerebral amyloid deposition), and calcium channel blockers (pretreatment for neuroprotective effects on stroke).

9.3. Dementia Stage

Patients at this stage have cognitive impairment severe enough to interfere with an independent social or occupational existence. They may have carotid stenosis, cardiac sources of embolism, intracranial small vessel stenosis, or other causes of stroke. Treatment measures include symptomatic (antidepressants, cholinergics, and nerve growth factors) and preventive (antihypertensives, aspirin, and ticlopidine) ones.

10. FUTURE DIRECTIONS

Vascular dementia has reached the stage of bewildering complexity preceding true understanding. Accepting a broad definition for vascular dementia and focusing on the early stages should allow longitudinal follow-up studies with emphasis on prevention and treatment. In addition, future advancement in three areas will improve our understanding in vascular dementia:

1. Functional neuroimaging;
2. Pathophysiology of ischemia and mechanisms of neuroprotection; and
3. Genetics of cerebrovascular diseases.

10.1. Functional Neuroimaging

The refinement of positron emission tomography has allowed noninvasive, in vivo examination of cerebral blood flow, oxygen uptake, and glucose metabolism in different brain regions *(14)*. Using this technique to study the physiological variables after stroke has provided new information on the ischemic penumbra, therapeutic window, and functional reorganization. The requirement of radionuclides generated from a cyclotron limits the availability of positron emission tomography to a few centers. The discovery of different magnetic properties between oxyhemoglobin and deoxyhemoglobin generated another noninvasive, in vivo technique of studying regional cerebral blood flow and its changes with activities; this is functional magnetic resonance imaging *(73)*. On the other hand, magnetic resonance spectroscopy enables noninvasive, in vivo investigation of biochemical changes in brain energy metabolites *(74)*. Thus, applying these new techniques in patients with vascular dementia allows for correlations among cerebral blood flow and metabolism, anatomical brain lesions, and neuropsychological performance.

10.2. Pathophysiology of Ischemia and Mechanisms of Neuroprotection

Recent studies on the molecular pathophysiological responses to ischemia reveal that the cellular cascade of events from onset of ischemia to cell death is complicated. In addition to early ischemic cell death after severe and prolonged ischemia, milder and/or repeated ischemia results in delayed cell death (apoptosis) and changes in protein synthesis. In general, protein synthesis is very sensitive to changes in blood flow, and profound, prolonged suppression of protein synthesis occurs even with mild ischemia *(27)*. This suppression of protein synthesis is selective, and genes including proto-oncogenes (like c-*fos* and c-*jun*) *(75)* and stress genes (like heat-shock genes family) *(76)* are preferentially transcribed and translated into protein products. Further understanding in the ischemic cellular pathophysiology and the intrinsic cellular protective mechanisms can lead to new interventions in stroke and vascular dementia.

10.3. Genetics of Cerebrovascular Diseases

Genetic factors are important in many human diseases. Although hereditary causes of vascular dementia are rare, advances in this area, as exemplified by the description and genetic identification of CADASIL, pave the way for progress in the pathophysiology of vascular dementia *(77)*.

ACKNOWLEDGMENTS

V. H. is a Career Investigator of the Heart and Stroke Foundation of Canada. R. T. F. C. is a recipient of a Research Fellowship from the Medical Council of Canada.

REFERENCES

1. Jorm, A. F., Korten, A. E., and Henderson, A. S. (1987) The prevalence of dementia: a quantitative integration of the literature, *Acta Psychiatr. Scand.* **76**, 465–479.
2. Kase, C. S. (1991) Epidemiology of multi-infarct dementia, *Alzheimer Dis. Assoc. Disord.* **5**, 71–76.
3. Skoog, I., Nilsson, L., Palmertz, B., Andreasson, L. -A., and Svanborg, A. (1993) A population-based study of dementia in 85-year-olds, *N. Engl. J. Med.* **328**, 153–158.
4. Kiyohara, Y., Yoshitake, T., Kato, I., Ohmura, T., Kawano, H., Ueda, K., and Fujishima, M. (1994) Changing patterns in the prevalence of dementia in a Japanese community: the hisayama study, *Gerontology* **40(Suppl. 2)**, 29–35.
5. Ueda, K., Kawano, H., Hasuo, Y., and Fujishima, M. (1992) Prevalence and etiology of dementia in a Japanese community, *Stroke* **23**, 798–803.
6. Forstl, H. and Beats, B. (1991) Translation, *Alzheimer Dis. Assoc. Disord.* **5**, 69,70.
7. Fisher, C. M. (1968) Dementia in cerebral vascular disease, in *Cerebral Vascular Diseases, 6th Princeton Conference* (Toole, J. F., Siekert, R. G., and Whisnant, J. P., eds.), Grune, New York, pp. 232–236.
8. Tomlinson, B. E., Blessed, G., and Roth, M. (1970) Observations on the brains of demented old people, *J. Neurol. Sci.* **11**, 205–242.
9. Hachinski, V. C., Lassen, N. A., and Marshall, J. (1974) Multi-infarct dementia. A cause of mental deterioration in the elderly, *Lancet* **2**, 207–210.
10. Blass, J. P., Hoyer, S., and Nitsch, R. (1991) A translation of Otto Binswanger's article, "The delineation of the generalized progressive paralyses," *Arch. Neurol.* **48**, 961–972.
11. Hachinski, V. (1991) Binswanger's disease: neither Binswanger's nor a disease, *J. Neurol. Sci.* **103**, 1.
12. Brust, J. C. M. (1988) Vascular dementia is overdiagnosed, *Arch. Neurol.* **45**, 799–801.
13. O'Brien, M. D. (1988) Vascular dementia is underdiagnosed, *Arch. Neurol.* **45**, 797,798.

14. Weiller, C. (1995) Recovery from motor stroke: human positron emission tomography studies, *Cerebrovasc. Dis.* **5**, 282–291.
15. Tatemichi, T. K. (1990) How acute brain failure becomes chronic—a view of the mechanisms of dementia related to stroke, *Neurology* **40**, 1652–1659.
16. Hachinski, V. C. (1990) The decline and resurgence of vascular dementia, *Can. Med. Assoc. J.* **142**, 107–111.
17. Erkinjuntti, T. and Hachinski, V. C. (1993) Rethinking vascular dementia, *Cerebrovascular Disease* **3**, 3–23.
18. Kotila, M., Waltimo, O., Niemi, M. L., and Laaksonen, R. (1986) Dementia after stroke, *Eur. Neurol.* **25**, 134–140.
19. Tatemichi, T. K., Foulkes, M. A., Mohr, J. P., Hewitt, J. R., Hier, D. B., Price, T. R., and Wolf, P. A. (1990) Dementia in stroke survivors in the stroke data bank cohort—prevalence, incidence, risk factors, and computed tomographic findings, *Stroke* **21**, 858–866.
20. O'Brien, M. D. (1994) How does cerebrovascular disease cause dementia? *Dementia* **5**, 133–136.
21. Tatemichi, T. K., Desmond, D. W., Paik, M., Figueroa, M., Gropen, T. I., Stern, Y., Sano, M., Remien, R., Williams, J. B. W., Mohr, J. P., and Mayeux, R. (1993) Clinical determinants of dementia related to stroke, *Ann. Neurol.* **33**, 568–575.
22. de Ser, T., Bermejo, F., Portera, A., Arredondo, J. M., Bouras, C., and Constantinidis, J. (1990) Vascular dementia. A clinicopathological study, *J. Neurol. Sci.* **96**, 1–17.
23. Roman, G. C., Tatemichi, T. K., Erkinjuntti, T., Cummings, J. L., Masdeu, J. C., Garcia, J. H., Amaducci, L., Orgogozo, J.-M., Brun, A., Hofman, A., Moody, D. M., O'Brien, M. D., Yamaguchi, T., Grafman, J., Drayer, B. P., Bennett, D. A., Fisher, M., Ogata, J., Kokmen, E., Bermejo, F., Wolf, P. A., Gorelick, P. B., Bick, K. L., Pajeau, A. K., Bell, M. A., DeCarli, C., Culebras, A., Korczyn, A. D., Bogousslavsky, J., Hartmann, A., and Scheinberg, P. (1993) Vascular dementia: diagnostic criteria for research studies—report of the NINDS-AIREN International Workshop, *Neurology* **43**, 250–260.
24. Garcia, J. H. and Brown, G. G. (1992) Vascular dementia: neuropathologic alterations and metabolic brain changes, *J. Neurol. Sci.* **109**, 121–131.
25. Cinotti, L., Croisile, B., Laurent, B., Le Bars, D., Malbezin, M., and Mauguiere, F. (1995) Assessment of cerebrovascular disease with positron emission tomography: attempt of an in vivo model for treatment evaluation of brain glucose metabolism, *Eur. Neurol.* **35(Suppl. 1)**, 17–22.
26. Brun, A., Fredriksson, K., and Gustafson, L. (1992) Pure subcortical arteriosclerotic encephalopathy (Binswanger's Disease): a clinicopathologic study, *Cerebrovascular Disease* **2**, 87–92.
27. Hossmann, K.-A. (1994) Viability thresholds and the penumbra of focal ischemia, *Ann. Neurol.* **36**, 557–565.
28. De Reuck, J., Decoo, D., Strijkmans, K., and Lemahieu, I. (1992) Does the severity of leukoaraiosis contribute to senile dementia, *Eur. Neurol.* **32**, 199–205.
29. Yao, H., Sadoshima, S., Kuwabara, Y., Ichiya, Y., and Fujishima, M. (1990) Cerebral blood flow and oxygen metabolism in patients with vascular dementia of the Binswanger type, *Stroke* **21**, 1694–1699.
30. Olszewski, J. (1962) Subcortical arteriosclerotic encephalopathy, *World Neurol.* **3**, 359–375.
31. Babikian, V. and Ropper, A. H. (1987) Binswanger's disease: a review, *Stroke* **18**, 2–12.
32. Loizou, L. A., Kendall, B. E., and Marshall, J. (1981) Subcortical arteriosclerotic encephalopathy: a clinical and radiological investigation, *J. Neurol. Neurosurg. Psychiat.* **44**, 294–304.
33. George, A. E., de Leon, M. J., Gentes, C. I., Miller, J., London, E., Budzilovich, G. N., Ferris, S., and Chase, N. (1986) Leukoencephalopathy in normal and pathologic aging: 1. CT of brain lucencies, *Am. J. Neuroradiology* **7**, 561–566.
34. Yamanouchi, H. (1991) Loss of white matter oligodendrocytes and astrocytes in progressive subcortical vascular encephalopathy of Binswanger type, *Acta. Neurol. Scand.* **83**, 301–305.

35. Hachinski, V. C., Potter, P., and Merskey, H. (1987) Leuko-Araiosis, *Arch. Neurol.* **44,** 21–23.
36. Munoz, D. G., Hastak, S. M., Harper, B., Lee, D., and Hachinski, V. C. (1993) Pathologic correlates of increased signals of the centrum ovale on magnetic resonance imaging, *Arch. Neurol.* **50,** 492–497.
37. Steingart, A., Hachinski, V. C., Lau, C., Fox, A. J., Diaz, F., Cape, R., Lee, D., Inzitari, D., and Merskey, H. (1987) Cognitive and neurologic findings in subjects with diffuse white matter lucencies on computed tomographic scan (Leuko-Araiosis), *Arch. Neurol.* **44,** 32–35.
38. Inzitari, D., Diaz, F., Fox, A., Hachinski, V. C., Steingart, A., Lau, C., Donald, A., Wade, J., Mulic, H., and Merskey, H. (1987) Vascular risk factors and Leuko-Araiosis, *Arch. Neurol.* **44,** 42–47.
39. Raiha, I., Tarvonen, S., Kurki, T., Rajala, T., and Sourander, L. (1993) Relationship between vascular factors and white matter low attenuation of the brain, *Acta Neurol. Scand.* **87,** 286–289.
40. Mineura, K., Sasajima, H., Kikuchi, K., Kowada, M., Tomura, N., Monma, K., and Segawa, Y. (1995) White matter hyperintensity in neurologically asymptomatic subjects, *Acta Neurol. Scand.* **92,** 151–156.
41. Steingart, A., Hachinski, V. C., Lau, C., Fox, A. J., Fox, H., Lee, D., Inzitari, D., and Merskey, H. (1987) Cognitive and neurologic findings in demented patients with diffuse white matter lucencies on computed tomographic scan (Leuko-Araiosis), *Arch. Neurol.* **44,** 36–39.
42. Markesbery, W. R. (1991) Comments on vascular dementia, *Alzheimer Dis. Assoc. Disord.* **5,** 149–153.
43. Wahlund, L.-O., Basun, H., Almkvist, O., Andersson-Lundman, G., Julin, P., and Saaf, J. (1994) White matter hyperintensities in dementia: does it matter? *Magn. Reson. Imaging* **12,** 387–394.
44. Almkvist, O., Wahlund, L.-O., Andersson-Lundman, G., Basun, H., and Backman, L. (1992) White-matter hyperintensity and neuropsychological functions in dementia and healthy aging, *Arch. Neurol.* **49,** 626–632.
45. Herholz, K., Heindel, W., Rackl, A., Neubauer, I., Steinbrich, W., Pietrzyk, U., Erasmi-Korber, H., and Heiss, W.-D. (1990) Regional cerebral blood flow in patients with leuko-araiosis and atherosclerotic carotid artery disease, *Arch. Neurol.* **47,** 392–396.
46. Wallin, A., Blennow, K., Fredman, P., Gottfries, C. G., Karlsson, I., and Svennerholm, L. (1990) Blood brain barrier function in vascular dementia, *Acta Neurol. Scand.* **81,** 318–322.
47. Mecocci, P., Parnetti, L., Reboldi, G. P., Santucci, C., Gaiti, A., Ferri, C., Gernini, I., Romagnoli, M., Cadini, D., and Senin, U. (1991) Blood-brain-barrier in a geriatric population: barrier function in degenerative and vascular dementias, *Acta Neurol. Scand.* **84,** 210–213.
48. Pantoni, L., Inzitari, D., Pracucci, G., Lolli, F., Giordano, G., Bracco, L., and Amaducci, L. (1993) Cerebrospinal fluid proteins in patients with leucoaraiosis: possible abnormalities in blood-brain barrier function, *J. Neurol. Sci.* **115,** 125–131.
49. Mattila, K. M., Pirttila, T., Blennow, K., Wallin, A., Viitanen, M., and Frey, H. (1994) Altered blood-brain-barrier function in Alzheimer's disease, *Acta Neurol. Scand.* **89,** 192–198.
50. Kuwabara, Y., Ichiya, Y., Otsuka, M., Masuda, K., Ichimiya, A., and Fujishima, M. (1992) Cerebrovascular responsiveness to hypercapnia in Alzheimer's dementia and vascular dementia of the Binswanger type, *Stroke* **23,** 594–598.
51. Cummings, J. L. (1983) Treatable dementias, in: The Dementias (Mayeux, R. and Rosen, W. G., eds), Raven, New York, pp. 165–183.
52. Cummings, J. L. (1994) Vascular subcortical dementias: clinical aspects, *Dementia* **5,** 177–180.
53. Gorelick, P. B. and Mangone, C. A. (1991) Vascular dementias in the elderly, *Clin. Geriatr. Med.* **7,** 599–615.
54. Loeb, C. (1995) Dementia due to lacunar infarctions: a misnomer or a clinical entity? *Eur. Neurol.* **35,** 187–192.
55. Saunders, A. M., Strittmatter, W. J., Schmechel, D., St. George-Hyslop, P. H., Pericak-Vance, M. A., Joo, S. H., Rosi, B. L., Gusella, J. F., Crapper-MacLachlan, D. R., Alberts, M. J., Hulette, C., Crain, B., Goldgaber, D., and Roses, A. D. (1993) Association of apolipoprotein E allele E4 with late-onset familial and sporadic Alzheimer's disease, *Neurology* **43,** 1467–1472.

56. Frisoni, G. B., Calabresi, L., Geroldi, C., Bianchetti, A., D'Acquarica, A. L., Govoni, S., Sirtori, C. R., Trabucchi, M., and Franceschini, G. (1994) Apolipoprotein E epsilon-4 allele in Alzheimer's disease and vascular dementia, *Dementia* **5,** 240–242.

57. Alberts, M. J. (1991) Genetic aspects of cerebrovascular disease, *Stroke* **22,** 276–280.

58. Tournier-Lasserve, E., Joutel, A., Melki, J., Weissenbach, J., Lathrop, G. M., Chabriat, H., Mas, J. L., Cabanis, E. A., Baudrimont, M., Maciazek, J., Bach, M. A., and Bousser, M. G. (1993) Cerebral autosomal dominant arteriopathy with subcortical infarcts and leukoencephalopathy maps to chromosome 19q12, *Nat. Genet.* **3,** 256–259.

59. Sourander, P. and Walinder, J. (1977) Hereditary multi-infarct dementia. Morphological and clinical studies of a new disease, *Acta Neuropathol.* **39,** 247–254.

60. Baudrimont, M., Dubas, F., Joutel, A., Tournier-Lasserve, E., and Bousser, M. G. (1993) Autosomal dominant leukoencephalopathy and subcortical ischemic stroke. A clinicopathological study, *Stroke* **24,** 122–125.

61. Naritomi, H. (1991) Experimental basis of multi-infarct dementia, *Alzheimer Dis. Assoc. Disord.* **5,** 103–111.

62. de la Torre, J. C., Fortin, T., Park, G. A. S., Butler, K. S., Kozlowski, P., Pappas, B. A., de Socarraz, H., Saunders, J. K., and Richard, M. T. (1992) Chronic cerebrovascular insufficiency induces dementia-like deficits in aged rats, *Brain Res.* **582,** 186–195.

63. de la Torre, J. C. and Fortin, T. (1994) A chronic physiological rat model of dementia, *Behav. Brain Res.* **63,** 35–40.

64. Hachinski, V. C., Lliff, L. D., Zilhka, E., Du Boulay, G. H., McAllister, V. L., Marshall, J., Ross Russell, R. W., and Symon, L. (1975) Cerebral blood flow in dementia, *Arch. Neurol.* **32,** 632–637.

65. Rosen, W. G., Terry, R. D., Fuld, P. A., Katzman, R., and Peck, A. (1980) Pathological verification of ischemic score in differentiation of dementias, *Ann. Neurol.* **7,** 486–488.

66. Fischer, P., Jellinger, K., Gatterer, G., and Danielczyk, W. (1991) Prospective neuropathological validation of Hachinski's ischaemic score in dementias, *J. Neurol. Neurosurg. Psychiatr.* **54,** 580–583.

67. Wetterling, T., Kanitz, R. D., and Borgis, K. J. (1994) The ICD-10 criteria for vascular dementia, *Dementia* **5,** 185–188.

68. Chui, H. C., Victoroff, J. I., Margolin, D., Jagust, W., Shankle, R., and Katzman, R. (1992) Criteria for the diagnosis of ischemic vascular dementia proposed by the state of California Alzheimer's disease diagnostic and treatment centers, *Neurology* **42,** 473–480.

69. Erkinjuntti, T. (1994) Clinical criteria for vascular dementia: the NINDS-AIREN criteria, *Dementia* **5,** 189–192.

70. Rockwood, K., Parhad, I., Hachinski, V., Erkinjuntti, T., Rewcastle, B., Kertesz, A., Eastwood, M. R., and Phillips, S. (1994) Diagnosis of vascular dementia: consortium of canadian centres for clinical cognitive research concensus statement, *Can. J. Neurol. Sci.* **21,** 358–364.

71. Hachinski, V. (1992) Preventable senility: a call for action against the vascular dementias, *Lancet* **340,** 645–648.

72. Hachinski, V. (1994) Vascular dementia: a radical redefinition, *Dementia* **5,** 130–132.

73. Frahm, J., Bruhn, H., Merboldt, K. D., and Hänicke, W. E. (1992) Dynamic MR imaging of human brain oxygenation during rest and photic stimulation, *J. Magn. Reson. Imaging* **2,** 501–506.

74. Gadian, D. G., Allen, K., van Bruggen, N., Busza, A. L., King, M. D., and Williams, S. R. (1993) Applications of NMR spectroscopy to the study of experimental stroke in vivo, *Stroke* **24(Suppl. I),** I-57–I-59.

75. Hsu, C. Y., An, G., Liu, J. S., Xue, J. J., He, Y. Y., and Lin, T. N. (1993) Expression of immediate early gene and growth factor mRNAs in a focal cerebral ischemia model in the rat, *Stroke* **24(Suppl. I),** I-78–I-81.

76. Sharp, F. R., Kinouchi, H., Koistinaho, J., Chan, P. H., and Sagar, S. M. (1993) HSP70 heat shock gene regulation during ischemia, *Stroke* **24(Suppl. I),** I-72–I-75.

77. Bowler, J. V. and Hachinski, V. (1994) Progress in the genetics of cerebrovascular disease: inherited subcortical arteriopathies, *Stroke* **25,** 1696–1698.

Piero Parchi and Pierluigi Gambetti

INTRODUCTION

Prion diseases are a group of neurodegenerative conditions of humans and animals that include sporadic, inherited, and transmitted forms. They are best characterized by their distinctive pathogenic mechanism, which is shared by all three forms. The central event in the pathogenesis of these diseases is thought to be a change in protein conformation that results in the conversion of a normal protein, identified as cellular prion protein (PrP^C), into an isoform that is partially resistant to proteases (PrP^{res}) *(1)*. The molecular events leading to this conformational change, however, remain largely unknown.

Prion diseases are among the most heterogeneous group of diseases of the nervous system (Tables 1–3) *(2)*. Genetic factors, such as mutation and amino acid substitutions in polymorphic sites of the prion protein gene (PRNP), heavily affect the phenotypic expression of prion diseases. Their high phenotypic variability also depends on the biology of prions, the infectious particles involved in these disorders. Distinct prions preparations, called strains or isolates, carry information, possibly encoded in the prion conformation, which is independent from the host genotype *(1,3,4)*. Each prion strain, when inoculated intracerebrally in syngenic animals, induces a disease with specific phenotypic characteristics *(1,3,4)*. It is believed that this property is the consequence of the prion's ability to target selective neuronal populations and subsequently spread within the brain from these cells *(1)*. As a consequence, different brain regions may be involved at different times during the course of the disease and, in turn, symptoms and signs that reflect the involvement of different brain regions may appear at onset or later in the course of the disease.

Despite their phenotypic variability, most subtypes of prion diseases are classified in one of the following three distinct phenotypes: Creutzfeldt-Jakob disease (CJD), fatal familial insomnia (FFI), and Gerstmann-Sträussler-Scheinker syndrome (GSS) *(2)*. A minority of cases, however, cannot be accommodated in any of these phenotypes and form a heterogeneous group. This group is essentially made up of the familial prion diseases associated with insertion mutations in PRNP *(2)*. The salient clinical and pathological features of the various subtypes of prion diseases belonging to the sporadic, familial, and iatrogenic forms, grouped according to whether they fit best the CJD, FFI, GSS, or the variable phenotype, are listed in Tables 1–3. In this chapter, we examine

From: Molecular Mechanisms of Dementia *Edited by: W. Wasco and R. E. Tanzi Humana Press Inc., Totowa, NJ*

Table 1
CJD and FFI Phenotypes

Genotype	Inheritance	Duration	Clinical and Pathological Features
			CJD
Wild-type 129 M/M PrPres 1 (CJDM/M1)	Sporadic	1–6 mo	Clinical: Rapidly progressive dementia often associated with visual signs or ataxia, myoclonus and PSW on EEG. Pathological: Mild to moderate spongiosis, gliosis, and neuronal loss in all layers of the cerebral cortex, striatum, thalamus, and molecular layer of cerebellum.
Wild-type 129 M/M PrPres 2	Sporadic	1–4 yr	Clinical: Dementia with slower progression than in CJDM/M1; no PSW on EEG; mild or absent cerebellar signs. Pathological: Spongiosis, gliosis, and neuronal loss in the cerebral cortex, striatum, and thalamus.
Wild-type 129 M/V PrPres 2	Sporadic	5–20 mo	Clinical: Ataxia and dementia with slower progression than in CJDM/M1; no PSW on EEG. Pathological: Widespread spogiosis, gliosis, and neuronal loss in limbic lobe, striatum, diencephalus, brainstem, and cerebellum with relative sparing of the neocortex in short-duration (<8 mo) cases; kuru-like amyloid plaques in the cerebellum.
Wild-type 129 V/V PrPres 2	Sporadic	4–20 mo	Clinical: Ataxia followed by late dementia, late or no PSW on EEG. Pathological: As in CJDM/V2 group, but with more severe pathology in the cerebellum and no kuru plaques.
D178N 129V	Familial	9–51 mo	Clinical: Dementia, myoclonus, extrapyramidal, and pyramidal signs, mild or no ataxia; slower progression than typical sporadic form (CJDM/M1), rare PSW on EEG. Pathological: Spongiosis, neuronal loss, and astrogliosis in the cerebral cortex (most severe), striatum, and thalamus (least severe); cerebellum relatively spared.
V180I 129M	Familial	1–2 yr	Clinical: Similar to the typical sporadic form (CJDM/M1) but with a slower progression. Pathological: Like typical sporadic form.
E200K 129M	Familial	2–41 mo	Clinical: Similar to the typical sporadic form (CJDM/M1), but with atypical signs, such as supranuclear palsy, spastic paresis, and neuropathy in some cases and less costant PSW on EEG. Prominent motor signs with only late dementia in some cases. Pathological: Similar to typical sporadic form, but with a relative sparing of the neocortex in some cases with short duration.
H208A-129M	Familial	2–4 mo	Clinical: Like typical sporadic form (CJDM/M1). Pathological: Like typical sporadic form.
V2101-129M	Familial	2–4 mo	Clinical: Like typical sporadic form (CJDM/M1). Pathological: Like typical sporadic form.
M232R-129M	Familial	NA	Clinical: Like typical sporadic form (CJDM/M1). Pathological: Like typical sporadic form.
			FFI
D178N 129M	Familial	6–45 mo	Clinical: Reduction of total sleep time, enacted dreams, increased sympathetic activity, myoclonus, ataxia, late dementia pyramidal, and extrapyramidal signs. Pathological: Preferential thalamic and olivary atrophy; spongiosis in the cerebral cortex in the subjects with a duration of symptoms >1yr.

NA, not available; PrP, prion protein.

Table 2
GSS Phenotype

Genotype	Inheritance	Duration	Clinical and pathological features
P102L-129M[a]	Familial	1–10 yr	Clinical: Slowly progressive cerebellar syndrome with late dementia, extrapyramidal and pyramidal signs; rare cases (shorter duration) overlap with CJD. Pathological: PrP amyloid deposits in the cerebellum and, to a lesser extent, in the cerebrum; variable degree of spongiosis, neuronal loss, and astrogliosis; no NFT.
P105L-129V	Familial	6–12 yr	Clinical: Spastic paraparesis progressing to quadriparesis; late dementia; no myoclonus and only mild cerebellar signs. Pathological: PrP amyloid deposits, neuronal loss, and gliosis in the cerebral cortex and, to a lesser extent, in the striatum and thalamus; no spongiform changes and NFT.
A117V-129V	Familial	1–11 yr	Clinical: Dementia, parkinsonism, pyramidal signs; occasional cerebellar signs. Pathological: Widespread PrP amyloid deposits in the cerebrum and, more rarely, in the cerebellum associated with variable degree of spongiform changes, neuronal loss and astrogliosis; no NFT.
Y145 STOP-129M	Familial	21 yr	Clinical: Slowly progressive dementia. Pathological: PrP amyloid deposits in the cerebral and cerebellar cortices associated with NFT in the neocortex, hippocampus, and subcortical nuclei; PrP amyloid angiopathy; no spongiosis.
F198S-129V	Familial	3–11 yr	Clinical: Like 102 GSS subtype, but with a more chronic course (no overlap with CJD). Pathological: Like 102 GSS subtype, but with more extensive PrP amyloid deposits, NFT in the cerebral cortex and subcortical nuclei, and inconspicuous spongiosis.
Q217R-129V	Familial	5–6 yr	Clinical: Slowly progressive dementia, cerebellar and extrapyramidal signs. Pathological: Like 198 GSS subtype, but with the most severe lesions in the cerebral cortex, thalamus, and amygdala.

NA, not available; PrP, prion protein; NFT, neurofibrillary tangles.
[a]The phenotype lacks prominent cerebellar signs when leucine (L) is present at position 219 on the same allele as the P102L mutation.

the presence of cognitive impairment in each of the phenotypes of prion diseases, and we discuss the possible mechanisms underlying the neuronal dysfunction causing dementia in these conditions. Although dementia and cortical pathology are usually prominent features of human prion diseases, they are not invariably present in all subtypes. Moreover, the cognitive deficit shows a high variability in the timing of appearance, rate of evolution, and accompanying neurological signs. Taking into account these notions and focusing on dementia, the various subtypes of human prion diseases can be operationally classified in two major groups according to whether or not they present with dementia in the early stage of the disease (Table 4). In addition, each subgroup can be further divided in subacute or chronic forms according to the disease's duration.

Table 3
Insertion Mutations: Variable Phenotype

Genotype	Inheritance	Duration	Clinical and pathological features
Ins 24 bp 129M	Apparently sporadic	4 mo	Clinical: Like typical sporadic CJD (CJDMM/1 = rapidly progressive dementia, myoclonus, and PSW on EEG). Pathological: NA.
Ins 48 bp 129M	Apparently sporadic	3 mo	Clinical: Like typical sporadic CJD (CJDMM/1). Pathological: Like typical sporadic CJD (spongiosis, gliosis, and neuronal loss in the cerebral cortex, striatum, thalamus, and cerebellum).
Ins 96 bp 129M	Apparently sporadic	4 mo	Clinical: Like typical sporadic CJD. Pathological: Like typical sporadic CJD (CJDMM/1). Patches of PrP immunoreactivity in the cerebellum.
Ins 120 bp- 129M	Familial	5,15 yr	Clinical: Slowly progressive dementia, myoclonus, cerebellar, pyramidal, and extrapyramidal signs. Pathological: Spongiosis, gliosis, and neuronal loss (no information on topography, severity, presence of PrP immunoreactivity).
Ins 144 bp- 129M	Familial	4–13 yr	Clinical: Similar to 120-bp insertion subtype. Pathological: Widespread atrophy, mild and patchy spongiosis or status spongiosus; patches of PrP immunoreactivity in the cerebellum.
Ins 168 bp- 129M	Familial	7,10 yr	Clinical: Similar to 120-bp insertion subtype. Pathological: Diffuse spongiosis, gliosis, and neuronal loss in one case, mild gliosis and neuronal loss, and no spongiosis in a second one (no information on presence of patches of PrP immunoreactivity in the cerebellum).
Ins 192 bp- 129V	Familial	3 mo– 5 yr	Clinical: Similar to 120-bp insertion subtype. Pathological: Spongiosis, gliosis, and neuronal loss (no information on topography and severity), PrP unicentric, and multicentric amyloid plaques in the cerebellum.
Ins 216 bp- 129M	Apparently sporadic	2.5 yr	Clinical: Similar to 120-bp insertion subtype. Pathological: patches of PrP immunoreactivity in the cerebellum, cerebral cortex, and striatum; no obvious neuronal loss, gliosis, or spongiosis.

NA, not available; PrP, prion protein.

2. PRESENCE OF DEMENTIA IN EACH INDIVIDUAL PRION DISEASE PHENOTYPE

2.1. The CJD Phenotype

The sporadic form of CJD is the most frequent, accounting for approx 85% of all human prion diseases. Sporadic CJD presents, in most cases, with a consistent clinical and pathological phenotype, which includes rapidly progressive dementia, myoclonus, and periodic sharp-waves electroencephalographic activity (Table 1). However, 20–30% of patients show significant variations in clinical and pathological features, as well as in the duration of the disease (5–7). This has led to the description of several clinicopathological variants. They include a more chronic and indolent form that

Table 4
Classification of Human Prion Disease According to the Timing of Dementia

Early dementia and cortical pathology		Late dementia and cortical pathology	
Subacute (<1 yr in most cases)	Chronic (>1 yr in most cases)	Subacute (<1 yr in most cases)	Chronic (>1 yr in most cases)
Sporadic CJD 129M/M PrP^{res} type 1	Sporadic CJD 129M/M PrP^{res} type 2	Sporadic CJD 129V/V PrP^{res} type 2 Early sign: ataxia	Sporadic CJD[a] 129M/V PrP^{res} type 2 Early signs: ataxia, memory loss
Iatrogenic CJD (dura mater grafts, corneal transplants)	Familial CJD D178N-129V	Iatrogenic CJD (peripheral contamination) Early sign: ataxia	GSS P102L-129M Early sign: ataxia
Familial CJD H208A-129M, V210I-129M, M232R-129M	Mixed phenotype with long PRNP insertions (>96 bp)	[a]Familial CJD 200 129M/M or M/V Early signs: ataxia, pyramidal signs, peripheral neuropathy	GSS P105L-129V Early sign: spastic paraparesis
Mixed phenotype with short PRNP insertions (<120 bp)	GSS A117V-129V, Y145STOP-129M	FFI D178N-129M Early signs: insomnia, dysautonomia, ataxia	GSS F198S-129V; Q217R-129V Early signs: ataxia, parkinsonism, memory loss

[a]Dementia can be an early feature in some cases of these groups.

progresses over years and that is clinically often indistinguishable from Alzheimer's disease, a form with early pathological involvement of the occipital cortex leading to cortical blindness (Heidenhain variant), and one with early and predominant ataxia (Brownell-Oppenheimer or ataxic variant). In addition, kuru-like, Congo red-positive, amyloid plaques are observed in about 5% of cases *(5)*. We have recently demonstrated that the clinical and pathological features of sporadic CJD correlate with the PRNP codon 129 haplotype and the size of the PrP^{res} fragment that is present in the brain *(6)*. On the basis of these data, we have proposed a novel classification of the sporadic form of CJD in four groups. Group 1 includes the typical CJD phenotype or myoclonic variant, and the Heidenhain variant. This group is linked to methionine homozygosity at codon 129 and to the presence of a PrP^{res} fragment of a size corresponding to 20–21 kDa, designated as "type 1" (CJDM/M1) *(6)*. The atypical and rarer variants all share a PrP^{res} fragment smaller in size than PrP^{res} "type 1" (18–19 kDa) designated as "type 2," and are linked to methionine (group 2) and valine (group 4) homozygosity as well as methionine/valine heterozygosity (group 3) at codon 129. Group 2 is characterized by dementia of long duration (CJDM/M2), group 3 is characterized by the presence of kuru plaques (CJDM/V2) *(6)*, and group 4 includes the ataxic variant (CJDV/V2).

In the familial forms of CJD, two mutations at codon 200 and 178 of PRNP have been consistently linked to the disease and influence its clinicopathological features (Table 1). The phenotype associated with the 178 mutation (CJD[178]) differs from the typical sporadic CJD phenotype (CJDM/M1) for the earlier onset, the longer duration of symptoms, and the absence of periodic sharp waves (PSW) on the EEG in the majority of subjects *(8)*. It is characterized by early dementia in all cases *(8)*. In contrast, the clinical features associated with the 200 mutation comprise prominent motor signs, such as ataxia, spastic paresis, and supranuclear gaze palsy, at onset associated with rapidly evolving dementia (*9*, Young and Parchi, unpublished observations). Also in this CJD variant, PSW on the EEG are not a constant finding *(10)*. Other point mutations at PRNP codons 180, 210, and 232 have been recently reported *(11,12)*. The phenotype linked to these mutations appears indistinguishable from that of the typical sporadic CJD phenotype (CJDM/M1) *(11,12)*. Finally, the iatrogenic form of CJD shows the same variability of phenotypic expression of the sporadic form *(2)*.

The cognitive profile in CJD has not been fully characterized because of the relative paucity of cases, the rapid course, and the variability of phenotypic expression. Although a certain degree of mental deterioration with memory loss is invariably present in all subtypes of CJD sometime during the course of the disease, signs of impairment of higher cortical function appear in about 75% of cases *(5)*. They may lack in the variants that involve predominantly subcortical brain regions in the early course (sporadic CJDV/V2 [group 2] and CJDM/V2 [group 3], iatrogenic CJD secondary to hormone administration and familial CJD with 200 mutation) (Table 4), and may not be seen in cases with a very rapid course, which are dominated by confusion and delirium leading to early stupor or coma.

In CJD, the early signs of cognitive decline usually include confusion and memory loss *(5,6)*. More rarely, the onset of the mental deterioration is marked by signs of cortical visual dysfunction, including visuospatial disorientation, visual agnosia, and simultanagnosia or aphasia *(5,6)*. When fully developed, the cognitive decline does not generally show a specific pattern and is characterized by a progressive course toward a global cortical dementia *(5)*. However, detailed neuropsychological studies of patients with the CJD variants are needed to exclude the existence of different patterns of cognitive impairment in CJD. There is, in fact, a difference in the topography of involvement of the cerebral cortex among some of the variants. For example, the most common sporadic CJD variant (CJD M/M1) is characterized by a prominent involvement of the posterior cortex, which, in contrast, is relatively spared in the sporadic CJDV/V2, CJDM/V2 subtypes *(6)*.

2.2. The FFI Phenotype

Despite its relative rarity and recent description, FFI is among the best characterized of the human prion diseases. The finding that FFI shares the same mutation of CJD[178], but has a significantly different phenotype, which is determined by the genotype at PRNP codon 129 (the methionine codon on the mutated allele is linked to FFI, the valine codon to CJD[178]), represents a striking example of the mechanisms regulating phenotypic expression in human prion diseases *(13)*. Moreover, FFI exemplifies well a prion disease that lacks early, significant dementia and cortical pathology in the majority of cases. The pathological hallmark of FFI is loss of neurons and astrogliosis in the thalamus, which are present in all subjects, independently of the duration of symptoms (Table 1). The inferior olives also show neuronal loss and gliosis in most cases. In contrast, the pathology of the cerebral cortex varies in proportion to the disease duration and is more severe in the limbic lobe than in the neocortex *(14)*. The entorhinal cortex and, to a lesser extent, the pyriform and paraolfactory cortices show spongiosis and/or gliosis in most subjects, which increase in severity according to the duration of the disease. The neocortex, instead, is virtually spared in the subjects with a duration of symptoms of <1yr; it is focally affected by spongiosis and gliosis in those with a clinical course between 12 and 20 mo and diffusely involved only in the subjects with the longest duration (>20 mo). These features of FFI have been further emphasized by the studies of the intracerebral distribution of PrP^{res} *(14)* and of the cerebral regional glucose metabolism *(15,16)* in patients with different disease duration. They both showed a predominant subcortical involvement in the subjects with a duration of about 1 yr or less, whereas in those with a duration of symptoms longer than 15–20 mo the cerebral cortex was also significantly affected. This finding argues, like in other prion diseases, for a spread of the disease process from subcortical structures to the cerebral cortex *(6,14)*.

Detailed behavioral and neuropsychological examinations have been performed in most patients *(17,18)*. The results indicate that three major features characterize the cognitive profile of FFI:

1. Deficit of attention and vigilance;
2. Amnesia; and
3. Impairment of temporal ordering of events.

In contrast, disturbances of language, praxis, and gnosic abilities are consistently absent.

A prominent feature of FFI patients is a peculiar fluctuation of vigilance, which progressively worsens during the course of the disease *(18–20)*. If left alone, patients lapse in an oneiric state, during which they are confused, appear to mimic the content of their dream, and confabulate *(18–20)*. Polysomnographic analysis showed that these episodes represent a loss of reciprocal integration between wakefulness and sleep states *(21)*.

The amnesiac disturbances are characterized by markedly impaired learning and long-term memory with preservation of immediate verbal and visual memory as well as semantic, retrograde, and procedural memory *(18)*. This kind of amnesia appeared to be owing to altered encoding and incorrect ordering of events probably related to a deficit in the early stages of treatment of information so that the message is neither properly coded nor adequately "consolidated" in the long-term store *(18)*. In conclusion, FFI patients present a peculiar picture of cognitive decline with progressively increasing fluctuations in the attention and vigilance associated with disturbances of memory and temporal organization. This cognitive profile includes characteristics of the confusional state and of the so-called subcortical dementia, and it is quite distinct from a cortical dementia. This is consistent with the finding that, in most subjects with FFI, the distribution of PrP^{res}, glucose hypometabolism, and histopathological lesions predominantly affect subcortical structures *(14,15)*.

2.3. The GSS Phenotype

The GSS phenotype has only been observed linked to PRNP mutations *(22)*. Currently, six-point mutations in PRNP have been found associated with GSS (Table 2).

All variants share a relatively chronic course (longer than 2 yr in most cases) and the presence of congo red-positive amyloid plaques containing PrP^{res} fragments. Despite this fact, they show striking phenotypic differences (Table 2). The onset can be characterized by ataxia (102, 117–129M/V mutations), spastic paraparesis (105 mutation), extrapyramidal signs (217 mutation), or dementia (145 and 117 mutations). Pathologically, the amyloid plaques can coexist with significant spongiform degeneration (102 mutation), neurofibrillary degeneration (145, 198, and 217 mutations), or amyloid angiopathy (145 mutation) *(22,23)*.

The codon 129 has been shown to influence age at onset and duration of the disease in the phenotype associated with the 198 mutation *(24)*. The role of the codon 129 polymorphism in association with other GSS mutations has not been determined.

In GSS, like in CJD, comprehensive neuropsychological studies are virtually lacking, and the description of the cognitive changes in the various kindreds has been limited to bedside mental status examinations. In a recent study, however, the cognitive profile has been studied by means of neuropsychological tests in three GSS patients carrying the 198 mutation and belonging to the Indiana kindred *(24a)*. The patients with disease duration of 3 yr or more had deficits in secondary memory, motor skills, intelligence, visuoperceptual skill, attention, speed of processing, and executive ability consistent with global dementia. In contrast, the patient with the shortest duration of symptoms of about 1 yr showed a more selective pattern of cognitive impairment characterized by disturbances of secondary memory, executive dysfunction, and manual motor impairment, which indicate subcortical, including cerebellar, involvement.

2.4. The Heterogenous Phenotype Associated with Insertion Mutations in PRNP

The PRNP gene has an unstable region of five variant octapeptide coding repeats between codons 51 and 91. Insertions ranging from 1 to 9 extrarepeats in this region have been found in 10 families and 8 affected individuals from uninformative families. The phenotype associated with the insertion mutations shows a high variability, particularly in the duration of the disease. The clinicopathological features range from a typical CJD phenotype of short duration to a chronic disease of several years without specific histopathological changes, and are therefore difficult to include in the spectrum of the CJD, GSS, and FFI phenotypes (Tables 1 and 3). Clinically, patients with insertion mutations usually present with memory loss associated with other features that indicate cortical involvement, such as frontal release signs, dysphasia, apraxia, visual disturbances, or personality disorders. After months or years, the cognitive impairment usually progresses to a global cortical dementia, and additional neurological features, such as cerebellar, extrapyramidal, and pyramidal signs, are commonly observed.

3. MOLECULAR MECHANISMS IN PRION DEMENTIA

The molecular mechanisms underlying neurologic dysfunction and structural changes in prion diseases have not been fully clarified.

The strongest notion about the pathogenesis of prion diseases comes from studies of animal models of scrapie and patients affected by CJD, FFI, and GSS, which have shown that the pathogenesis of these conditions is strictly related to the intracerebral formation and accumulation of PrP^{res} derived from the constitutively expressed PrP^c.

PrP^res fragments, often differing in size and proportion of glycosylated forms, have indeed been detected intracerebrally in all major variants of human and animal prion diseases *(6,25–33)*. Although the presence of PrP^res as the hallmark of prion diseases has become widely accepted, a major question still concerns the precise pathogenic role of the abnormal protein. More precisely, it is not known whether PrP^res is the fundamental cause of neuronal dysfunction and neuropathology, or a byproduct of a more subtle and yet unrecognized pathogenic process. For example, the possibility that it is not the deposition of PrP^res, but rather the lack of PrP^c availability for the cell that is directly linked to neuronal dysfunction in prion diseases is still open *(34,35)*. However, many lines of evidence provide strong support to the notion that PrP^res formation and accumulation are the cause of neuronal dysfunction and of the neuropathology in prion diseases:

1. In both humans and animals, the intracerebral deposition of the abnormal protein precedes the appearance of histopathological changes, and the deposition of PrP^res is always spatially related to the presence of lesions *(4,6,14,36,37)*.
2. Immunochemicals and ultrastructural studies have clearly shown that PrP^res primarily accumulates in the neuropil and, more specifically, on the plasmalemma of dendrites, axons, and synapses *(38,39)*. Preliminary findings indicate that this process is associated with a loss of synaptophisin immunoreactivity, suggesting that PrP^res deposition causes a loss of contacts at the levels of the dendritic spines and axons *(40)*.
3. The study of correlation among cerebral glucose metabolism, PrP^res distribution, and histopathology in FFI-affected subjects with a relatively short duration has shown a widespread cerebral hypometabolism in most cases with a much better correlation with the distribution of PrP^res than that of the histopathological lesions *(16)*.
4. A PrP synthetic peptide homologous to a PrP^res fragment isolated from the cerebral cortex of a patient with a GSS variant induces cell death by apoptosis in rat hippocampal neurons in vitro *(41)*.

Recent findings showing that the expression of PrP^c is required for the neurotoxicity of PrP^res both in vivo *(34)* and in vitro *(42)* have added further complexity to the issue. The most likely explanation of this observation is that PrP^res is pathogenic only to cell expressing PrP^c either because it initiates conversion of PrP^c to PrP^res at the cell surface interfering with the membrane function and/or because it is neurotoxic only when it is internalized by way of association with PrP^c, which is known to be endocytosed efficiently at the plasma membrane *(43)*.

The issue of the molecular basis of neuronal dysfunction in prion diseases is further complicated by the lack of correlation between the severity and variety of clinical symptoms and the extent of histopathological lesions. Indeed, the type and severity of structural abnormalities in the brain of the subjects affected by prion diseases show a wide range, which includes virtually absent neuropathology and extremely severe brain damage. When present, the lesions are also variable in type, and none of the lesions are invariably detected in all subtypes of prion diseases. Therefore, it seems that the critical level for the appearance of neuronal dysfunction is variable in these conditions: in some instances, it probably precedes the appearance of morphological abnormalities and is mainly dysfunctional; in others, it is predominantly the consequence of neuronal structural damage. Recent studies have begun to address this issue at the molecular level. They have disclosed at least three potential mechanisms that may explain the protean phenotypic expression of human prion diseases.

First, it has been shown that the PrP^res^ fragments found in brain extracts from patients with prion diseases are heterogenous and differ in size and ratio of glycoforms among subjects with different phenotypic expressions of the disease and different PRNP genotype *(6,32)*. In addition, it has been shown that these truncated forms of PrP^res^ are formed in vivo and reflect different conformations of PrP^res^ and/or distinct ligand interactions *(31,32,44)*. Therefore, it has been hypothesized that the different PrP^res^ fragments associated with the various subtypes of prion diseases may have distinct neurotoxic effects and be responsible, at least in part, for the heterogeneity of phenotypic expression of these conditions *(32)*.

In this regard, it is of interest that, while all subjects affected by familial and sporadic CJD and FFI present in the brain PrP^res^ fragments of a size between 19 and 21 kDa, which are truncated at the N-terminal of PrP but contain an intact C-terminal, the major constituents of the amyloid plaques that distinguish the GSS phenotype are smaller fragments of about 7–11 kDa, which lack the C-terminal portion of PrP^res^ and the glycosylated isoforms *(45)*. The only exception to this rule is the GSS variant linked to the 102 mutation, which seems to include in the plaques a fragment that is not C-terminally truncated *(45,46)*. Interestingly, the phenotype of this GSS variant is the one that overlaps most with the CJD phenotype *(45,47)*. These observations suggest that the type of PrP^res^ fragment that accumulates in the brain is a major molecular determinant of phenotypic expression of human prion diseases. Different fragments may not only have different neurotoxicity, but also cause distinct lesions as a consequence of their different properties, such as aggregability *(48)*.

In view of the chronic course of GSS patients who more consistently show amyloid plaques, it has also been suggested that the formation of fragments with high tendency of aggregation and the formation of plaques may give relative protection and less neuronal dysfunction with respect to such forms as CJD, where the PrP^res^ deposition is usually more diffuse *(49)*.

A second potential factor that may explain the phenotypic variability of prion diseases comes from studies of the regional distribution of PrP^res^ in FFI and CJD. It has been found that, in FFI, the amounts of PrP^res^ that accumulate intracerebrally are, on average, 5–10 times less than those detected in sporadic and, to a lesser extent, familial CJD *(6,14)*. This observation may explain the absence or mildness of severity of spongiform degeneration in the FFI phenotype. There is, in fact, a good correlation between the amount of PrP^res^ and the presence and severity of spongiform degeneration in both FFI and sporadic CJD *(6,14,37)*. The findings that PrP^res^ accumulates in different amounts among the different subtypes of prion diseases indicate that not only the characteristics of PrP^res^, but also the rate and the overall amount of accumulation of the abnormal protein are determinants of the phenotypic expression of prion diseases.

Finally, a third mechanism of phenotypic modulation, which is strictly related to those already mentioned, has been recently suggested by studies of the effect of PRNP mutations on the metabolism of PrP in vitro. It has been demonstrated that the D178N mutation results in instability of the mutant protein, which predominantly affects the unglycosylated form *(50)*. As a consequence, the mutant protein at the cell surface is, in contrast to the wild-type protein, predominantly composed of glycosylated isoforms. Since it has been shown that the PrP^c^ reaches the cell surface when it is converted to PrP^res^ *(51)*, and that the conversion process exclusively or predominantly affects the mutant protein *(52)*, the altered processing of the mutant protein might influence the phenotypic expression of the disease by determining the characteristic of the PrP^{res} fragment and its rate of accumulation. It is likely that other mutations linked to familial prion diseases would alter the processing of PrP^c and influence the disease phenotype by a similar mechanism.

4. CONCLUSIONS

Prion diseases pose a great challenge to the study of the molecular mechanisms of dementia. Owing to the relative rarity and rapid course of the majority of the prion diseases, a rigorous and systematic characterization of the cognitive impairment in these diseases has been rarely conducted. Moreover, in contrast to Alzhemer's disease, prion diseases are characterized by a great variability in the clinical and pathological features, which is mirrored by a variability in the timing of appearance and cognitive profile of the dementia. Several lines of evidence indicate that the phenotypic variability of prion diseases is largely controlled by the PRNP haplotype and the characteristics of the PrP^{res} fragments associated with the various subtypes of prion diseases. In addition, complex interactions may occur between PrP^C and PrP^{res} that might affect the function of PrP^C. According to recent evidence, PrP^C plays a role in the modulation of the GABA$_A$ receptor-mediated synaptic inhibition and of long-term potentiation, a form of synaptic plasticity associated with learning and memory, as well as in the regulation of the sleep–wake cycle *(53,54)*.

Some of the very same reasons that make the study of cognitive impairment in prion diseases so challenging might also prove highly rewarding. The clarification of the pathogenic mechanisms of PrP^{res} and of its derivatives, of the effects that PrP^{res} may have on PrP^C, and of the functions of PrP^C may provide important and novel clues to the understanding of the basic mechanisms of dementia.

ACKNOWLEDGMENTS

This work was supported by NIH grants AG08155, AG08992, AG08012, and the Britton fund.

REFERENCES

1. Prusiner, S. B. and DeArmond, S. J. (1994) Prion diseases and neurodegeneration, *Ann. Rev. Neurosci.* **17,** 311–319.
2. Parchi, P. and Gambetti, P. (1995) Human prion diseases, *Curr. Opinion Neurol.* **8,** 286–293.
3. Fraser, H. and Dickinson, A. G. (1973) Scrapie in mice. Agent-strain differences in the distribution and intensity of grey matter vacuolation, *J. Comp. Pathol.* **83,** 23–40.
4. Hecker, R., Taraboulos, A., Scott, M., Pan, K. M., Yang, S. L., Torchia, M., Jendroska, K., DeArmond, S. J., and Prusiner, S. B. (1992) Replication of distinct scrapie prion isolates is region specific in brains of transgenic mice and hamsters, *Genes Dev.* **6,** 1213–1228.
5. Brown, P., Gibbs, C. J., Rodgers-Johnson, P., Asher, D. M., Sulima, M. P., Bacote, A., Goldfarb, L. G., and Gajdusek, D. C. (1994) Human spongiform encephalopathy: The National Institutes of Health series of 300 cases of experimentally transmitted disease, *Ann. Neurol.* **35,** 513–529.
6. Parchi, P., Castellani, R., Capellari, S., Ghetti, B., Young, K., Chen, S. G., Farlow, M., Dickson, D. W., Sima, A. A. F., Trojanowski, J. Q., Petersen, R. B., and Gambetti, P. (1996) Molecular basis of phenotypic variability in sporadic Creutzfelt-Jakob disease, *Ann. Neurol.* **39,** 767–778.

7. Richardson, E. P. and Masters, C. L. (1995) The nosology of Creutzfeldt-Jakob disease and conditions related to the accumulation of PrP^{CJD} in the nervous system, *Brain Pathol.* **5**, 33–41.
8. Brown, P., Goldfarb, L. G., Kovanen, J., Haltia, M., Cathala, F., Sulima, M., Gibbs, C. J., and Gajdusek, D. C. (1992) Phenotypic characteristics of familial Creutzfeldt-Jakob disease associated with the codon 178 Asn PRNP mutation, *Ann. Neurol.* **31**, 282–285.
9. Bertoni, J. M., Brown, P., Goldfarb, L. G., Rubenstein, R., and Gajdusek, D. C. (1992) Familial Creutzfeldt-Jakob disease (codon 200 mutation) with supranuclear palsy, *JAMA* **268**, 2413–2415.
10. Tietjen, G. E. and Drury, I. (1990) Familial Creutzfeldt-Jakob disease without periodic EEG activity, *Ann. Neurol.* **28**, 585–588.
11. Pocchiari, M., Salvatore, M., Cutruzzola, F., Genuardi, M., Allocatelli, C. T., Masullo, C., Macchi, G., Alema, G., Galgani, S., Xi, Y. G., Petraroli, R., Silvestrini, M. C., and Brunori, M. (1993) A new point mutation of the prion protein gene in Creutzfeldt-Jakob disease, *Ann. Neurol.* **34**, 802–807.
12. Kitamoto, T. and Tateishi, J. (1994) Human prion diseases with variant prion protein, *Phil. Trans. R. Soc. Lond. B.* **343**, 391–398.
13. Goldfarb, L. G., Petersen, R. B., Tabaton, M., Brown, P., LeBlanc, A. C., Montagna, P., Cortelli, P., Julien, J., Vital, C., Pendlebury, W. W., Haltia, M., Willis, P. R., Hauw, J. J., McKeever, P. E., Monari, L., Schrank, B., Swergold, G. D., Autilio-Gambetti, L., Gajdusek, C., Lugaresi, E., and Gambetti, P. (1992) Fatal familial insomnia and Familial Creutzfeldt Jakob disease: disease phenotype determined by a DNA polymorphism, *Science* **258**, 806–808.
14. Parchi, P., Castellani, R., Cortelli, P., Montagna, P., Chen, S. G., Petersen, R. B., Manetto, V., Vnencak-Jones, C. L., McLean, M. J., Sheller, J. R., Lugaresi, E., Autilio-Gambetti, L., and Gambetti, P. (1995) Regional distribution of protease-resistant prion protein in Fatal Familial Insomnia, *Ann Neurol.* **38**, 21–29.
15. Perani, D., Cortelli, P., Lucignani, G., Montagna, P., Tinuper, P., Gallassi, R., Gambetti, P., Lenzi, G. L., Lugaresi, E., and Fazio, F. (1993) [^{18}F] FDG PET in Fatal familial insomnia: the functional effects of thalamic lesions, *Neurology* **43**, 2565–2569.
16. Perani, D., Parchi, P., Cortelli, P., Montagna, P., Grassi, F., Castellani, R., Gambetti, P., Lugaresi, E., and Fazio, F. (1995) Relationship between protease-resistant prion protein distribution and in vivo regional cerebral metabolism in Fatal Familial Insomnia (FFI), *Neurology* **45**, A406.
17. Gallassi, R., Morreale, A., Gambetti, P., and Lugaresi, E. (1992) Fatal familial insomnia: neuropsychological study of a disease with thalamic degeneration, *Cortex* **28**, 175–187.
18. Gallassi, R., Morreale, A., Montagna, P., Cortelli, P., Avoni, P., Castellani, R., Gambetti, P., and Lugaresi, L. (1996) Fatal familial insomnia: behavioral and cognitive features, *Neurology* **46**, 935–939.
19. Lugaresi, E., Medori, R., Montagna, P., Baruzzi, A., Cortelli, P., Lugaresi, A., Tinuper, P., Zucconi, M., and Gambetti, P. (1986) Fatal familial insomnia and dysautonomia with selective degeneration of thalamic nuclei, *N. Engl. J. Med.* **315**, 997–1003.
20. Montagna, P., Cortelli, P., Tinuper, P., Sforza, E., Avoni, P., Gallassi, R., Morreale, A., Roiter, I., Perani, D., Lucignani, G., Fazio, F., and Lugaresi, E. (1994) Fatal familial insomnia: A disease that emphasizes the role of the thalamus in the regulation of sleep and vegetative functions, in *Fatal Familial Insomnia: Inherited Prion Diseases, Sleep, and the Thalamus* (Guilleminault, C., Lugaresi, E., Montagna, P., and Gambetti, P., eds.), Raven, New York, pp. 1–14.
21. Tinuper, P., Montagna, P., Medori, R., Cortelli, P., Zucconi, M., Baruzzi, A., and Lugaresi, E. (1989) The thalamus participates in the regulation of the sleep-waking cycle. A clinico-pathological study in Fatal Familial Thalamic degeneration, *Electroencephalogic Clin. Neurophysiol.* **73**, 117–120.
22. Ghetti, B., Dlouhy, S. R., Giaccone, G., Bugiani, O., Frangione, B., Farlow, M. R., and Tagliavini, F. (1995) Gerstmann-Sträussler-Scheinker disease and the Indiana kindred, *Brain Pathol.* **5**, 61–75.

23. Ghetti, B., Piccardo, P., Spillantini, M. G., Ichimiya, Y., Porro, M., Perini, F., Kitamoto, T., Tateishi, J., Seiler, C., Frangione, B., Bugiani, O., Giaconne, G., Prelli, F., Goedert, M., Dlouhy, S. R., and Tagliavini, F. (1996) Vascular variant of prion protein cerebral amyloidosis with τ-positive neurofibrillary tangles: The phenotype of the stop codon 145 mutation in PRNP, *Proc. Natl. Acad. Sci. USA* **93**, 744–748.

24. Dlouhy, S. R., Hsiao, K., Farlow, M. R., Foroud, T., Conneally, P. M., Johnson, P., Prusiner, S. B., Hooles, M. E., and Ghetti, B. (1992) Linkage of the Indiana kindred of Gerstmann-Sträussler-Scheinker disease to the prion protein gene, *Nature Genet.* **1**, 64–67.

24a. Unverzagt, F. W., Farlow, M. R., Norton, J., Dlouhy, S. R., Young, K., and Ghetti, B. Neurophysiological function in patients with Gerstmann-Sträussler-Scheinker disease from the Indiana Kindred (F198S), in press.

25. Bolton, D. C., McKinley, M. P., and Prusiner, S. B. (1982) Identification of a protein that purifies with the scrapie protein, *Science* **218**, 1309,1310.

26. Kascsak, R. J., Rubenstein, R., Merz, P. A., Carp, R. I., Robakis, N. K., Wisniewski, H. M., and Diringer, H. (1986) Immunological comparison of scrapie-associated fibrils isolated from animals infected with four different scrapie strains, *J. Virol.* **59**, 676–683.

27. Rubenstein, R., Merz, P. A., Kascsak, R. J., Carp, R. I., Scalici, C. L., Fama, C. L., and Wisniewski, H. M. (1987) Detection of scrapie-associated fibrils (SAF) and SAF proteins from scrapie-affected sheep, *J. Infect. Dis.* **156**, 36–42.

28. Hope, J., Ritchie, L., Farquhar, C., Somerville, R., and Hunter, N. (1989) Bovine spongiform encephalopathy: a scrapie-like disease of British cattle, *Prog. Clin. Biol. Res.* **317**, 659–667.

29. Brown, P., Coker-Vann, M., Pomeroy, K., Franko, M., Asher, D. M., Gibbs, C. J., and Gajdusek, D. C. (1986) Diagnosis of Creutzfeldt-Jakob disease by western blot identification of marker protein in human brain tissue, *N. Engl. J. Med.* **314**, 547–551.

30. Bockman, J. M., Kingsbury, D. R., McKinley, M. P., Bendheim, P. E., and Prusiner, S. B. (1985) Creutzfeldt-Jakob disease prion proteins in human brains, *N. Engl. J. Med.* **312**, 73–78.

31. Bessen, R. A. and Marsh, R. F. (1994) Distinct PrP properties suggest the molecular basis of strain variation in transmissible mink encephalopathy, *J. Virol.* **68**, 7859–7868.

32. Monari, L., Chen, S. C., Brown, P., Parchi, P., Petersen, R. B., Mikol, J., Gray, F., Cortelli, P., Montagna, P., Ghetti, B., Goldfarb, L. G., Gajdusek, D. C., Lugaresi, E., Gambetti, P., and Autilio-Gambetti, L. (1994) Fatal Familial Insomnia and Familial Creutzfeldt-Jakob disease: Different prion proteins determined by a DNA polymorphism, *Proc. Natl. Acad. Sci. USA*, **91**, 2839–2842.

33. Tagliavini, F., Prelli, F., Ghiso, J., Bugiani, O., Serban, D., Prusiner, S. B., Farlow, M. R., Ghetti, B., and Frangione, B. (1991) Amyloid protein of Gertsmann-Strausser-Scheinker disease (Indiana kindred) is an 11kd fragment of prion protein with an N-terminal glycine at codon 58, *EMBO J.* **10**, 513–519.

34. Brandner, S., Isenmann, S., Raeber, A., Fischer, M., Sailer, A., Kobayashi, Y., Marino, S., Weissmann, C., and Aguzzi, A. (1996) Normal host prion protein necessary for scrapie-induced neurotoxicity, *Nature* **379**, 339–343.

35. Collinge, J., Whittington, M. A., Sidle, K. C., Smith, C. J., Palmer, M. S., Clarke, A. R., and Jefferys, J. G. R. (1994) Prion protein is necessary for normal synaptic function, *Nature* **370**, 295–297.

36. Jendroska, K., Heinzel, F. P., Torchia, M., Stowring, L., Kretzschmar, H. A., Kon, A., Stern, A., Prusiner, S. B., and DeArmond, S. J. (1991) Proteinase-resistant prion protein accumulation in Syrian hamster brain correlations with regional pathology and scrapie infectivity, *Neurology* **41**, 1482–1490.

37. Castellani, R., Parchi, P., Stahl, J., Capellari, S., Cohen, M., and Gambetti, P. (1996) Early pathological and biochemical changes in Creutzfeldt-Jakob disease: study of brain biopsies, *Neurology* **46**, 1690–1693.

38. Kitamoto, T., Shin, R. W., Doh-ura, K., Tomokane, N., Miyazono, M., Muramoto, T., and Tateishi, J. (1992) Abnormal isoform of prion proteins accumulates in the synaptic struc-

tures of the central nervous system in patients with Creutzfeldt-Jakob disease, *Am. J. Pathol.* **140,** 1285–1294.

39. Jeffrey, M., Goodsir, C. M., Bruce, M., McBride, P. A., Scott, J. R., and Halliday, W. G. (1994) Correlative light and electron microscopy studies of PrP localization in 87V scrapie, *Brain Res.* **656,** 329–343.

40. Clinton, J., Forsyth, C., Royston, M. C., and Roberts, G. W. (1993) Synaptic degeneration is the primary neuropathological feature in prion disease: a preliminary study, *NeuroReport* **4,** 65–68.

41. Forloni, G., Angeretti, N., Chiesa, R., Monzani, E., Salmona, M., Bugiani, O., and Tagliavini, F. (1993) Neurotoxicity of a prion protein fragment, *Nature* **362,** 543–546.

42. Brown, D. R., Herms, J., and Kretzschmar, H. A. (1994) Mouse cortical cells lacking cellular PrP survive in culture with a neurotoxic PrP fragment, *NeuroReport* **5,** 2057–2060.

43. Shyng, S. L., Huber, M. T., and Harris, D. A. (1993) A prion protein cycles between the cell surface and an endocytic compartment in cultured neuroblastoma cells, *J. Biol. Chem.* **268,** 15,922–15,928.

44. Chen, S. G., Teplow, D. B., Parchi, P., Teller, J. K., Gambetti, P., and Autilio-Gambetti, L. (1995) Truncated forms of the human prion protein in normal brain and in prion diseases, *J. Biol. Chem.* **270,** 19,173–19,180.

45. Ghetti, B., Piccardo, P., Frangione, B., Bugiani, O., Giaccone, G., Young, K., Prelli, F., Farlow, M. R., Dloughy, S. R., and Tagliavini, F. (1996) Prion protein amyloidosis, *Brain Pathol.* **6,** 127–145.

46. Piccardo, P., Ghetti, B., Dickson, D. W., Vinters, H. V., Giaccone, G., Bugiani, O., Tagliavini, F., Young, K., Phil, D., Dloughy, S. R., Seiler, C., Jones, C. K., Lazzarini, A., Golbe, L. I., Zimmerman, T. R., Perlman, S. L., McLachlan, D. C., St. George-Hyslop, P. H., and Lennox, A. (1995) Gertsmann-Straussler-Scheinker disease (PRNP P102L): Amyloid deposits are best recognized by antibodies directed to epitopes in PrP region 90-165, *J. Neurol. Exp. Neurol.* **54,** 790–801.

47. Hainfellner, J. A., Brantner-Inthaler, S., Cervenakova, L., Brown, P., Kitamoto, T., Tateishi, J., Diringer, H., Liberski, P. P., Regele, H., Feucht, M., Mayr, N., Wessely, P., Summer, K., Seitelberger, F., and Budka, H. (1995) The original Gertsmann-Sträussler-Scheinker family of Austria: Divergent clinicopathological phenotypes but constant PrP genotype, *Brain Pathol.* **5,** 201–211.

48. Tagliavini, F., Prelli, F., Verga, L., Giaccone, G., Sarma, R., Gorevic, P., Ghetti, B., Passerini, F., Ghibaudi, E., Forloni, G., Salmona, M., Bugiani, O., and Frangione, B. (1993) Synthetic peptides homologous to prion protein residues 106–147 form amyloid-like fibrils in vitro, *Proc. Natl. Acad. Sci. USA* **90,** 9678–9682.

49. Castano, E. M. and Frangione, B. (1995) Non-Alzheimer's disease amyloidoses of the nervous system, *Curr. Opinion Neurol.* **8,** 279–285.

50. Petersen, R. B., Parchi, P., Richardson, S. L., Urig, C. B., and Gambetti, P. (1996) Effect of the D178N mutation and the codon 129 polymorphism on the metabolism of the prion protein, *J. Biol. Chem.* **271,**21, 12,661–12,668.

51. Caughey, B. and Raymond, G. J. (1991) The scrapie-associated form of PrP is made from a cell surface precursor that is both protease- and phospholipase-sensitive, *J. Biol. Chem.* **266,** 18,217–18,223.

52. Chen, S. G., Parchi, P., Brown, P., Roos, R. P., Vnencak-Jones, C. L., and Gambetti, P. (1996) Fatal familial insomnia and familial Creutzfeldt-Jakob disease: abnormal prion protein (PrP^{res}) encoded by the mutant allele, *J. Neuropath. Exp. Neurol.* **55,**5, A124.

53. Collinge, J., Whittington, M. A., Sidle, K. C. L., Smith, C. J., Palmer, M. S., Clarke, A. R., and Jeffreys, J. G. R. (1994) Prion protein is necessary for normal synaptic function, *Nature* **370,** 295–297.

54. Tobler, I., Gaus, S. E., Deboer, T., Achermann, P., Fischer, M., Rülicke, T., Moser, M., Oesch, B., McBride, P. A., and Manson, J. C. (1996) Altered circadian activity rhythms and sleep in mice devoid of prion protein, *Nature* **380,** 639–642.

Index